HEALTH BEHAVIOR
AND
HEALTH EDUCATION

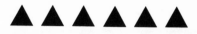

Karen Glanz
Frances Marcus Lewis
Barbara K. Rimer
Editors

HEALTH BEHAVIOR AND HEALTH EDUCATION

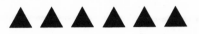

Theory,
Research,
and Practice

Jossey-Bass Publishers
San Francisco • Oxford • 1991

HEALTH BEHAVIOR AND HEALTH EDUCATION
Theory, Research, and Practice
by Karen Glanz, Frances Marcus Lewis, and Barbara K. Rimer, Editors

Library of Congress Cataloging-in-Publication Data

Health behavior and health education.

(The Jossey-Bass health series)
1. Health behavior.   2. Health education.   I. Glanz,
Karen.   II. Lewis, Frances Marcus.   III. Rimer, Barbara K.
IV. Series.
RA776.9.H434   1990   613   90-4016
ISBN 1-55542-243-8

Manufactured in the United States of America

The paper in this book meets the guidelines for
permanence and durability of the Committee on
Production Guidelines for Book Longevity of the
Council on Library Resources.

JACKET DESIGN BY WILLI BAUM

FIRST EDITION
    HB Printing   10 9 8 7 6 5 4 3

Code 9048

The Jossey-Bass
Health Series

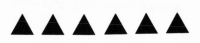

Contents

Tables and Figures

xiii

Chapter 6

Chapter 8

Chapter 9

Chapter 10

Chapter 12

Chapter 13

Chapter 14

Chapter 15

This book is dedicated to the cherished memory of Jack Kirscht, scholar, teacher, and friend, whose work has greatly advanced the understanding and development of theories of health behavior. He has been an inspiration to generations of students and colleagues, among whom we are fortunate to be counted.

To John, David, Steven, Deloris, Alex,
Dr. Huggins, Muriel, Laurel;
Bernard, Joan, Irv, and Kermit

Foreword

If it is true that there is nothing so practical as a good theory, then one must wonder why so much practice in health education is atheoretical. I suspect the answer to this paradox lies in the quality of teaching about behavioral and educational theory in the health professions. The difficulty of teaching social and behavioral theory can be laid to the wide-ranging theories to be mastered and the race to stay abreast of new developments and applications of the theories in research and practice.

The editors of this volume have taken an important step in giving professors, students, and practitioners a head start in this race. They have enlisted the help of authors who are working on the cutting edge of theory development and testing in the health sciences. The authors are themselves seasoned investigators and experienced practitioners sensitive to the hard political and economic realities of trying to maintain fidelity in the application of theory in the field.

The virtual explosion of new research in health promotion in very recent years and the continued logarithmic growth of patient education and health behavior research have advanced the credibility of these enterprises in the health professions and in health policy by leaps. Witness the number of articles on health education and health behavior topics in the *Journal of the American Medical Association* and in *Morbidity and Mortality Weekly Reports* in recent years compared with the number a decade ago as evidence of their policy relevance.

This book does a great service by positioning health education in its most meaningful place within the broad scope of health promotion. In sorting out the terminology of health education and health promotion, the editors of this book have settled on the term *health education* in conjunction with health behavior to characterize the scope of the book. Acknowledging that the term *health promotion* has been defined more broadly in national and international health policies, they also note that the history of health education includes numerous early references to these broader organizational, economic, and environmental targets of health education. In the final analysis, as the editors note, the two terms are inextricably intertwined.

One might say that unless we develop and apply the art and science of health education, we have no hope of promoting health in a democratic society. This book is an excellent map and compass for those who would pursue either the research and development or the application path, and especially for those who would pursue both.

Menlo Park, California   Lawrence W. Green
March 1990   Vice President
                                 Henry J. Kaiser Family Foundation

Preface

Health education programs can help participants prevent disease, enhance health, and manage chronic illnesses, as well as help improve the well-being of organizations and communities. These benefits are most likely to occur when the program or intervention is directed by a theory of health behavior. Theories of health behavior can help health professionals identify the targets for behavior change as well as the methods for accomplishing such change. Theories also inform the evaluation of change efforts by helping to identify the outcomes to be measured and the timing and methods of study to be used.

Theory-driven health education programs and interventions require an understanding of the components of health behavior theory as well as the operational or practical forms of the theory. However, to date, no text has provided an in-depth analysis of the theories of health behavior relevant to health education. Instead, health educators and students and teachers of health education have had to rely primarily on journal articles, esoteric reference materials, or textbooks that offer topical, not analytical, treatment of the theories.

While the most effective behavior change interventions are likely to be those that are informed by theory, students of health education are often left to integrate for themselves the worlds of theory and application. In order for the field of health education to build on conceptually sound research and practice, there is a need to synthesize what has been done and to link explicitly theory, research, and practice applications.

Increasingly, a diverse group of health and other helping professionals must respond to pressing public health problems, sometimes without formal training in health education theory and practice. Until now, no single book has addressed a broad range of theories of health-related behavior and clearly demonstrated their application to health education. The aim of *Health Behavior and Health Education* is to bring together important health behavior theories that are related to individuals as well as to communities, research based on these theories, and examples of health education practice that are derived from theory and have been tested through research. This book makes theory and practice accessible to both novices and seasoned health educators and makes conceptual frameworks accessible to scientists whose work emphasizes theory and research.

The ultimate purpose of *Health Behavior and Health Education* is to advance the science and practice of health education through the informed application of theories of health behavior. The book aims to achieve this goal in three ways: by analyzing the key components of social-behavioral theories relevant to health education and health behavior; by describing and analyzing current applications of these theories in health education interventions; and by delineating the needed future directions for theory, research, and practice in health education. The book also can promote improved health education practice through a fuller understanding of health behavior in its many contexts and thus facilitate more effective integration of theory and practice.

Audience

Health Behavior and Health Education speaks to graduate students, practitioners, and scientists who spend part or all of their time in the broad arena of health education; this audience will find that the text assists them both to understand the theories and to apply them in practical settings. The practitioner as well as the student of health education will find this text a helpful reference for the development and evaluation of theory-driven health education programs and interventions, and the researcher should recognize the areas in which empirical support is deficient and theory testing is required, which will help to set the research agenda for health behavior and health education.

This book is intended to assist all professionals who value the need to influence health behavior positively. Their fields include health education, medicine, nursing, health psychology, nutrition and dietetics, dentistry, pharmacy, exercise science, clinical psychology, occupational and physical therapy, and behavioral medicine.

Overview of the Book

The authors of this book understand both theory and its application in a variety of settings that characterize the diverse practice of health education, including work sites, hospitals, ambulatory care settings, schools, and communities, and they also represent expertise in a variety of health problem areas, such as helping people stop smoking, increasing use of screening, and improving community health. The chapters, written expressly for this book, address theories of behavior at the level of the individual, dyad, group, and community.

The book is organized into five parts. Part One defines key terms and concepts. The next three parts reflect important units of health education practice: the individual, the interpersonal or group level, and the community or aggregate level. Each of these parts has several chapters. Part Two focuses on theories of individual health behavior, and its chapters focus on variables *within the individual* participants in health education that influence their health behavior. Four bodies of theory are reviewed in separate chapters: the Health Belief Model, the Theory of Reasoned Action and Multiattribute Utility Models, Attribution Theory, and Consumer Information Processing. Part Three examines interpersonal theories, which emphasize elements in the *interpersonal* environment that affect individuals' health behavior. Three chapters focus on Social Learning Theory; social support, participation, and control; and interpersonal influence. Part Four covers models for the *community or aggregate level* of change, and includes chapters on community organization, adoption and diffusion of innovations, organizational change, social marketing, and media advocacy. Finally, Part Five presents future directions for theory, research, and practice in health education.

The major emphasis of *Health Behavior and Health Education* is on the analysis and application of health behavior theories to health education practice. Each core chapter in Parts Two, Three, and Four has two sections. The first section defines and analyzes the central concepts of the specific behavioral science theory and its derivative conceptual framework. In this section, some major hypotheses or assumptions derived from the theory are presented, empirical support for these propositions is briefly reviewed, and directions for research in health behavior and health education are summarized. In the second section of each core chapter, the authors analyze applications of the theory in health education programs that are aimed at changing health behavior. Through these applications, the reader will understand how the theory has shaped interventions and with what results. The applications reflect the many issues and problems that health education addresses and the many settings in which health education occurs.

To facilitate the reader's understanding of theory, research, and practice, each of the three central parts of the book concludes with a chapter that offers the editors' perspectives on the theories discussed and their application through health education interventions. Strengths, weaknesses, areas for future research, and promising strategies are highlighted.

No single book can be truly comprehensive and still be concise and readable. Decisions about which theories to include were made with both an appreciation of the evolution of health education and a vision of its future. Throughout the decision-making process, we were cognizant of selecting theories that had a substantial collection of research studies behind them, and we chose theories that have been well developed in their use for health education. We purposely chose to emphasize theories that encompass a range from the individual to the societal level. Of necessity, some promising evolving theories were not included.

Health Behavior and Health Education grew out of the editors' own experiences, frustrations, and needs, as well as their desire to synthesize the diverse literatures and to draw clearly the linkages between theory, research, and the practice of health education. We have sought to present theory, research, and practice as they interrelate and to make each accessible and practical. In this way, we hope that practitioners will benefit from the large base of theory and research and that professionals concerned primarily with theory and research will develop a keener appreciation of the practice of health education.

Acknowledgments

We owe deep gratitude to all the authors whose work is represented in this book. They worked diligently with us to produce an integrated volume, and we greatly appreciate their willingness to tailor their contributions to realize the vision of the book. Their collective depth of knowledge and experience across the broad range of theories and topics far exceeds the expertise that the editors can claim.

Kenneth Beck, Carol D'Onofrio, and Godfrey Hochbaum provided timely and insightful reviews of the chapters at a crucial stage in the book's development. Alis Valencia and Becky McGovern at Jossey-Bass provided valuable guidance throughout.

The editors are indebted to their colleagues and students who, over the years, have taught them the importance of both health behavior theories and their cogent and precise representation. The foundations for this work began during our training and were further nurtured during our years of work at Stanford University, the University of Michigan, The Johns Hopkins University School of Hygiene and Public Health, Temple University, and the University of Washington.

We particularly want to acknowledge the following individuals: David Brinberg, Robert Croyle, Michael Eriksen, Joel Rudd, the behavioral research staff at Fox Chase Cancer Center, John Lowe, and Robert Denniston.

Completion of this manuscript would not have been possible without the continuous assistance of Mary A. Fernandez, Siobhan LaCreta, and Kathy Smith.

We also wish to express our thanks to our colleagues, friends, and families, whose patience, good humor, and encouragement sustained us through our work on this book.

For this volume, we, the editors, have chosen to list our names in alphabetical order.

March 1990   Karen Glanz
                                          Philadelphia, Pennsylvania

                                          Frances Marcus Lewis
                                          Seattle, Washington

                                          Barbara K. Rimer
                                          Philadelphia, Pennsylvania

The Editors

Karen Glanz is professor in the Department of Health Education at Temple University in Philadelphia, and adjunct professor at Temple University School of Medicine. She received her B.A. degree (1974) in Spanish and her M.P.H. (1977) and Ph.D (1979) degrees in health behavior and health education, all from the University of Michigan.

Glanz's research and academic interests have been in the areas of health promotion program development and evaluation, nutrition behavior and education, patient compliance, medical education, and employee health promotion. She has served as an advisor and consultant to numerous public and private health, education, and business organizations. In 1984 she received the Early Career Award of the Public Health Education Section of the American Public Health Association. Glanz's scholarly contributions consist of more than forty journal articles and book chapters. She serves on the editorial boards of *Health Education Research,* the *Journal of Nutrition Education,* and *Patient Education and Counseling.*

Glanz was visiting professor at Teachers College, Columbia University in 1982 and spent 1987 to 1988 as a visiting scholar in the division of epidemiology at the University of Minnesota School of Public Health.

Frances Marcus Lewis is professor in the Department of Community Health Care Systems at the University of Washington. She is also an American Cancer Society Oncology Nursing Professor. She received her B.S.N. degree (1967) from Loretto Heights

College and her M.N. degree (1968) from the University of Washington. She received her M.A. (1975) in sociology and her Ph.D. (1977) in sociology of education from Stanford University. She completed her postdoctoral training (1978) in health education at The Johns Hopkins University School of Hygiene and Public Health.

Lewis's research interests are primarily in the areas of program evaluation; adjustment to chronic and life threatening illness; patient and family education; community health promotion; and health care systems. Her scholarly contributions include more than forty professional papers and several book chapters. She coauthored (with L. W. Green) the book *Evaluation and Measurement in Health Education and Health Promotion* (1986).

Lewis serves as a member of the Cancer Control Grant Review Committee of the National Cancer Institute. She is on the editorial boards of *Evaluation: A Journal of Applied Social Research, Health Education Quarterly, Family and Community Health,* and *Public Health Nursing.*

Barbara K. Rimer is Director of Behavioral Research at Fox Chase Cancer Center in Philadelphia. She received her B.A. degree (1970) in English and her M.P.H. degree (1973) in health education and health administration from the University of Michigan, and her Dr. P.H. degree (1982) in health education from The Johns Hopkins University School of Hygiene and Public Health.

Rimer's principal research activities have been in cancer control, focusing especially on smoking cessation among women and older adults, and on increasing the utilization of mammography among older women. She has published more than thirty-five peer-reviewed articles and book chapters. With colleagues, she has published most recently in *Cancer Research, Radiology, Health Education Quarterly, Journal of the American Board of Family Practice,* and *Journal of Compliance in Health Care.*

Rimer serves as an advisor and consultant to state and federal government health agencies and was a contributing author to the 1990 *Surgeon General's Report on Smoking and Health.* She recently served as the editor of a special issue on cancer control for *Health Education Research* and is on the journal's editorial board.

The Contributors

Tom Baranowski is associate professor in the Division of Sociomedical Sciences of the Department of Preventive Medicine and Community Health at the University of Texas Medical Branch in Galveston.

William B. Carter is professor in the Department of Health Services, School of Public Health and Community Medicine, University of Washington, and associate director, Northwest Health Services Research and Development, at the Seattle Veterans Administration Medical Center.

Lawren H. Daltroy is associate director of the RBB Multipurpose Arthritis Center, Brigham and Women's Hospital, in Boston, and instructor of medicine at Harvard Medical School.

Robert M. Goodman is assistant professor in the Department of Health Promotion and Education in the School of Public Health, University of South Carolina.

Nancy Haley is associate chief, Division of Nutrition and Endocrinology, and section head, Section of Clinical Biochemistry, at the American Health Foundation in New York City.

David H. Hickam is associate professor, Department of Medicine, Oregon Health Sciences University; coordinator of the Health Services Research and Development Program; and a staff physician at the Portland Veterans Administration Medical Center.

Barbara A. Israel is associate professor in the Department of Health Behavior and Health Education at the University of Michigan School of Public Health.

Sandra K. Joos is an investigator in the Health Services Research and Development Program at the Portland Veterans Administration Medical Center and adjunct assistant professor in the Department of Psychiatry at Oregon Health Sciences University.

John P. Kirscht (deceased) was professor of Health Behavior and Health Education, and of Epidemiology, at the University of Michigan School of Public Health.

Cassie Landers is research scientist, Division of Health Promotion Research, at the American Health Foundation in New York City.

Meredith Minkler is professor and chair of Community Health Education in the School of Public Health, University of California, Berkeley.

William D. Novelli is president of Porter/Novelli, a nationwide public relations agency with public health, not-for-profit, and corporate clients.

Mario A. Orlandi is chief, Division of Health Promotion Research, at the American Health Foundation in New York City.

Guy S. Parcel is director, Center for Health Promotion Research and Development, School of Public Health, University of Texas Health Sciences Center at Houston.

Cheryl L. Perry is associate professor of Epidemiology and chair of Community Health Education in the School of Public Health, University of Minnesota.

Irwin M. Rosenstock is FHP Endowed Professor and director of the Center for Health Behavior Studies at California State University, Long Beach.

Joel Rudd is associate professor in the School of Family and Consumer Resources at the University of Arizona.

Susan J. Schurman is codirector of the Joint Labor Management Relations Center at the Institute of Labor and Industrial Relations, University of Michigan.

Allan B. Steckler is professor in the Department of Health Behavior and Health Education at the School of Public Health, University of North Carolina, Chapel Hill.

Lawrence Wallack is associate professor of Community Health Education in the School of Public Health, University of California, Berkeley.

Raymond Weston is research scientist, Division of Health Promotion Research, at the American Health Foundation in New York City.

HEALTH BEHAVIOR
AND
HEALTH EDUCATION

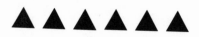

PART ONE

HEALTH EDUCATION
AND HEALTH BEHAVIOR:
THE FOUNDATIONS

Chapter 1

The Editors

▲ ▲ ▲

The Scope of Health Education: Parameters of a Maturing Field

The roles of health educators are nearly limitless. Health education professionals may counsel people at risk for AIDS about safe sex; help children avoid tobacco, alcohol, and drugs; assist adults to stop smoking; aid patients in managing their illnesses; or organize communities or advocate policy changes aimed at fostering health improvement. Health education professionals may also forge and test the fundamental theories that drive research and practice in health education. A premise of *Health Behavior and Health Education* is that a dynamic exchange between theory, research, and practice produces effective health education.

Perhaps never before have those concerned with health behavior and health education been faced with more challenges and opportunities than they are today. Kanfer and Schefft (1988, p. 7) observe that "as technology and science advance, the greatest mystery of the universe and the least conquered force of nature remains the human being and his actions and human experiences." The body of research in health behavior and health education has grown rapidly over the past two decades, and health education is recognized increasingly as a way to meet public health objectives and improve the success of public health and medical interventions. While this increasing literature improves the science base of health education, it also challenges those in the field to master and be facile with an almost overwhelming body of knowledge.

Health education is, by its very nature, eclectic. It is strengthened by being inclusive rather than exclusive. Health education is at the intersection of the biological and behavioral sciences. It draws on the theoretical perspectives, research, and practice tools of such diverse disciplines as psychology, sociology, anthropology, communications, nursing, and marketing. Yet, health education is also dependent on epidemiology, statistics, and medicine. This leaves the individual health education professional with the task of synthesizing large and diverse literatures.

Health education practice is strengthened by the close collaboration among professionals of different disciplines, each concerned with the behavioral and social intervention process, but each contributing a unique perspective. Psychology brings to health education a rich legacy of over 100 years of research and practice on individual differences, motivation, learning, persuasion, and attitude and behavior change (Matarazzo and others, 1984). Physicians are important collaborators and are in key roles to effect change in health behavior. Likewise, nurses and social workers bring to health education their particular expertise in working with individual patients, groups of patients, and patients' families to facilitate learning and behavior change. Other health, education, and human service professionals contribute their special expertise as well.

The Changing Context of Health and Disease, and Health Education

Americans are living longer than ever before. By the year 2010, 20 percent of the population will be sixty-five years of age or older. The major causes of death in the United States and other developed countries are now chronic diseases, such as heart disease, cancer, and stroke (U.S. Department of Health, Education, and Welfare, 1979). At least in part, these are life-style diseases. For example, one in six deaths in the United States is caused by smoking (U.S. Department of Health and Human Services, 1988). Dietary practices play a direct role in five of the ten leading causes of death and contribute to three others through excess alcohol consumption (*Surgeon General's Report on Nutrition and Health*, 1988). Life-style diseases are, by and large, the result of behavior and can often be altered by positive changes in behavior.

During the past twenty years, there has been a dramatic increase in public, private, and professional interest in preventing disability and death in the United States through changes in individual behaviors, such as smoking cessation, weight reduction, increased exercise, dietary change, injury prevention, protected sexual activity, and participation in screening and disease control programs. Much of this interest in health promotion and disease prevention has been stimulated by the epidemiologic transition from infectious to chronic diseases as leading causes of death, the aging of the population, rapidly escalating health care costs, and data linking individual behaviors to increased risk of morbidity and mortality. More recent developments, such as the AIDS epidemic, have also contributed (McLeroy, Bibeau, Steckler, and Glanz, 1988).

The publication in 1974 of the Lalonde report in Canada—*A New Perspective on the Health of Canadians* (Lalonde, 1974)—and the 1979 publication of *Healthy People* in the United States (U.S. Department of Health, Education, and Welfare, 1979) heralded the commitment of governments to health promotion. Both recognized the contributions of health education to improved health. In the United States, federal initiatives were spurred by the development of the *Health Objectives for the Nation* (U.S. Department of Health and Human Services, 1980). In Canada, the 1984 Ottawa Charter renewed and expanded the concept of health promotion as a public concern (Epp, 1986).

The increased interest in behavioral determinants of health and disease has drawn attention to the importance of health behavior change and spawned numerous training programs and public and commercial service programs. Research programs have been established to identify and test the most effective methods for achieving individual behavior change. More precise quantification of personal health behaviors and improved health outcomes has grown from the partnerships between behavioral scientists and biomedical health specialists (Breslow and Somers, 1977; Matarazzo and others, 1984). The field of psychology, with its emphasis on individual behavior, has been central to many of the research studies published during this period.

Within the field of health education, some critics have reacted to these trends with dismay, noting that they advance victim-blaming ideologies and fail to address the broader social determinants of health (see, for example, Allegrante and Green, 1981; Freudenberg, 1984–1985; Minkler, 1989). Advocates of system-level changes to improve health have called for implementation of a broad vision of health promotion as defined in recent national and international health policies and programs (Minkler, 1989). These recent calls for moving health education toward social action are well within the tradition of health education. They indicate the extent to which the popularization of individual behavior change approaches and research on individuals and small groups has dominated the health education landscape in recent years.

Over the past thirty years, outstanding leaders in health education repeatedly stressed the importance of political, economic, and social factors as determinants of health. Mayhew Derryberry (1960, p. 11) noted that "health education . . . requires careful and thorough consideration of the present knowledge, attitudes, goals, perceptions, social status, power structure, cultural traditions, and other aspects of whatever public is to be addressed." In 1966, Dorothy Nyswander spoke of the importance of attending to social justice and individuals' sense of control and self-determination (Nyswander, 1966). These ideas were reiterated later when William Griffiths (1972, p. 13) stressed that "health education is concerned not only with individuals and their families, but *also with the institutions and social conditions* that impede or facilitate individuals toward achieving optimum health" (italics added).

The view of health education as an instrument of social change has been eclipsed in recent years by the visibility and popularity of individually focused behavior change approaches. Undoubtedly, increased action directed toward the broad social agenda that has long been espoused as essential to health education will depend partly on the training of professionals, employment opportunities, and funding for research in these areas. Additional important influences include dissemination of the results of successful action programs and research (for example, Brown, 1983; Minkler, 1985). This volume purposefully includes chapters on community and societal influences on health behavior and strategies to effect community and social policy changes. In this context, definitions of health education and health promotion are discussed and recognized as overlapping and intertwined.

Health Education, Health Promotion, and Health Behavior

Health Education and Health Promotion

Health education is defined in many ways. According to Griffiths (1972, p. 12), "Health education attempts to close the gap between what is known about optimum health practice and that which is actually practiced." Simonds (1976, p. 107) defined health education as aimed at "bringing about behavioral changes in individuals, groups, and larger populations from behaviors that are presumed to be detrimental to health, to behaviors that are conducive to present and future health."

Subsequent definitions of health education emphasize voluntary, informed behavior changes. In 1980, Green defined health education as "any combination of learning experiences designed to facilitate voluntary adaptations of behavior conducive to health" (Green and others, 1980, p. 7). The Role Delineation Project defined health education as "the process of assisting individuals, acting separately or collectively, to make informed decisions about matters affecting their personal health and that of others" (National Task Force on the Preparation and Practice of Health Educators, 1983, p. 50).

Health education evolved from three settings: communities, schools, and patient care settings. Kurt Lewin's pioneering work in group process and his developmental field theory during the 1930s and 1940s comprise the intellectual roots of much of today's health education practice. One of the earliest models developed to explain health behavior, the Health Belief Model, was developed during the 1950s initially to explain behavior related to tuberculosis screening (Hochbaum, 1958).

Health education includes not only instructional activities but also organizational efforts, policy directives, economic supports, environmental activities, and community-level programs. McLeroy, Bibeau, Steckler, and Glanz (1988) have identified five distinct sets of factors comprising an ecological perspective as integral to health education and health promotion:

1. Intrapersonal factors—characteristics of the individual, such as knowledge, attitudes, behavior, self-concept, and skills. This includes the developmental history of the individual

2. Interpersonal processes and primary groups—formal and informal social network and social support systems, including family, work group, and friendship networks

3. Institutional factors—social institutions with organizational characteristics and formal (and informal) rules and regulations for operation

4. Community factors—relationships among organizations, institutions, and informal networks within defined boundaries

5. Public policy—local, state, and national laws and policies

Health education covers the continuum from disease prevention and promotion of optimal health to the detection of illness to treatment, rehabilitation, and long-term care. Health education is delivered in almost every conceivable setting—universities, schools, hospitals, pharmacies, grocery stores and shopping centers, community organizations, voluntary health agencies, work sites, churches, prisons, health maintenance organizations, migrant labor camps, advertising agencies, and health departments and at all levels of government. These diverse settings are discussed later in this chapter.

The definition of *health promotion* has been proposed by some leaders as being broader than *health education* because some of the methods integral to health promotion do not embrace an "educational philosophy" (Green, 1984). From this perspective, health promotion is a broader endeavor than health education and subsumes health education within its boundaries. Green (1984) defines health promotion as "health education and related organizational, economic, and environmental supports conducive to health." The World Health Organization Working Group (1984) defines health promotion as a process of enabling people to improve their health by synthesizing personal choice and social responsibility. This definition was expanded by the Ottawa Charter (Epp, 1986), which adds that health promotion includes creating healthy policies and supportive environments, and reorienting health services beyond clinical and curative care. Health promotion, thus, is "a combination of health education and health advocacy" (Minkler, 1989, p. 22).

While greater precision of terminology can be achieved by drawing a clear distinction between *health education* and *health promotion,* to do so is to ignore long-standing tenets of health education and its broad social mission. That mission was articulated years before the nomenclature of "health promotion" was introduced, much less accepted in common parlance. Moreover, it seems that the terms are often used interchangeably in the field of practice and higher education, by both professionals and the lay public. Hence, in their technical use, these terms usually differ in emphasis, with *health promotion* intended to underscore the broader social structural context of health behavior more clearly than *health education.* As with all language, however, these terms must ultimately be understood in terms of their common usage by scientists and practitioners—as closely linked and overlapping, with a common historical and philosophical foundation.

Health Behavior

The central concern of health education is health behavior. It is included in every definition of health education and is the crucial dependent variable in research on the impact of health education intervention strategies. Positive changes in health behavior are the ultimate aims of health education programs; if behaviors change but health is not subsequently improved, the result is a paradox that must be resolved by examining other issues (see, for example, Lorig and Laurin, 1985).

Gochman proposes a working defintion of *health behavior* that includes not only observable, overt actions but also the mental events and feeling states that can be reported and measured. His definition, including determinants of behavior as well as behavior itself, broadly circumscribes the *field* of health behavior: "those personal attributes such as beliefs, expectations, motives, values, perceptions, and other cognitive elements; personality characteristics, including affective and emotional states and traits; and overt

behavior patterns, actions and habits that relate to health maintenance, to health restoration, and to health improvement" (Gochman, 1982, p. 169).

Gochman's definition is consistent with and embraces the
definitions of specific categories of overt health behavior proposed
by Kasl and Cobb in their seminal articles (1966a, 1966b). Kasl and
Cobb define three categories of health behavior as follows:

> *Preventive health behavior:* any activity undertaken by
> an individual who believes himself to be healthy,
> for the purpose of preventing or detecting illness in
> an asymptomatic state
>
> *Illness behavior:* any activity undertaken by an indi-
> vidual who perceives himself to be ill, to define the
> state of his health, and to discover a suitable remedy
> (Kasl and Cobb, 1966a, p. 246)
>
> *Sick-role behavior:* any activity undertaken by an indi-
> vidual who considers himself to be ill, for the pur-
> pose of getting well. It includes receiving treatment
> from medical providers, generally involves a whole
> range of dependent behaviors, and leads to some
> degree of exemption of one's usual responsibilities
> (Kasl and Cobb, 1966b, p. 531).

In this book, the term *health behavior* is reserved for a variety
of overt behaviors, or actions. However, the definition set forth by
Gochman, which includes the presumed determinants (and sometimes results) of behavior, applies to the scope of *health behavior
research* as represented in this volume.

Settings and Audiences for Health Education

During the past century and more specifically during the past few
decades, the scope and methods of health education have broadened
and diversified dramatically. This book reflects an *inclusive* definition of health education, one that encompasses health education
and health promotion. This section briefly reviews the range of
settings and audiences of health education today.

Settings: Where Is Health Education Provided?

Today, health education is omnipresent. Five major settings are particularly relevant to health education: schools, communities, work sites, health care settings, and the consumer marketplace.

Schools. Health education in the schools includes classroom teaching, teacher training, and changes in the school environment that support healthy behaviors (Parcel, Simons-Morton, and Kolbe, 1988). To support long-term health enhancement initiatives, theories of organizational change are used to encourage adoption of comprehensive smoking control programs in schools (see Chapter Fourteen).

Communities. Community-based health education draws on social relationships and organizations to reach large populations with media and interpersonal strategies. Models of community organization enable program planners both to gain support for and to design suitable health education messages and delivery mechanisms (see Chapter Twelve). Several large community intervention studies of cardiovascular disease (CVD) risk reduction in the 1970s and 1980s incorporated theory and research precepts applicable to many community settings (Farquhar and others, 1984; Lasater and others, 1984).

Work Sites. Since its emergence in the mid-1970s, work site health promotion has grown and spawned new tools for health educators. Because people spend so much time at work, the workplace is situated ideally as both a source of stress and a source of social support (see Chapter Nine). Effective work site programs can harness social support as a buffer to stress, with the goal of improved worker health and health practices. Today, many businesses, particularly large corporations, provide health promotion programs for their employees (Fielding and Piserchia, 1989).

Health Care Settings. Health education for patients, their families, and the surrounding community and in-service training for health care providers are all part of health care today. The changing nature of health service delivery has stimulated greater emphasis on health education in physicians' offices, health maintenance organizations, public health clinics, and hospitals. Health education in these settings focuses on preventing or detecting disease and managing acute and chronic illnesses (Pender, 1987).

The Consumer Marketplace. The advent of home health and self-care products, as well as the use of "health" appeals to sell consumer goods, has created new opportunities for health education *and* for misleading consumers about the potential health effects of items they purchase. Social marketing, with its roots in consumer behavior theory, is used increasingly by health educators to enhance the salience of health messages and to improve their persuasive impact. Theories of Consumer Information Processing (CIP) provide a framework for understanding why people do or do not pay attention to, understand, and make use of nutrient labels on packaged food products (see Chapter Six).

Audiences: Who Are the Targets of Health Education?

For health education to be effective, it should be designed with an understanding of the target audiences, their health and social characteristics, and their beliefs, attitudes, values, skills, and past behaviors. These audiences consist of people who may be reached as individuals, in groups, through organizations, or as communities or sociopolitical entities. They may be health professionals, clients, or patients. This section discusses two dimensions along which potential target audiences can be characterized: life cycle stage and sociodemographic characteristics.

Life Cycle Stage. Health education is provided for people at every stage of the life cycle, from childbirth education whose beneficiaries are not yet born to self-care education and rehabilitation for the very old. Developmental perspectives help guide the choice of interventions and research methods.

- Children may have misperceptions about health and illness, such as that illnesses are a punishment for bad behavior. Knowledge of children's cognitive development helps provide a framework for understanding these beliefs and ways to respond to them.

- Adolescents may feel invulnerable to accidents and chronic diseases. The Health Belief Model (see Chapter Three) is a useful framework for understanding the factors that may predispose youth to drive after drinking.
- Older adults may attribute symptoms of cancer to the inexorable process of aging. Beliefs such as this must be considered in program planning, implementation, and evaluation (Rimer and others, 1983; Keintz, Rimer, Fleisher, and Engstrom, 1988).

Sociodemographic Characteristics. Sociodemographic characteristics such as gender, age, race, marital status, place of residence, employment, and educational level are cornerstones of describing health education audiences. These factors, while generally not *modifiable* within health education programs, are useful in guiding the tailoring of strategies and educational materials. Printed educational materials should be tailored to the educational and reading levels of particular target audiences and be consistent with their ethnic and cultural backgrounds.

Health Education Foundations and
Theory, Research, and Practice

This chapter has discussed the dynamic nature of health education today in the context of changing patterns of disease and trends in health promotion and disease prevention. It has provided definitions of health education, health promotion, and health behavior and described the broad and diverse parameters of this maturing field. The interrelationships and importance of theory, research, and practice are set against a backdrop of the important, growing, and complex challenges in health education and health behavior.

References

Allegrante, J., and Green, L. W. "When Health Policy Becomes Victim Blaming." *New England Journal of Medicine,* 1981, *306,* 1528–1529.

Breslow, L., and Somers, A. "The Lifetime Health Monitoring Program." *New England Journal of Medicine*, 1977, *296*, 601–610.

Brown, E. R. "Community Organization Influence on Local Public Health Care Policy: A General Research Model and Comparative Case Study." *Health Education Quarterly*, 1983, *10*, 205–233.

Derryberry, M. "Health Education—Its Objectives and Methods." *Health Education Monographs*, 1960, *8*, 5–11.

Epp, L. *Achieving Health for All: A Framework for Health Promotion in Canada.* Toronto: Health and Welfare Canada, 1986.

Farquhar, J. W., and others. "The Stanford Five City Project: An Overview." In J. D. Matarazzo and others (eds.), *Behavioral Health: A Handbook of Health Enhancement and Disease Prevention.* New York: Wiley, 1984.

Fielding, J. E., and Piserchia, P. V. "Frequency of Worksite Health Promotion Activities." *American Journal of Public Health*, 1989, *79*, 16–20.

Freudenberg, N. "Training Health Educators for Social Change." *International Quarterly of Community Health Education*, 1984–85, *5*, 37–52.

Gochman, D. S. "Labels, Systems, and Motives: Some Perspectives for Future Research." *Health Education Quarterly*, 1982, *9*, 167–174.

Green, L. W. "Health Education Models." In J. D. Matarazzo and others (eds.), *Behavioral Health: A Handbook of Health Enhancement and Disease Prevention.* New York: Wiley, 1984.

Green, L. W. "The Theory of Participation: A Qualitative Analysis of Its Expression in National and International Health Policies." *Advances in Health Education and Promotion*, 1986, *1*, 211–236.

Green, L. W., and others. *Health Education Planning: A Diagnostic Approach.* Mountain View, Calif.: Mayfield, 1980.

Griffiths, W. "Health Education Definitions, Problems, and Philosophies." *Health Education Monographs*, 1972, *31*, 12–14.

Hochbaum, G. M. *Public Participation in Medical Screening Programs: A Sociopsychological Study.* Public Health Service Publication no. 572, 1958.

Kanfer, F. H., and Schefft, B. *Guiding the Process of Therapeutic Change.* Champaign, Ill.: Research Press, 1988.

Kasl, S. V., and Cobb, S. "Health Behavior, Illness Behavior, and

Sick-Role Behavior: I. Health and Illness Behavior." *Archives of Environmental Health,* 1966a, *12,* 246-266.

Kasl, S. V., and Cobb, S. "Health Behavior, Illness Behavior, and Sick-Role Behavior: II. Sick-Role Behavior." *Archives of Environmental Health,* 1966b, *12,* 531-541.

Keintz, M. K., Rimer, B., Fleisher, L., and Engstrom, P. "Educating Older Adults About Their Increased Cancer Risk." *Gerontologist,* 1988, *28,* 487-490.

Lalonde, M. *A New Perspective on the Health of Canadians: A Working Document.* Toronto: Health and Welfare Canada, 1974.

Lasater, T., and others. "Lay Volunteer Delivery of a Community-Based Cardiovascular Risk Factor Change Program: The Pawtucket Experiment." In J. D. Matarazzo and others (eds.), *Behavioral Health: A Handbook of Health Enhancement and Disease Prevention.* New York: Wiley, 1984.

Lorig, K., and Laurin, J. "Some Notions About Assumptions Underlying Health Education." *Health Education Quarterly,* 1985, *12,* 231-243.

McLeroy, K. R., Bibeau, D., Steckler, A., and Glanz, K. "An Ecological Perspective on Health Promotion Programs." *Health Education Quarterly,* 1988, *15,* 351-377.

Matarazzo, J.D., and others (eds.). *Behavioral Health: A Handbook of Health Enhancement and Disease Prevention.* New York: Wiley, 1984.

Minkler, M. "Building Supportive Ties and Sense of Community Among the Inner City Elderly: The Tenderloin Senior Outreach Project." *Health Education Quarterly,* 1985, *12,* 303-314.

Minkler, M. "Health Education, Health Promotion, and the Open Society: An Historical Perspective." *Health Education Quarterly,* 1989, *16,* 17-30.

National Task Force on the Preparation and Practice of Health Educators, Inc. *A Framework for the Development of Competency-Based Curricula for Entry Level Health Educators.* New York: National Task Force on the Preparation and Practice of Health Educators, 1983.

Nyswander, D. "The Open Society: Its Implications for Health Educators." *Health Education Monographs,* 1966, *1,* 3-13.

Parcel, G., Simons-Morton, B. G., and Kolbe, L. J. "Health Promotion: Integrating Organizational Change and Student Learning Strategies." *Health Education Quarterly,* 1988, *15,* 435–450.

Pender, N. J. *Health Promotion in Nursing Practice.* (2nd ed.) Norwalk, Conn.: Appleton and Lange, 1987.

Rimer, B., and others. "Planning a Cancer Control Program for Older Citizens." *Gerontologist,* 1983, *23,* 384–389.

Simonds, S. K. "Health Education in the Mid-1970s: State of the Art." In *Preventive Medicine USA.* New York: Prodist, 1976.

Surgeon General's Report on Nutrition and Health. Public Health Service Publication no. 88-50210, 1988.

U.S. Department of Health, Education, and Welfare. *Healthy People: The Surgeon General's Report on Health Promotion and Disease Prevention.* Public Health Service Publication no. 79-55071, 1979.

U.S. Department of Health and Human Services. *Promoting Health and Preventing Disease: Health Objectives for the Nation.* Washington, D.C.: U.S. Government Printing Office, 1980.

U.S. Department of Health and Human Services. *Reducing the Health Consequences of Smoking: 25 Years of Progress. A Report of the Surgeon General.* Centers for Disease Control Publication no. 89-8411, prepublication version, 1988.

World Health Organization Working Group. *Report of the Working Group on Concepts and Principles of Health Promotion.* Copenhagen: World Health Organization, 1984. (Later published in *Health Promotion,* 1986, *1,* 73–76.)

Chapter 2

The Editors

▲ ▲ ▲

Theory, Research, and Practice in Health Education: Building Bridges and Forging Links

Theory, Research, and Practice: Interrelationships

Aristotle distinguished between *theoria* and *praxis*. *Theoria* signifies those sciences and activities that are concerned with knowing for its own sake, whereas *praxis* corresponds to the ways in which we now commonly speak of action or doing. This contrast between theory and practice (Bernstein, 1971, p. ix) permeates Western philosophical and scientific thought from Aristotle to Marx and on to Dewey and other contemporary twentieth-century philosophers. Dewey attempted to resolve the dichotomy by focusing on the similarities and continuities between theoretical and practical judgments and inquiries. He described "experimental knowing" essentially as an art that involves a conscious, directed manipulation of objects and situations. "The craftsman perfects his art, not by comparing his product to some 'ideal' model, but by the cumulative results of experience—experience which benefits from tried and tested procedures but always involves risk and novelty" (Bernstein, 1971, p. 218). Dewey thus described empirical investigation, that is, research, as the ground between theory and practice and the testing of theory in action.

Although the perception of theory and practice as a dichotomy has a long tradition in intellectual thought, we follow in Dew-

17

ey's tradition and focus on the similarities and continuities rather than on the differences. Theory, research, and practice are a continuum along which the skilled professional can move with ease. Theory and research are not solely the province of the academic, just as practice is not solely the field of the practitioner. Researchers and practitioners may differ in their priorities, but the relationship between research and its application can and should move in both directions. "The search for truth and for an ultimate understanding of the forces that make humans think, feel, and act as they do is the long-term goal" (Kanfer and Schefft, 1988, p. 14).

The task of health education is both to understand health behavior and to transform knowledge about behavior into useful strategies for health enhancement. Research in health education has an inherently applied cast; it is motivated and driven by service to existing or anticipated health concerns of individuals, groups, communities, and societies. As Rosenstock suggests in Chapter Three, we should test our theories iteratively in the real world. When we do so, theory, research, and practice begin to converge. The theories and research in this book are treated in light of their applicability and not as *basic* health behavior research.

Health Behavior and Health Education aims to help educators, whatever their background, understand some of the most important theoretical underpinnings of health education and use theory to inform research and practice. To function effectively in the increasingly complex world of health education, one needs a broad-based understanding of theory, research, and practice. "Health educators cannot limit themselves to the simple replication of well-researched programs. For one thing, we do not yet have enough programs of that kind. More importantly, people and communities are too complex and changeable for such an approach" (Kling, 1984, p. 342).

The authors of *Health Behavior and Health Education* believe that "there is nothing so useful as a good theory" (Lewin, 1935). Each chapter demonstrates the practical value of theory; each synthesizes what was learned through conceptually sound research and practice and draws the linkages between theory, research, and practice.

Professionals charged with responsibility for health education are, by and large, interventionists. They are action oriented. They use their knowledge to design and to implement programs to improve health. This is true whether they are working to encourage positive changes in individual or community behavior. It is equally true of most health education research. Such research is conducted primarily in the real world, not in isolated laboratories. Usually, in the process of attempting to change behavior or policies, researchers must do precisely what practitioners do—develop and deliver interventions. At some level, both practitioners and researchers are accountable for results, whether these are measured in terms of participants' satisfaction with programs or changes in awareness, knowledge, attitudes, beliefs, health behaviors; institutional norms; community integration; or more distal results, including morbidity, mortality, and quality of life. Health educators may assess these results anecdotally, or they may conduct more rigorous evaluations.

The design of interventions that yield desired changes can best be done with an understanding of theories of behavior change and an ability to use them skillfully in practice. Most health educators work in situations in which resources are limited, which makes judgments about the choice of intervention very important. There may be no second chance to reach a critical target audience.

A synthesis of theory, research, and practice will advance what is known about health behavior. A health educator without theory is like a mechanic, or a mere technician, whereas the professional who understands theory and research comprehends the "why?" and can design and craft well-tailored interventions. He or she does not blindly follow a cookbook recipe but constantly creates the recipe anew, depending on the circumstances (Kreuter, 1988). In health education, the circumstances include the nature of the target audience, the setting, resources, goals, and constraints.

Understanding theory also gives the health educator the power to measure more carefully and astutely in order to assess the impact of interventions. Learning from successive interventions strengthens not only the knowledge base of the individual health professional. Over time, this cumulative learning contributes to the knowledge base of all. In their continuum, theory, research, and practice nurture and are nurtured by each other.

The health educator in a health maintenance organization

who understands the importance of Social Learning Theory may be able to design better interventions to help patients lose weight or stop smoking. The community health educator who understands the principles of media advocacy and social marketing can make far better use of the mass media than one who does not. A working knowledge of community organization can help the educator identify and mobilize key individuals and groups to develop or maintain a health education program. The physician who understands interpersonal influence can communicate more effectively with patients. The psychologist who understands Multiattribute Utility Theory will know how to design better exercise and weight control interventions.

What Is Theory?

A theory is a set of interrelated propositions containing concepts that describe, explain, predict, or control behavior (Kerlinger, 1986). A fully developed formal theory—more an ideal than a reality—is a completely closed deductive system of propositions that identifies the interrelationships among the concepts and is a systematic view of the phenomena (Kerlinger, 1986; Blalock, 1969, p. 2). In reality, there is no such system in the social sciences or health education; it can only be approximated (Blalock, 1969, p. 2). Theory has been defined in a variety of ways, each consistent with Kerlinger's definition. Table 2.1 summarizes several definitions of theory.

No single theory dominates research or practice in health education, and for good reasons. The goals, resources, policies, and limitations of the individual provider and the organization cast a net over the potentially modifiable factors for a particular situation. Different theories are best suited to different units of practice, such as individuals, groups, and organizations. Health behavior and the guiding concepts for influencing it are far too complex to be explained by a single, unified theory. Effective health education depends on marshaling the most appropriate theory and practice strategies for a given situation. For example, when one is attempting to overcome women's personal barriers to obtaining mammograms, the Health Belief Model may be useful. When trying to

Table 2.1. Definitions of Theory.

Definition	Source
A set of interrelated constructs (concepts), definitions, and propositions that present a systematic view of phenomena by specifying relations among variables, with the purpose of explaining and predicting the phenomena	Kerlinger, 1986, p. 9
A systematic explanation for the observed facts and laws that relate to a particular aspect of life	Babbie, 1989, p. 46
A formal and abstract statement about a selected aspect of reality	Kar, 1986, pp. 157–158
Knowledge writ large in the form of generalized abstractions applicable to a wide range of experiences	McGuire, 1983, p. 2
A set of relatively abstract and general statements which collectively purport to explain some aspect of the empirical world	Chafetz, 1978, p. 2
An abstract, symbolic representation of what is conceived to be reality—a set of abstract statements designed to "fit" some portion of the real world	Zimbardo, Ebbesen, and Maslach, 1977, p. 53

change physicians' mammography practices by instituting reminder systems, organizational change theories are more suitable.

Theories explain. Explanation involves a delineation of the ways, processes, or mechanisms by which health behavior is affected. Bandura's Social Learning Theory represents one of the most formally developed theories of behavior today. It identifies the determinant or explanatory variables and their interrelationships, as well as the methods for inducing changes in the determinant variables. Ajzen and Fishbein's Theory of Reasoned Action is also a highly developed theory of behavior. It not only identifies and defines key variables that affect a person's intentions to act but also identifies the sequence of variables and their interrelationships that predict the behavioral intention. Both of these theories have been applied to health behavior.

By telling us about the what, how, when, and why, theories can inform programs in health education. By delineating the elements of a theory, the theory can guide the development of a health education intervention. The *what* tells us the elements we should consider as the targets for the intervention. For example, the Health Belief Model suggests that to increase the practice of AIDS prevention behaviors, people must feel susceptible to AIDS. Even though various theoretical models of health behavior may reflect the same general ideas (Cummings, Becker, and Maile, 1980), each theory employs a unique vocabulary to articulate the specific factors considered to be important. The *why* tells us about the processes by which changes occur in the target variables. The *when* tells us about the timing and sequencing of our interventions in order to achieve maximum effects. The *how* tells us the methods or ways we should focus our interventions; it includes the specific means of inducing changes in the explanatory variables.

Theories vary in the extent to which they have been conceptually developed and empirically tested. Bandura (1986, p. xii) points out that "theories are interpreted in different ways depending on the stage of development of the field of study. In advanced disciplines, theories integrate laws; in less advanced fields, theories specify the determinants governing the phenomena of interest." The term *theory* must be used in the latter sense in *Health Behavior and Health Education* because the field is still relatively young.

Principles, Concepts, and Variables. Theories go beyond principles. Principles are general guidelines for action (Green and Lewis, 1986). They are broad and nonspecific and may actually distort realities or results based on research. Principles may be based on precedent or history, *or* they may be based on research. At their worst, principles are so broad that they invite multiple interpretations and are therefore unreliable. At their best, principles are based on accumulated research. In their best form, principles provide hypotheses and serve as our most informed hunches about how or what we should do to obtain a desired outcome in a target population. In their weakest form, principles are like horoscopes: Anyone can derive whatever meaning he or she wants from them.

Concepts are the major components of a theory; they are the building blocks or primary elements of a theory. Concepts vary in the extent to which they have meaning or can be understood outside the context of a specific theory. When concepts were developed or adopted for use in a particular theory, they are called constructs (Kerlinger, 1986). The term *subjective normative belief* is an example of a construct within Ajzen and Fishbein's (1980) Theory of Reasoned Action; the specific construct is understood only within the context of that theory. Another example of a construct is the term *perceived susceptibility* in the Health Belief Model (see Chapter Three).

Variables are the empirical counterparts or operational definitions of concepts (Green and Lewis, 1986). They specify how a concept is to be measured. For example, the concept of subjective norm in the Theory of Reasoned Action might be measured on a seven-point scale ranging from "definitely should" to "definitely should not" carry out a particular behavior.

Paradigms for Theory and Research in Health Education. A paradigm is a basic schema that organizes our broadly based view of something (Babbie, 1989, p. 47). Paradigms are widely recognized scientific achievements that, for a time, provide model problem-solving approaches to a community of practitioners. They include theory, application, and instrumentation and comprise models that represent coherent traditions of scientific research (Kuhn, 1962). Paradigms gain status because they are more successful at solving pressing problems than are their competitors (Kuhn, 1962).

Paradigms create boundaries within which the search for answers occurs; they do not answer particular questions, but they do direct the search for answers to questions (Babbie, 1989, p. 47). Paradigms circumscribe or delimit what is important to examine in a given field of inquiry. The collective judgments of scientists define the dominant paradigm that constitutes the body of science (Wilson, 1952, p. 21).

In health education and health behavior, as well as in this text, the dominant perspective that supports the largest body of theory and research is that of *logical positivism,* or *logical empiricism.* This basic view, developed in the Vienna Circle from 1924 to 1936, has two central features: (1) an emphasis on the use of induction, or sensory experience, feelings, and personal judgments as the source of knowledge, and (2) the view that deduction is the standard for verification or confirmation of theory so that theory must be tested through empirical methods and systematic observation of phenomena (Runes, 1984). Logical empiricism reconciles the deductive and inductive extremes; it prescribes that the researcher begin with a hypothesis deduced from a theory and then test it, subjecting it to the jeopardy of disconfirmation through empirical test (McGuire, 1983, p. 7; Thompson, 1985).

An alternative world view in health education relies more heavily on induction and is often identified as a *qualitative* perspective. This perspective argues that the organization and explanation of events must be revealed in the course of events through a process of discovery rather than organized into prescribed conceptual categories before a study begins. As such, data collection methods such as standardized questionnaires and predetermined response categories have a limited place. Ethnography, phenomenology, and grounded theory are examples of approaches using a qualitative perspective (Strauss, 1987; Mullen and Iverson, 1986).

McGuire has proposed a contextualist epistemology that is consistent with some of logical empiricism's premises but extends beyond it. The contextualist position agrees that a theoretically derived hypothesis should "precede and guide a scientist's empirical observations and that empirical confrontation is essential for developing the hypothesis's scientific meaning and validity (McGuire, 1983, p. 7). The contextualist perspective departs from logical empiricism by maintaining that "all theories, even mutually contradictory ones, are right" (p. 7). In other words, contextualism asserts that the research process seeks to clarify the *contexts,* or circumstances, under which a hypothesis is true rather than its absolute rightness or wrongness. It seeks an understanding of *what works best under which conditions.* This view implies that scientists should represent the meaning of theories by making explicit their limiting assumptions or the conditions under which the predicted results will occur. The contextualist perspective is central to this volume, with its goal of summarizing the various theories that inform health education activities for a wide variety of settings, audiences, and topics.

Selection of Theories for This Book

No single theory or conceptual framework dominates research or practice in health education today. Instead, there is a multitude of theories from which to choose. McGuire (1984) identifies sixteen possible theories that could be used in the creation of public health communication campaigns. A recent review of 116 theory-based articles published between 1986 and 1988 in two major health education journals, *Health Education Quarterly* and *Health Education Research*, revealed fifty-one distinct theoretical formulations. Many of the articles employed one or more of three important theories: Social Learning Theory (twenty-three articles), Theory of Reasoned Action (nineteen articles), and the Health Belief Model (sixteen articles). However, even the most frequently mentioned—Social Learning Theory—accounted for less than one-quarter of the articles (Glanz, 1988). For the unprepared, the choices can be overwhelming; but for those who understand the commonalities and differences among theories of health behavior and health education, the growing knowledge base can provide a firm foundation upon which to build. We hope that *Health Behavior and Health Education* will provide and strengthen that foundation for readers.

Theories that gain recognition in a discipline shape the field, help define the scope of practice, and influence the training and socialization of its professionals. The theories included in *Health Behavior and Health Education* were selected to provide readers with a range of theories representing different units of intervention, for example, the individual, group, and community. They were also chosen because they represent, as with the Health Belief Model and Social Learning Theory, dominant theories of health behavior and health education. Others were chosen, as in the case of social marketing and Consumer Information Processing Theory, to acquaint readers with promising theoretical formulations that are likely to become increasingly useful to professionals concerned with health behavior change.

The selection of theories for inclusion in this book is the result of some difficult decisions. First, the theory must meet basic criteria of adequacy for research and practice. Another consideration is that *current* health education research must be employing the theory. For example, we include the Health Belief Model rather than Lewin's Field Theory. In addition, the theory must be explicit and be more narrowly focused than a broad schema for program development.

The adequacy of a theory is most often assessed in terms of three criteria (McGuire, 1983): (1) its *internal consistency* in not yielding mutually contradictory derivations, (2) the extent to which it is *parsimonious*, or broadly relevant while using a manageable number of concepts, and (3) its *plausibility* in fitting with prevailing theories in the field. The unique identification and "naming" of a theory rests on its *novelty;* a "new" theory must be more than just a minor variation on a familiar theme (McGuire, 1983).

Theories are further judged in the context of activities of practitioners and researchers. Practitioners apply the pragmatic criterion of *usefulness* of a theory. Researchers make scientific judgments of a theory's *ecological validity*, or the extent to which it conforms to observable reality when empirically tested (McGuire, 1983).

Three criteria that tend to limit the scope of theoretical frameworks most readily available for use in health education also helped to define the content of this book. One is that the theory must have a history of testing on health-related behavior or use as a basis for health education interventions. The second criterion is that there must be at least promising, if not substantial, empirical evidence supporting the theory's validity in predicting or changing health behavior. Third, the theory should have potential for effective use by health education practitioners.

Because of the eclectic and derivative nature of health education theory, adaptations and refinements of theories of health behavior and health education occur in response to both scientists' and practitioners' concerns. A circularity exists between theory and practice. As Roberts (1959, p. 160) astutely noted three decades ago, "The theoretical base of our profession must be augmented and modified by continuing, careful analysis of documented practice and from collaborative action research."

In some cases, the "purpose" rather than the theory is the identifying title for a chapter—as in the case of Chapter Nine on

Interpersonal Influence, which describes several theories of social influence and weighs their utility for health education. Chapter Twelve on Community Organization is named for the resultant intervention strategies rather than for the convergent theoretical bases that form the foundation for community organization work.

The editors of this book recognize the lack of consensus regarding the definition and classification of theories. We have taken a liberal, ecumenical stance toward theory. And we concede that the lowest common denominator of the theoretical models herein might be that they are all *conceptual or theoretical frameworks,* or broadly conceived perspectives used to organize ideas. Nevertheless, we have not abandoned the term *theory* because it accurately describes the spirit of the volume, the goal to be attained for developing frameworks, and the tools for refining health education research and practice.

Building Bridges and Forging Links

Practitioners of health education at once benefit from and are challenged by the eclectic and derivative nature of their endeavor: A multitude of theoretical frameworks and models from the social sciences are available for their use, but the best choices and direct translations may not be immediately evident. There is an inherent danger in a book like this: One can begin to think that the links between theory, research, and health education practice are easily forged. They are not. Several issues are particularly relevant in creating these links.

Theories developed for and tested under controlled experimental conditions may require modification to permit their application to a field setting. Interpretation and adaptation of a theory are always requisites of field application. Extensions of health behavior theories to health education are not always obvious or clear. In their current form, some theories may not have direct applicability to health education interventions. Further, the assumptions underlying a theory may not fit with the constraints of the field setting.

Science is by definition cumulative, and the same applies to the science base that supports long-standing as well as innovative health education interventions. The gift of theory is that it provides the conceptual underpinnings to well-crafted research and informed practice. "The scientist values research by the size of its contribution to that huge, logically articulated structure of ideas which is already, though not yet half built, the most glorious accomplishment of mankind" (Medawar, 1967).

In this book, we aim to demystify theory and to communicate theory and theoretically inspired research alongside their implications for practice. The ultimate test of these ideas and this information rests on its use over time. Like any long-term behavior, this will require social support, supportive environments, and periodic reinforcement. The mutual benefits will be for practitioners, researchers, and the participants in health education programs.

Limitations of This Book

No text can be all-inclusive. This is certainly true of *Health Behavior and Health Education*. There are important theories and conceptual frameworks that could not be included because of space limitations. These include Self-Regulation Theory (Leventhal, Zimmerman, and Gutmann, 1984), Protection Motivation Theory (Rogers, 1975), Prospect Theory (Slovic and Lichtenstein, 1968), the Transtheoretical Model (Prochaska and DiClemente, 1983), and more familiar classical theories such as Field Theory (Lewin, 1935) and Cognitive Consistency (Festinger, 1957). Some of these are described within the historical origins of the various theories discussed in this book. Others will be discussed in the synthesis and perspectives chapters.

This book is not intended to be a how-to guide or manual for program planning and development in health education. Other books in health education (Dignan and Carr, 1987; Green and others, 1980), nursing (Pender, 1987), medicine (Vanderschmidt, Koch-Weser, and Woodbury, 1987), psychology (Kanfer and Goldstein, 1975), and nutrition education (Snetselaar, 1983) serve that purpose, and the reader is directed to those sources for more on the "nuts and bolts" of practice.

Neither is this volume intended to serve as an in-depth treatise on research methods in health behavior and health education. Instead, it demonstrates by example how theories are operationalized in a modest number of examples. The reader who wishes more guidance regarding applied research for studies of health education will find ample resources in books on social science research methodology (Babbie, 1989; Kidder, 1984; Kerlinger, 1986) and on evaluation and measurement in health education and health promotion (Dignan, 1986; Green and Lewis, 1986; Windsor, Baranowski, Clark, and Cutter, 1984).

The editors hope that readers will emerge with a critical appreciation of theory and with the curiosity to pursue not only the theories presented in *Health Behavior and Health Education* but other promising theories as well. Thus, *Health Behavior and Health Education* should be regarded as the starting point, not the end.

Theories—or conceptual frameworks—can be, and *are*, useful because they enrich, inform, and complement the practical technologies of health education. Thus the readers of this book should "pass with relief from the tossing sea of Cause and Theory to the firm ground of Result and Fact" (Churchill, 1898). As the ocean meets the shore, so we hope you will find that theory, research, and practice in health education stretch out to converge in a single landscape.

References

Ajzen, I., and Fishbein, M. *Understanding Attitudes and Predicting Social Behavior.* Englewood Cliffs, N.J.: Prentice-Hall, 1980.

Babbie, E. *The Practice of Social Research.* (5th ed.) Belmont, Calif.: Wadsworth, 1989.

Bandura, A. *Social Foundations of Thought and Action: A Social Cognitive Theory.* Englewood Cliffs, N.J.: Prentice-Hall, 1986.

Bernstein, R. *Praxis and Action.* Philadelphia: University of Pennsylvania Press, 1971.

Blalock, H. M., Jr. "Theory Building and Causal Inferences." In H. M. Blalock, Jr., and A. B. Blalock (eds.), *Methodology in Social Research.* New York: McGraw-Hill, 1968.

Blalock, H. M., Jr. *Theory Construction, From Verbal to Mathematical Constructions.* Englewood Cliffs, N.J.: Prentice-Hall, 1969.

Chafetz, J. *A Primer on the Construction of Theories in Sociology.* Itasca, Ill.: Peacock, 1978.

Churchill, W. *The Malakand Field Force.* 1898.

Cummings, K. M., Becker, M. H., and Maile, M. C. "Bringing the Models Together: An Empirical Approach to Combining Variables Used to Explain Health Actions." *Journal of Behavioral Medicine,* 1980, *3*, 123–145.

Dignan, M. B. *Measurement and Evaluation of Health Education.* Springfield, Ill.: Thomas, 1986.

Dignan, M. B., and Carr, P. A. *Program Planning for Health Education and Health Promotion.* Philadelphia: Lea & Febiger, 1987.

Festinger, L. *A Theory of Cognitive Dissonance.* Stanford, Calif.: Stanford University Press, 1957.

Glanz, K. "Can Health Education Research and Practice Be More Successful by Using Behavioral Theory?" Paper presented at American Public Health Association annual meeting, Boston, Nov. 14, 1988.

Green, L. W., and Lewis, F. M. *Evaluation and Measurement in Health Education and Health Promotion.* Mountain View, Calif.: Mayfield, 1986.

Green, L. W., and others. *Health Education Planning: A Diagnostic Approach.* Mountain View, Calif.: Mayfield, 1980.

Kanfer, F. H., and Goldstein, A. P. *Helping People Change.* New York: Pergamon Press, 1975.

Kanfer, F. H., and Schefft, B. *Guiding the Process of Therapeutic Change.* Champaign, Ill.: Research Press, 1988.

Kar, S. B. "Introduction: Theoretical Foundations of Health Education and Promotion." *Advances in Health Education and Promotion,* 1986, *1*, 157–163.

Kerlinger, F. N. *Foundations of Behavioral Research.* (3rd ed.) New York: Holt, Rinehart & Winston, 1986.

Kidder, L. *Research Methods in Social Relations.* (4th ed.) Ann Arbor, Mich.: Society for the Psychological Study of Social Issues, 1984.

Kling, B. "Health Education Practice and the Literature." *Health Education Quarterly,* 1984, *11*, 341–347.

Kreuter, M. "The Practical Outcomes of Theory-Based Health Education Practice." Paper presented at American Public Health Association annual meeting, Boston, Nov. 14, 1988.

Kuhn, T. S. *The Structure of Scientific Revolution.* Chicago: University of Chicago Press, 1962.

Leventhal, H., Zimmerman, R., and Gutmann, M. "Compliance: A Self-Regulation Perspective." In D. Gentry (ed.), *Handbook of Behavorial Medicine.* New York: Guilford Press, 1984.

Lewin, K. *A Dynamic Theory of Personality.* New York: McGraw-Hill, 1935.

McGuire, W. J. "A Contextualist Theory of Knowledge: Its Implications for Innovation and Reform in Psychological Research." *Advances in Experimental Social Psychology,* 1983, *16*, 1–47.

McGuire, W. J. "Public Communication as a Strategy for Inducing Health Promoting Behavioral Change." *Preventive Medicine,* 1984, *13*, 299–313.

Medawar, P. B. *The Art of the Soluble.* New York: Methuen, 1967.

Mullen, P. D., and Iverson, D. "Qualitative Methods," In L. W. Green and F. M. Lewis, *Measurement and Evaluation in Health Education and Health Promotion.* Mountain View, Calif.: Mayfield, 1986.

Pender, N. J. *Health Promotion in Nursing Practice.* (2nd ed.) Norwalk, Conn.: Appleton and Lange, 1987.

Prochaska, J. O., and DiClemente, C. C. "Stages and Processes of Self-Change of Smoking: Toward an Integrative Model of Change." *Journal of Consulting and Clinical Psychology,* 1983, *51*, 390–395.

Roberts, B. J. "Decision Making: An Illustration of Theory Building." Presidential address, 10th annual meeting of the Society of Public Health Educators, Atlantic City, N.J., Oct. 18, 1959.

Rogers, R. "A Protection Motivation Theory of Fear Appeals and Attitude Change." *Journal of Psychology,* 1975, *91*, 93–114.

Runes, D. *Dictionary of Philosophy.* Totawa, N.J.: Rowman and Allanheld, 1984.

Slovic, P., and Lichtenstein, S. "Relative Importance of Probabilities and Payoffs in Risk Taking." *Journal of Experimental Psychology,* 1968, *78*, pt. 2.

Snetselaar, L. G. *Nutrition Counseling Skills: Assessment, Treatment, and Evaluation.* Rockville, Md.: Aspen Research, 1983.

Strauss, A. L. *Qualitative Analysis for Social Scientists.* Cambridge, England: Cambridge University Press, 1987.

Thompson, J. L. "Practical Discourse in Nursing: Going Beyond Empiricism and Historicism." *Advances in Nursing Science,* 1985, 7, 59–71.

Vanderschmidt, H. F., Koch-Weser, D., and Woodbury, P. A. (eds.). *Handbook of Clinical Prevention.* Baltimore, Md.: Williams & Wilkins, 1987.

Wilson, E. B. *An Introduction to Scientific Research.* New York: McGraw-Hill, 1952.

Windsor, R. A., Baranowski, T., Clark, N., and Cutter, G. *Evaluation of Health Promotion and Education Programs.* Mountain View, Calif.: Mayfield, 1984.

Zimbardo, P. G., Ebbesen, E. B., and Maslach, C. *Influencing Attitudes and Changing Behavior.* (2nd ed.) Reading, Mass.: Addison-Wesley, 1977.

▲ ▲ ▲

PART TWO

MODELS OF
INDIVIDUAL HEALTH BEHAVIOR

Individuals are one of the essential units of health education theory, research, and practice. This does not mean that the individual is the only or necessarily the most important unit of intervention. But all other units, whether they are groups, organizations, communities or larger units, are composed of individuals. To explain human behavior and to influence it, those concerned with health behavior and health education must understand the individual.

A wide range of health professionals, including health educators, physicians, psychologists, and nurses, focus all or most of their efforts on changing the health behavior of individuals. To intervene effectively and to make informed judgments about how to measure the success of such interventions, health professionals must have an understanding of the role of the individual in health behavior. This section of *Health Behavior and Health Education* helps the reader achieve a greater understanding of theories that focus primarily on individual health behavior.

Lewin's (1935) seminal Field Theory was one of the early and most far-reaching theories of behavior, and most contemporary theories of health behavior owe a major intellectual debt to Lewin. During the 1940s and 1950s, we began to learn more about how individuals make decisions concerning health and what determines health behavior. Rosenstock and Hochbaum, from their vantage point at the United States Public Health Service, began their pioneering work to understand why individuals participated in screening programs for tuberculosis. The Health Belief Model emerged from their efforts as one of the foundations of contemporary health behavior and health education (Janz and Becker, 1984). Rosenstock reviews the evolution of the Health Belief Model in Chapter Three. In the last twenty years, considerable progress has been made in understanding the determinants of individuals' health-related behaviors and ways to stimulate positive behavior changes. Value Expectancy Theories, which include both the Health Belief Model and the Theory of Reasoned Action (Chapter Two), matured during this time. Together with Attribution Theory and Consumer Information Processing, these theories form the basis for Part Two of this book.

Rosenstock explains in Chapter Three that the Health Belief Model is used to understand why people accept preventive health services and why they do or do not adhere to other kinds of health care regimens. The Health Belief Model spawned literally hundreds of health education research studies and provided the conceptual basis for many interventions and research studies in the years since it was formulated. It has been used across the health continuum, from prevention to detection to illness and sick-role behavior (Becker and Maiman, 1975; Janz and Becker, 1984). It is among the most widely applied theoretical foundations for the study of health behavior change. The Health Belief Model is appealing and useful to a wide range of professionals concerned with behavior change. Physicians, dentists, nurses, psychologists and health educators have all used the Health Belief Model in designing and evaluating interventions to alter health behavior.

Rosenstock explains how the model is used to understand health behavior and to design and test interventions. He describes the original study in which the model was first formulated—the study of people's responses to free screening for tuberculosis. While tuberculosis is less of a problem today than it was in 1950, many current health education interventions are aimed at enhancing adherence to screening and early detection measures such as mammography and cholesterol screening.

In Chapter Four, Carter discusses two Value Expectancy Theories, the Theory of Reasoned Action and Multiattribute Utility

Theory. This family of theories has had a major influence on both research and practice in health behavior and health education. As Carter shows, Value Expectancy Theories provide a way to define and assess the elements of health decisions. The Theory of Reasoned Action and Multiattribute Utility Theory provide direction for intervention when supplemented by other theories.

The Theory of Reasoned Action, as developed by Fishbein and Ajzen (1975), proposes that behavioral intentions and behaviors result from a rational process. The theory has been used to intervene in many health behaviors, including smoking, weight control, family planning, and the marketing of commercial products (Jaccard and Davidson, 1972; Ajzen and Fishbein, 1980; McCarty, 1981; Lowe and Frey, 1983). Recently, these theories have been used by AIDS researchers in developing interventions to help people at high risk to lower their risk of infection.

Multiattribute Utility Theory models predict behavior from a person's evaluation of the consequences or outcomes associated with both performing and not performing a given behavior. Multiattribute Utility Theory models also can be used to influence personal health decisions. For example, Multiattribute Utility Theory is being used to help people select among different kinds of smoking cessation programs.

Carter explicates Decision-Making Theory and Multiattribute Utility Theory through the use of two examples. In the first, he shows how the theories were used to design an intervention to promote acceptance of influenza vaccination. In the second, he demonstrates how the models were used to design an intervention for the primary prevention of sexually transmitted diseases. His applications also illustrate how practical decision aids can be constructed from information collected by means of Multiattribute Utility Theory models.

In Chapter Five, Lewis and Daltroy review Attribution Theory, which describes the processes by which individuals explain events in their lives as they try to make sense of the world around them. This theory proposes that individuals develop personal cognitive explanations about factors affecting their levels of health or illness. These cognitions, in turn, influence individuals' health-related behaviors. The authors discuss the evolution of Attribution

Theory and its key assumptions and integrate the works of Weiner (1979) and Abramson, Seligman, and Teasdale (1978). On the basis of substantial empirical literature, they propose a schema for organizing interventions on attributions. Attribution Theory has proven to be a useful theoretical foundation in understanding individual health behaviors, such as alcohol use, and how people respond to symptoms and diagnoses of illness. It has important potential as a basis for health education interventions.

In their applications, Lewis and Daltroy analyze two important problems relevant to Attribution Theory. First, they discuss how people adjust to life-threatening or chronic illnesses through attributions about disease causation and their beliefs about controllability. They also consider how attributions about drug effects and side effects affect patients' perceptions about potential side effects.

Researchers concerned with behavior change have long been interested in questions of how people seek, use, and process information. Information is at the heart of or at least central to most behavior change interventions. Chapter Six focuses on ways in which individuals use information for health action. Rudd and Glanz review the origins and context of Consumer Information Processing Theory and its major assumptions. Consumer Information Processing is part of the larger Theory of Information Processing, which has had a profound influence on our understanding of how people process information. Rudd and Glanz present Bettman's consumer choice model as applicable to the study of consumer health behavior. The reader will appreciate both the possibilities and limitations of human information processing. In their applications, the authors focus on two salient health issues, the use of nutrition information for making food choices and the use of quality of care information in selecting health care providers.

Together, the chapters in Part Two provide the reader with an appreciation of the complexity of human behavior and the many ways of understanding and influencing health-related behaviors.

References

Abramson, L. Y., Seligman, M.E.P., and Teasdale, J. D. "Learned Helplessness in Humans: Critique and Reformulation." *Journal of Abnormal Psychology*, 1978, *87*, 49–74.

Ajzen, I., and Fishbein, M. *Understanding Attitudes and Predicting Social Behavior.* Englewood Cliffs, N.J.: Prentice-Hall, 1980.

Becker, M. H., and Maiman, L. A. "Sociobehavioral Determinants of Compliance with Health and Medical Care Recommendations." *Medical Care,* 1975, *13,* 10-24.

Fishbein, M., and Ajzen, I. *Belief, Attitude, Intention and Behavior: An Introduction to Theory and Research.* Reading, Mass.: Addison-Wesley, 1975.

Jaccard, J. J., and Davidson, A. R. "Toward an Understanding of Family Planning Behaviors: An Initial Investigation." *Journal of Applied Social Psychology,* 1972, *2,* 228-235.

Janz, N. K., and Becker, M. H. "The Health Belief Model: A Decade Later." *Health Education Quarterly,* 1984, *11,* 1-47.

Lewin, K. *A Dynamic Theory of Personality.* New York: McGraw-Hill, 1935.

Lowe, R. H., and Frey, J. D. "Predicting Lamaze Childbirth Intentions and Outcomes: An Extension of the Theory of Reasoned Action to a Joint Outcome." *Basic and Applied Social Psychology,* 1983, *4,* 353-372.

McCarty, D. "Changing Contraceptive Usage Intention: A Test of the Fishbein Model of Intention." *Journal of Applied Social Psychology,* 1981, *11,* 192-211.

Weiner, B. "A Theory of Motivation for Some Classroom Experiences." *Journal of Educational Psychology,* 1979, *71,* 3-25.

Chapter 3

Irwin M. Rosenstock

The Health Belief Model:
Explaining Health Behavior
Through Expectancies

Theoretical and Programmatic Origins

The Health Belief Model (HBM) was initially developed in the 1950s by a group of social psychologists at the U.S. Public Health Service in an effort to explain the widespread failure of people to participate in programs to prevent or to detect disease (Hochbaum, 1958; Rosenstock, 1960, 1966, 1974). Later, the model was extended to apply to people's responses to symptoms (Kirscht, 1974) and to their behavior in response to diagnosed illness, particularly compliance with medical regimens (Becker, 1974). For more than three decades, the model has been one of the most influential and widely used psychosocial approaches to explaining health-related behavior.

Although the model evolved gradually in response to very practical programmatic concerns that will be described presently, its basis in psychological theory is provided as an aid to understanding its rationale as well as its strengths and weaknesses.

During the early 1950s, academic social psychology was engaged in developing an approach to understanding behavior that grew out of a confluence of learning theories derived from two major sources: Stimulus Response (S-R) Theory (Thorndike, 1898; Watson, 1925; Hull, 1943) and Cognitive Theory (Kohler, 1925; Tolman, 1932; Lewin, 1935, 1936, 1951; Lewin, Dembo, Festinger, and

Sears, 1944). S-R theory itself represents a marriage of classical conditioning theory (Pavlov, 1927) and instrumental conditioning theory (Thorndike, 1898).

In simple terms, S-R theorists believe that learning results from events (termed *reinforcements*) that reduce physiological drives that activate behavior. In the case of punishment, behavior that avoids punishment is learned because it reduces the tension set up by the punishment. The concept of drive reduction, however, is not necessary to S-R theory. Skinner (1938) formulated the widely accepted hypothesis that the frequency of a behavior is determined by its consequences (or reinforcements). For Skinner, the mere temporal association between a behavior and an immediately following reward is sufficient to increase the probability that the behavior will be repeated. Such behaviors are termed operants; they operate on the environment to bring about changes resulting in reward or reinforcement. In this view, no mentalistic concept such as reasoning or thinking is required to explain behavior. While Skinner does not deny the existence of the mind, he omits it from his theory, believing that behavioral response can be fully explained by reinforcement contingencies alone.

Cognitive theorists emphasize the role of subjective hypotheses or expectations held by the subject (for example, Lewin, Dembo, Festinger, and Sears, 1944). In this perspective, behavior is a function of the subjective *value* of an outcome and of the subjective probability or *expectation* that a particular action will achieve that outcome. Such formulations are generally termed value expectancy theories. (See Chapter Four for an analysis of other value expectancy theories.) Mental processes, such as thinking, reasoning, hypothesizing, or expecting, are critical components of all cognitive theories. Cognitive theorists, along with behaviorists, believe that reinforcements, or consequences of behavior, are important, but for cognitive theorists, reinforcements operate by the influencing expectations (or hypotheses) regarding the situation rather than by influencing behavior directly (Bandura, 1977a).

When value expectancy concepts were gradually reformulated in the context of health-related behavior, the translations were as follows: (1) the desire to avoid illness or to get well (value) and (2) the belief that a specific health action available to a person will prevent (or ameliorate) illness (expectancy). The expectancy was further delineated in terms of the individual's estimate of personal susceptibility to and severity of an illness and of the likelihood of being able to reduce that threat through personal action.

The development of the Health Belief Model grew out of real concerns with the limited success of various programs of the Public Health Service in the 1950s. One such early example was the failure of large numbers of eligible adults to participate in tuberculosis screening programs provided at no charge, in mobile X-ray units conveniently located in various neighborhoods. The concern of the program operators was with explaining people's behavior by illuminating those factors that were inhibiting positive responses. In studying this problem, Hochbaum (1958) focused less on why people did not come in for screening and more on why they did come in. The emphasis was thus placed as much on the forces that drive behavior as on those that inhibit behavior.

Beginning in 1952, Hochbaum studied more than 1,200 adults in three cities, assessing their "readiness" to obtain X rays, which included their beliefs that they were susceptible to tuberculosis and their beliefs in the personal benefits of early detection. Perceived susceptibility to tuberculosis itself comprised two elements: first, the respondents' beliefs about whether contracting tuberculosis was not only a mathematical possibility but a realistic possibility for them personally; and second, the extent to which they accepted the fact that one may have tuberculosis in the absence of all symptoms. Hochbaum and his colleagues believed then, and still believe, that people's ability to accept the possibility that they may be undergoing a pathological process in the complete absence of symptoms may be rare, but yet it seems crucial to the decision to seek screening for health-related reasons. The failure to believe in the possibility of having asymptomatic pathology may help explain poor response to cancer screening programs and noncompliance with antihypertensive medical regimens.

The measure of perceived benefits also included two elements: whether respondents believed that X rays could detect tuberculosis prior to the appearance of symptoms and whether they believed that early detection and treatment would improve the prognosis. For the group of people who exhibited both beliefs, that is, belief in their own susceptibility to tuberculosis and the belief that overall benefits would accrue from early detection, 82 percent had had at least one voluntary chest X ray during a specified period preceding the interview. Of the group exhibiting neither of these beliefs, only 21 percent had obtained a voluntary X ray during the criterion period. In short, four out of five people who exhibited both beliefs (susceptibility and benefits) took the predicted action, while four of five people who accepted neither of the beliefs had not taken the action. Thus, Hochbaum demonstrated with considerable precision that a particular action to screen for a disease was strongly associated with the two interacting variables: perceived susceptibility and perceived benefits.

The belief in one's susceptibility to tuberculosis appeared to be the more powerful variable studied. For the individuals who exhibited this belief without accepting the benefits of early detection, 64 percent had obtained prior voluntary X rays. Of the individuals accepting the benefits of early detection without accepting their susceptibility to the disease, only 29 percent had prior voluntary X rays. Hochbaum also thought that the readiness to take action (perceived susceptibility and benefits) could only be potentiated by other factors, particularly by "cues" to instigate action, such as bodily events, or by environmental events such as media publicity. He did not, however, study the role of cues empirically. Indeed, while the concept of cues as a trigger mechanism is appealing, it has been most difficult to study in explanatory surveys; a cue can be as fleeting as a sneeze or the barely conscious perception of a poster.

Components of the Health Belief Model

Over the years since Hochbaum's survey, many investigations have helped expand and clarify the Health Belief Model and extend it beyond screening behaviors to include all preventive actions, illness behaviors, and sick-role behaviors (see summaries in Rosenstock, 1974; Kirscht, 1974; Becker, 1974; Becker and Maiman, 1980; Janz and Becker, 1984). In general, it is now believed that individuals will take action to ward off, to screen for, or to control ill-health conditions if they regard themselves as susceptible to the condition, if they believe it to have potentially serious consequences, if they believe that a course of action available to them would be beneficial in reducing either their susceptibility to or the severity of the condition, and if they believe that the anticipated barriers to (or costs of) taking the action are outweighed by its benefits. The following definitions and commentary specify the key variables in greater detail.

Perceived Susceptibility. The dimension of perceived susceptibility refers to one's subjective perception of the risk of contracting a health condition. In the case of medically established illness, the dimension has been reformulated to include acceptance of the diagnosis, personal estimates of resusceptibility, and susceptibility to illness in general.

Perceived Severity. Feelings concerning the seriousness of contracting an illness or of leaving it untreated include evaluations of both medical and clinical consequences (for example, death, disability, and pain) and possible social consequences (such as effects of the conditions on work, family life, and social relations).

Many investigators have found it useful to label the combination of susceptibility and severity as *perceived threat.*

Perceived Benefits. While acceptance of personal susceptibility to a condition also believed to be serious (perceived threat) is held to produce a force leading to behavior, it does not define the particular course of action that is likely to be taken. This is hypothesized to depend upon beliefs regarding the effectiveness of the various available actions in reducing the disease threat, or the perceived *benefits* of taking health action. Thus, an individual exhibiting an optimal level of beliefs in susceptibility and severity would not be expected to accept any recommended health action unless that action was perceived as feasible and efficacious.

Perceived Barriers. The potential negative aspects of a particular health action, or perceived barriers, may act as impediments to undertaking the recommended behavior. A kind of nonconscious, cost-benefit analysis is thought to occur wherein the individual weighs an action's effectiveness against perceptions that it may be expensive, dangerous (having negative side effects or iatrogenic outcomes), unpleasant (painful, difficult, upsetting), inconvenient, time-consuming, and so forth.

Thus, "The combined levels of susceptibility and severity provided the energy or force to act and the perception of benefits (less barriers) provided a preferred path of action" (Rosenstock, 1974, p. 332).

Other Variables. It is believed that diverse demographic, sociopsychological, and structural variables may, in any given instance, affect the individual's perception and thus indirectly influence health-related behavior. Specifically, sociodemographic factors, particularly educational attainment, are believed to have an indirect effect on behavior by influencing the perception of susceptibility, severity, benefits, and barriers.

In various early formulations of the HBM, such concepts as health concern or motive and cue to action were occasionally introduced. While such variables have frequently been discussed and may ultimately prove to be important, they have not been systematically studied. With but one exception, these variables have been omitted from consideration in this chapter. Larson, Olsen, Cole, and Shortell (1979) and Larson and others (1982) have examined the role of cues in encouraging preventive health behavior. Their work is described in greater detail later in this chapter.

Self-Efficacy. In 1977 Bandura introduced the concept of self-efficacy, or efficacy expectation, as distinct from outcome expectation (Bandura, 1977a, 1977b, 1986), which we now believe must be added to the HBM in order to increase its explanatory power (Rosenstock, Strecher, and Becker, 1988). Outcome expectation, defined as a person's estimate that a given behavor will lead to certain outcomes, is quite similar to the HBM concept of perceived benefits. Self-efficacy is defined as "the conviction that one can successfully execute the behavior required to produce the outcomes" (Bandura, 1977a, p. 79). For example, in order for people to quit smoking for health-related reasons, they must believe that cessation will benefit their health (outcome expectation) and also that they are capable of quitting (efficacy expectation).

It is not difficult to see why self-efficacy was never explicitly incorporated into early formulations of the HBM. The original focus of the early model was on circumscribed preventive actions, usually of a one-shot nature, such as accepting a screening test or an immunization, actions that generally were simple behaviors for most people to perform. Because it is likely that most prospective members of target groups for those programs had adequate self-efficacy for performing those simple behaviors (which often involved receiving a service), that dimension was not even recognized.

The situation is vastly different, however, in working with life-style behaviors requiring long-term changes. The problems involved in modifying lifelong habits of eating, drinking, exercising, and smoking are obviously far more difficult to surmount than are those for accepting a one-time immunization or screening test. The former requires a good deal of confidence that one can, in fact, alter such life-styles before successful change is possible. Thus, for behavior change to succeed, people must (as the original HBM theorizes) feel threatened by their current behavioral patterns (perceived susceptibility and severity) and believe that change of a specific kind will be beneficial by resulting in a valued outcome at acceptable cost, but they must also feel themselves competent (self-efficacious) to implement that change. A growing body of literature supports the importance of self-efficacy in helping to account for initiation and maintenance of behavioral change (Bandura, 1977b; Bandura, 1986; Marlatt and Gordon, 1985), although only a few published studies have specifically addressed health-related life-style practices (see Strecher, DeVellis, Becker, and Rosenstock, 1986, for a review of these).

The HBM, originally developed to explain health-related behavior, focused on cognitive variables. Efforts to change cognitions about health matters, however, have often involved attempts to arouse affect—fear—through threatening messages (Leventhal, 1970). According to Protection Motivation Theory (Rogers, 1975), the most persuasive communications are those that arouse fear while enhancing perceptions of the severity of an event, the likelihood of exposure to that event, *and* the efficacy of responses to that threat. More recently, Rogers (1983) has incorporated self-efficacy into his theory. This view of the joint role of fear and reassurance in persuasive communications is generally accepted.

It is clear that the cognitive components of protection motivation theory are quite similar, if not actually identical, to key HBM variables. Incorporating the fear variable gives added dimension to the explanatory theory by proposing one method for fostering cognitive and behavioral change.

As a convenient way of summarizing the components of the Health Belief Model, we may subsume the key variables under three categories, which are summarized in Table 3.1

Evidence For and Against the Model

In 1974, *Health Education Monographs* devoted an entire issue to "The Health Belief Model and Personal Health Behavior" (Becker, 1974). That monograph summarized findings from research on the HBM to understand why individuals did or did not engage in a wide variety of health-related actions; the monograph provided considerable support for the model in explaining behavior pertinent to prevention and behavior in response to symptoms or to diagnosed disease.

During the decade following publication of the monograph, the HBM continued to be a major organizing framework for explaining and predicting acceptance of health and medical care rec-

Table 3.1. Key Components of the Health Belief Model, 1989.

I. Threat
A. Perceived susceptibility to an ill-health condition (or acceptance of a diagnosis)
B. Perceived seriousness of the condition
II. Outcome expectations
A. Perceived benefits of specified action
B. Perceived barriers to taking that action
III. Efficacy expectations: conviction about one's ability to carry out the recommended action (self-efficacy)

Note: Sociodemographic factors such as education, age, sex, race, ethnicity, and income are believed to influence behavior indirectly by affecting perceived threat, outcome expectations, and efficacy expectations.

ommendations. Accordingly, Janz and Becker (1984) provided an updated critical review of HBM studies conducted between 1974 and 1984, which also combined the new results with earlier findings to permit an overall assessment of the model's performance. Space limitations do not permit more than a brief summary of the findings of the detailed reviews of 1974 and 1984; the interested reader should consult Becker (1974) and Janz and Becker (1984) for details.

The 1984 review applied stringent criteria for inclusion. Only studies published between 1974 and 1984 were included, each study had to have at least one behavioral outcome, only findings relating the four HBM dimensions to behavior were reported, and only studies related to medical conditions and to adults were included. Dental studies and studies of children were excluded. Because of the stringent inclusion criteria, the 1984 review was limited to twenty-nine HBM-related investigations published during the period 1974–1984; however, the 1984 review also tabulated the findings from seventeen studies conducted prior to 1974 and provided a summary of all forty-six HBM studies (eighteen prospective, twenty-eight retrospective). Twenty-four studies examined preventive health behaviors (PHB), nineteen explored sick-role behaviors (SRB), and three addressed clinic utilization. A "significance ratio" was constructed, and it divided the number of positive, statistically significant findings for an HBM dimension by the total number of studies reporting significance levels for that dimension.

The preventive health behaviors (including screening behaviors) that were reviewed in detail included influenza inoculation, Tay-Sachs carrier status screening program, practice of breast self-examination, and attendance at screening programs for high blood pressure. Preventive health behaviors included seat belt use, exercise, nutrition, smoking, visits to physicians for checkups, and fear of being apprehended while under the influence of alcohol. Sick-role behaviors included compliance with antihypertensive regimens, diabetic regimens, end-stage renal disease regimens, medication regimens for parents to give their children with otitis media, weight loss regimens, and medication regimens for parents to give to asthmatic children.

Summary results provide substantial empirical support for the HBM, with findings from prospective studies at least as favorable as those obtained from retrospective research. "Perceived barriers" was the most powerful single predictor of the HBM dimensions across all studies and behaviors. While both "perceived susceptibility" and "perceived benefits" were important overall, "perceived susceptibility" was a stronger predictor of preventive health behavior than sick-role behavior, and the reverse was true for "perceived benefits." Overall, "perceived severity" was the least powerful predictor; however, this dimension was strongly related to sick-role behavior.

Critique of the HBM

Several recurrent critiques have been made against the validity or utility of the HBM. One perennial criticism may well be leveled against the whole field of social psychology. This criticism holds that the belief-behavior relationship has never been uniformly established. It is of course true that behavior cannot always be accounted for by reference to beliefs. It is also true that beliefs often do account for variance in behavior, and the previously cited review offers many examples of significant predictions of behavior from beliefs (Janz and Becker, 1984). It has, however, rarely, if ever, been argued that beliefs are in themselves sufficient conditions for action. Researchers must seek out that constellation of conditions, including beliefs, which accounts for major variations in behavior. What would seem to be needed is further research to specify the conditions under which specific beliefs and behaviors are causally related and the conditions under which they are not. To reject approaches to explaining behavior that emphasize the role of beliefs seems tantamount to throwing out the baby with the bathwater.

A second, related criticism is that direct attempts to modify beliefs are often unsuccessful and that some alternative approaches are needed. This is certainly a valid comment but it is difficult to interpret it as a defect in the HBM. Kirscht and Rosenstock pointed out as early as 1974 that "the model does not presuppose or imply a strategy for change. We may assume that direct persuasion to modify beliefs is an obvious tactic, but perhaps a much broader view of belief change is necessary. It may be that modification of the structure of the medical care system is an effective method for changing beliefs about the efficacy of medical care. Second, environmental and structural changes may well have long-term effects on health beliefs" (Rosenstock and Kirscht, 1974, p. 472).

A third criticism follows directly from the second and holds that both individual *and* socioenvironmental factors should be targeted for health interventions. Perhaps the most comprehensive statement of this position is provided in a 1988 paper proposing an ecological perspective for health promotion (McLeroy, Bibeau, Steckler, and Glanz, 1988). This model proposes an emphasis on five factors, the first of which would include the Health Belief Model: (1) intrapersonal factors, (2) interpersonal processes, (3) institutional factors, (4) community factors, and (5) public policy, including law.

Proponents of the HBM would take little issue with the importance of using the entire array of factors described by the authors in efforts to promote health. Overenthusiastic proponents of the HBM may on occasion have attempted to explain more than such a model could possibly explain, but it is important to remind the reader that "the HBM is a *psychosocial* model; as such, it is limited to accounting for as much of the variance in individuals' health-related behaviors as can be explained by their attitudes and beliefs. It is clear that other forces influence health actions as well" (Janz and Becker, 1984, p. 44).

Some behaviors (such as cigarette smoking or toothbrushing) have a substantial habitual component that supersedes any continuing psychosocial decision-making process. Other health-related behaviors are undertaken for what are ostensibly nonhealth reasons (for example, dieting to improve appearance). Finally, economic and/or environmental factors may prevent the individual from undertaking a preferred course of action. However, these concerns excepted, the Janz and Becker review supports the view that health programs should attend to the attitude and belief dimensions of the HBM in addition to other likely influences on health-related behaviors.

While the role of environmental factors is important, we should not lose sight of the critical role of intrapersonal factors. Where societal changes have been mandated in the absence of a focus on individual motivational and belief factors, problems have arisen. Social engineering undeniably can modify behavior, but one must be wary of side effects. Witness the impact of the Eighteenth Amendment to the U.S. Constitution in 1919, which prohibited the manufacture, sale, or transportation of intoxicating liquors, and the legally mandated automobile seat belt interlock system imposed during the mid-1970s. In the latter case, public opposition was so great that Congress was quickly forced to rescind the law. In the case of the "Prohibition" amendment, ultimately repealed in 1933, not only did the law fail to reduce consumption of alcohol, but the amendment set off perhaps the greatest crime wave in U.S. history to that date in efforts to subvert the law.

Even engineering approaches to behavior must consider social-psychological realities. While individuals may be "engineered" into preventive or compliant practices today, how will they behave tomorrow in different situations? The belief consequences of change strategies may influence the long-term maintenance of behavior. Further, as Bandura (1977a) has argued in his discussion of reciprocal determinism, alterations in the environment often occur as a consequence of personal decisions. These changes may well influence the incentives to maintain a particular behavior. Moreover, decisions are made by somebody or somebodies. The beliefs of the decision makers have played a role in the decision. While the beliefs may not be those of the ultimate consumer, a strategy of belief change in the decision makers may be a necessary step in producing an effect down the line.

These considerations highlight the importance of including a consideration of intrapsychic factors in any effort to modify behavior by altering the social or physical environment.

A fourth criticism of the HBM relates to its lack of quantification. A fully useful model would provide numerical coefficients to the perceptions of susceptibility, severity, benefits, and barriers (and now self-efficacy) and would specify a mathematical relationship among them (for example, multiplicative or additive). It is hardly exculpatory to note that other models do not provide more adequate quantification. It is undeniable that the HBM variables have not been satisfactorily quantified beyond an ordinal scale (and frequently only on a nominal scale), nor have most investigators tested the joint relationships among the variables. With only a few exceptions (for example, Becker and others, 1977), research on the HBM has generally focused more on substance than on method. It is, however, gratifying to note that increasing, though unfortunately, desultory, attention has been given to measuring and improving the psychometric properties (reliability and validity) of measures of HBM variables (Maiman and others, 1977; Cummings, Jette, and Rosenstock, 1978). Clearly, much remains to be done in quantifying the HBM.

A fifth criticism is that by focusing on the individual determinants of health behaviors, there is a danger that victim-blaming will be encouraged. This might be true if one adopted a moralistic view of responsibility for a problem. Those who are prone to blame victims do not need much justification for doing so. It has, however, been argued (Rosenstock, 1988) that it is possible to assign "blame" for health problems to factors outside the individual while placing responsibility on the individual for problem solutions. The client or patient is thus not blamed for having the problem but is expected to assume responsibility for solving the problem. This has been termed a "compensatory" model of helping and coping, derived from work by Brickman and others (1982). This model appears to be appropriate to the prevention of relapse to unhealthful behaviors (Marlatt and Gordon, 1985). It seems reasonable to assign responsibility to the ex-smoker, to the recovering alcoholic, and to the former drug user for maintaining their new life-styles, without blaming them for having had the problems in the first place.

The HBM clearly had its roots in a threat-avoidance logic (preventing or detecting serious disease). One may properly question the applicability of the model to health promotion, which presumably begins with healthy people who seek to maintain or enhance their healthy state. One must further distinguish between actions undertaken for health-related reasons and actions undertaken for nonhealth reasons. Clearly, many diet and exercise enthusiasts are at least in part striving to prevent or delay the onset of heart disease, or stroke, or cancer, or diabetes. In such cases, behavior to promote health is essentially identical with behavior to prevent disease and consequently can be explained by traditional HBM variables just as other preventive or screening behaviors can.

While much of health promotive behavior does seem to be

explainable by a disease prevention approach, there remain a great many people who are asymptomatic and apparently unworried about any particular disease but who wish to achieve or maintain high levels of fitness, vigor, career advancement, or physical attractiveness for their own sake. One could translate such behavior as efforts to avoid the consequences of low levels of fitness, vigor, success, or attractiveness. It seems more profitable, however, to return to the general value expectancy model for an explanation of such behavior. What do people value and what are their expectations concerning the likelihood of maximizing those values? The challenge for health workers is to assist such people to find achievement of those values that are consonant with good health practices.

Applications of the Model

To illustrate the ways in which the HBM may be applied, two examples are presented, one dealing with weight loss in obese children and the other with acceptance of an influenza immunization among an at-risk group. These examples have been included because they represent clear-cut efforts to use all of the HBM variables to understand client behavior, both in the context of the at-risk or sick-role situation (obesity) and in a preventive situation (immunization). Moreover, each example includes both an explanatory component and an intervention component. Finally, each intervention is one that could reasonably be incorporated into a typical health care setting at little additional cost beyond what is now allocated to patient information and education.

Obesity. Becker and others (1977) studied factors influencing mothers' adherence to a diet prescribed for their obese children (ranging in age from 19 months to 17 years, with a mean age of 11.5 years). Interviews of 182 low socioeconomic status (SES) mothers, all but 11 of whom were black, were conducted over a two-year period and concerned their health beliefs and motives. Multiple-item scales were used to assess each HBM dimension prior to the mothers' receiving instruction and a weight-reduction plan from a dietitian. Each child's weight change was measured by the dietitian at four follow-up visits spaced two weeks apart. In addition, a general compliance measure, long-term clinic appointment keeping, was calculated for each child by dividing appointments kept by appointments made during a twelve-month period.

Perceived susceptibility was measured by a mother's perception of how easily her child might get sick, how likely her child was to develop each of eight specified illnesses or conditions, and by an index combining the general and specific vulnerability measures. All measures proved to be significant predictors of weight loss at all of the follow-up visits.

Perceived severity was assessed by determining a mother's degree of worry about the kinds of illnesses her child might get and by responses to the question "If your child were to get (each of the eight illnesses used in the susceptibility measure), how worried do you think you would be?" (Becker and others, 1977, p. 355). The severity measures were even more highly predictive of weight loss than the measures of susceptibility.

"Perceived benefits" was measured primarily by respondents' feelings about control over obesity and its consequences. For example, when asked what things a person can do to keep from having heart trouble, those who mentioned diet-related actions (such as weight, cholesterol) were scored high on benefits. A locus of control type of question was also asked to ascertain mothers' acceptance or rejection of the statement that "there isn't much anyone can do about how much he or she weighs," and who attributed the child's overweight to circumstances over which they had control. Responses reflecting an internal orientation were judged to be high on perceived benefits. All of these measures were predictive of weight loss, although three measures of faith in medical information and medical care proved to be unrelated to weight loss

"Perceived barriers" was measured by a number of discrete items concerning perceived safety of the diet, expected difficulty in achieving weight loss, whether the child had ever been on a diet before, mothers' opinions about the relative ease of the current diet compared to others, reported family problems, whether the mother found it relatively easy or difficult to get through the day and whether or not the mother reported that she would not miss clinic appointments for any reason. Results for the barriers dimension were more complex than for the other variables. Except for the item on expected difficulty in losing weight, each item was significantly correlated with one or another measure of weight loss and clinic appointment-keeping. Some items predicted early weight loss over the course of follow-up visits, whereas others predicted delayed weight loss.

Concerning sociodemographic factors, only age of child and mothers' marital status were associated with weight loss. Mothers of older children were better compliers, and married mothers were most likely to be successful in achieving weight loss in their children compared to the widowed, divorced, and never married.

The researchers conducted a multiple regression analysis in which weight change measures were regressed against belief measures. Together, the independent variables accounted for 49 percent of the variance in weight change on the first follow-up visit and dropped to 22 percent of variance by the fourth visit. Thus, health beliefs may be most important at the beginning of a regimen, but over time and concurrent experience with the diet, as well as experience with weight change outcomes, other variables may become important as well.

The same research also tested the efficacy of two levels of fear-arousing communication in enhancing regimen compliance. Subjects were randomly assigned to one of three groups: receipt of a "high fear" message and booklet concerning obesity and its possibly unfavorable consequences, receipt of a "low fear" message and booklet with similar (but less threatening) information, or no intervention at all (the control group).

The group exposed to the high-fear message lost the most weight and did not regain weight between follow-up visits. The low-fear group also lost weight, though it regained some weight between visits. The control group showed no weight loss over the course of the experiment.

Because the fear-arousal interventions were significantly associated with weight loss, analyses were performed to explore the influence of the study intervention on health beliefs. These analyses demonstrated that when the effects of the intervention were controlled, the HBM variables remained significant predictors of weight change. It was not possible to assess whether the intervention modified any of the health beliefs because they were measured only once, before the intervention.

Influenza Vaccination. Larson, Olsen, Cole, and Shortell (1979) applied the HBM in the context of obtaining influenza vaccination by people thought to be at high risk for serious complications from influenza infection (individuals over sixty-five years of age and patients with such chronic problems as diabetes or heart, bronchopulmonary, or renal disease). The target group was the clientele of the Family Medical Center at the University of Washington Medical Center. Following a flu epidemic, self-administered questionnaires to assess health beliefs and vaccination status were completed by 241 patients (a response rate of 75 percent); 232 were ultimately usable in the analysis.

The published paper reports findings for "perceived severity of influenza," "perceived susceptibility to influenza," "perceived efficacy of vaccine," "perceived expensiveness of vaccine," "self-reported inconvenience," and "satisfaction" (p. 1210). Self-reported inconvenience was not significantly associated with vaccination status, but all of the other HBM dimensions were significantly correlated with vaccination behavior, leading the investigators to conclude that "this study has demonstrated that health beliefs regarding susceptibility, severity, and [vaccine] efficacy are important factors in utilization of influenza vaccine" (p. 1211).

In a subsequent, related intervention study (Larson and others, 1982), a randomized trial of various postcard reminder "cues" was conducted to improve understanding of health-related behavior and to find better strategies for improving influenza vaccination compliance. Data were gathered on 283 high-risk patients (over sixty-five years of age or with certain chronic diseases) who received (1) a "neutral" postcard announcing the availability of vaccine, (2) a "personal" card without reference to any of the HBM variables, (3) a "Health Belief Model" card, or (4) no postcard. The personal card carried the client's name, used the personal pronoun in announcing the availability of the vaccine, and was signed by the physician. The HBM card, which was not personalized, specifically mentioned the target group's increased likelihood of contracting influenza, the seriousness of the disease in such people, and the efficacy of the vaccine in reducing the risk with almost no chance of adverse side effects. The neutral card merely mentioned the availability of the vaccine.

The highest rate of vaccination occurred among recipients of the Health Belief Model postcard (which had not been personalized). After adjusting for age and prior vaccination experience, the vaccination rate was found to be significantly higher for people who received the Health Belief Model postcard (51 percent) than for those who received no postcard (20 percent) or who received a neutral postcard (25 percent). Those receiving the personal card had higher vaccination rates than neutrals and controls (41 percent) but considerably lower rates than those receiving the HBM card. Impersonal reminder postcards emphasizing elements of the Health Belief Model were thus clearly shown to help increase vaccination rates.

HBM: Its Implications for Health Education Practice

This chapter has described both strengths and limitations in the HBM as formulated to date. It is hoped that future theory-building and theory-testing research will direct efforts more toward strengthening the model where it is weak than toward repeating what has already been established. More work is needed on experimental interventions to modify health beliefs and health behavior than on surveys to reconfirm already established correlations. More work is also needed to specify and measure factors that need to be added to the model to increase its predictive power. The addition of self-efficacy to the traditional HBM should improve explanation and prediction, particularly in the area of life-style practices.

This review has provided limited but important evidence that HBM variables are associated with health-related behavior and that manipulation of the health belief variables can lead to increased compliance with health recommendations. It is timely for professionals who are attempting to influence health-related behaviors to make use of the health belief variables, including self-efficacy in their program planning, both in needs assessment and in program strategies. Programs to deal with a health problem should be based in part on knowledge of how many and which members of the target population feel susceptible to a serious health problem (or believe they currently have the problem) and believe that the threat could be reduced by some action on their part, at an acceptable cost. Further, health professionals should obtain an important additional piece of information: the extent to which patients or clients feel competent (self-efficacious) to carry out the prescribed action(s), sometimes over long periods of time.

The collection of data on health beliefs, including self-efficacy, along with other data pertinent to the group or community setting, permits the planning of more effective programs than would otherwise be possible. Interventions can then be targeted to the specific needs identified by such assessment. This is true whether we are dealing with the problems of individual patients, with groups of clients, or with entire communities. For example, if we find that people accept their susceptibility to cancer and fear the consequences of the disease but also believe that there are no cures for cancer or that the cures may be worse than the disease, we can tailor interventions to increase perceived benefits and to reduce perceived barriers. Other belief combinations call for different program emphases.

Changes in knowledge and beliefs will surely continue to be required in efforts to achieve behavior change. However, an analysis of the literature linking self-efficacy to health behavior (Strecher, DeVellis, Becker, and Rosenstock, 1986) indicates that in the realm of chronic disease control, much more emphasis is likely to be needed on skill training to enhance self-efficacy. Specifically, self-efficacy can be enhanced by breaking the complexities of the target behavior into components that are relatively easy to manage (Bandura, 1977b). This requires a careful examination of the target behavior and identification of specific aspects of the behavior that call for skill development. Specific behaviors must then be arranged in a series so that they may be consecutively mastered, with initial tasks being easier than subsequent tasks (Nicki, Remington, and MacDonald, 1985). Moreover, self-efficacy may be increased by setting short-term rather than long-term goals for some desired achievement (Bandura and Simon, 1977; Bandura and Schunk, 1981). As clients demonstrate progressive movement toward attainment of their goals, their successes should be reinforced verbally by the provider, while any lapses in behavior should be treated as opportunities to analyze and subsequently control the factors that caused the lapse (Marlatt and Gordon, 1985).

Developing awareness of specific situations in which efficacy may be low and rehearsing the desired behavior in these situations appears to enhance self-efficacy (Gilchrist and Schinke, 1983). Other methods of enhancing efficacy include relaxation training to reduce anxiety during the behavior change process (Gilchrist and Schinke, 1983; Kaplan, Atkins, and Reinsch, 1984) and verbal reinforcement to enhance self-efficacy (Nicki, Remington, and MacDonald, 1985; Chambliss and Murray, 1979a, 1979b; Blittner, Goldberg, and Merbaum, 1978). The work of Ewart, Taylor, Reese, and Debusk (1984) suggests that counseling from a credible source may be effectively used to generalize specific task-related efficacy expectations to other behaviors.

In planning programs to influence the behavior of large groups of people for long periods of time, the role of the HBM, including self-efficacy, must be considered in context. Permanent changes in behavior can rarely be wrought solely by direct attacks on belief systems. Even more, where the behavior of large groups is the target, interventions at societal levels (for example, social networks, work organizations, the physical environment, the legislature) along with interventions at the individual level will likely prove more effective than single-level interventions. Yet, we should never lose sight of the fact that a crucial way station on the road to improved health involves the beliefs and behavior of each of a series of individuals.

References

Bandura, A. *Social Learning Theory.* Englewood Cliffs, N.J.: Prentice-Hall, 1977a.

Bandura, A. "Self-Efficacy: Toward a Unifying Theory of Behavior Change." *Psychological Review,* 1977b, *84,* 191–215.

Bandura, A. *Social Foundations of Thought and Action.* Englewood Cliffs, N.J.: Prentice-Hall, 1986.

Bandura, A., and Schunk, D. H. "Cultivating Competence, Self-Efficacy, and Intrinsic Interest Through Proximal Self-Motivations." *Journal of Personality and Social Psychology,* 1981, *41,* 586-598.

Bandura, A., and Simon, K. M. "The Role of Proximal Intentions in Self-Regulation of Refractory Behavior." *Cognitive Therapy and Research,* 1977, *1,* 177-193.

Becker, M. H. (ed.). "The Health Belief Model and Personal Health Behavior." *Health Education Monographs,* 1974, *2,* 324-473.

Becker, M. H., and Maiman, L. A. "Strategies for Enhancing Patient Compliance." *Journal of Community Health,* 1980, *6,* 113-135.

Becker, M. H., and others. "The Health Belief Model and Prediction of Dietary Compliance: A Field Experiment." *Journal of Health and Social Behavior,* 1977, *18,* 348-366.

Blittner, M., Goldberg, J., and Merbaum, M. "Cognitive Self-Control Factors in the Reduction of Smoking Behavior." *Behavior Therapy,* 1978, *9,* 553-561.

Brickman, P., and others. "Models of Helping and Coping." *American Psychologist,* 1982, *37,* 368-384.

Chambliss, C. A., and Murray, E. J. "Cognitive Procedures for Smoking Reduction: Symptom Attribution Versus Efficacy Attribution." *Cognitive Therapy and Research,* 1979a, *3,* 91-95.

Chambliss, C. A., and Murray, E. J. "Efficacy Attribution: Locus of Control and Weight Loss." *Cognitive Therapy and Research,* 1979b, *3,* 349-353.

Cummings, K. M., Jette, A. M., and Rosenstock, I. M. "Construct Validation of the Health Belief Model." *Health Education Monographs,* 1978, *6,* 394-405.

Ewart, C. K., Taylor, C. B., Reese, L. B., and Debusk, R. F. "Effects of Early Postmyocardial Infarction Exercise Testing on Self-Perception and Subsequent Physical Activity." *American Journal of Cardiology,* 1984, *41,* 1076-1080.

Gilchrist, L. D., and Schinke, S. P. "Coping with Contraception: Cognitive and Behavioral Methods with Adolescents." *Cognitive Therapy and Research,* 1983, *7,* 379-388.

Hochbaum, G. M. *Public Participation in Medical Screening Programs: A Sociopsychological Study.* Public Health Service Publication no. 572, 1958.

Hull, C. L. *Principles of Behavior*. East Norwalk, Conn.: Lange, 1943.

Janz, N. K., and Becker, M. H. "The Health Belief Model: A Decade Later." *Health Education Quarterly*, 1984, *11*, 1-47.

Kaplan, R. M., Atkins, C. J., and Reinsch, S. "Specific Efficacy Expectations Mediate Exercise Compliance in Patients with COPD." *Health Psychology*, 1984, *3*, 223-242.

Kirscht, J. P. "The Health Belief Model and Illness Behavior." *Health Education Monographs*, 1974, *2*, 387-408.

Kohler, W. *The Mentality of Apes*. San Diego, Calif.: Harcourt Brace Jovanovich, 1925.

Larson, E. B., Olsen, E., Cole, W., and Shortell, S. "The Relationship of Health Beliefs and a Postcard Reminder to Influenza Vaccination." *Journal of Family Practice*, 1979, *8*, 1207-1211.

Larson, E. B., and others. "Do Postcard Reminders Improve Influenza Vaccination Compliance?" *Medical Care*, 1982, *20*, 639-648.

Leventhal, H. "Findings and Theory in the Study of Fear Communications." In L. Berkowitz (ed.), *Advances in Experimental Social Psychology*. Vol 5. Orlando, Fla.: Academic Press, 1970.

Lewin, K. *A Dynamic Theory of Personality*. New York: McGraw-Hill, 1935.

Lewin, K. *Principles of Topological Psychology*. New York: McGraw-Hill, 1936.

Lewin, K. "The Nature of Field Theory." In M. H. Marx (ed.), *Psychological Theory*. New York: Macmillan, 1951.

Lewin, K., Dembo, T., Festinger, L., and Sears, P. S. "Level of Aspiration." In J. Hunt (ed.), *Personality and the Behavior Disorders*. New York: Ronald Press, 1944.

McLeroy, K. R., Bibeau, D., Steckler, A., and Glanz, K. "An Ecological Perspective on Health Promotion Programs." *Health Education Quarterly*, 1988, *15*, 351-377.

Maiman, L. A., and others. "Scales for Measuring Health Belief Model Dimensions: A Test of Predictive Value, Internal Consistency, and Relationships Among Beliefs." *Health Education Monographs*, 1977, *5*, 215-230.

Marlatt, G. A., and Gordon, J. R. (eds.). *Relapse Prevention*. New York: Guilford Press, 1985.

Nicki, R. M., Remington, R. E., and MacDonald, G. A. "Self-Efficacy, Nicotine-Fading/Self-Efficacy Monitoring and Cigarette Smoking Behavior." *Behaviour Research and Therapy*, 1985, *22*, 477-485.

Pavlov, I. *Conditioned Reflexes*. Oxford, England: Oxford University Press, 1927.

Rogers, R. W. "A Protection Motivation Theory of Fear Appeals and Attitude Change." *Journal of Psychology*, 1975, *91*, 93-114.

Rogers, R. W. "Cognitive and Physiological in Fear Appeals and Attitude Change: A Revised Theory of Protection Motivation." In J. Cacioppo and R. Petty (eds.), *Social Psychophysiology*. New York: Guilford Press, 1983.

Rosenstock, I. M. "What Research in Motivation Suggests for Public Health." *American Journal of Public Health*, 1960, *50*, 295-301.

Rosenstock, I. M. "Why People Use Health Services." *Milbank Memorial Fund Quarterly*, 1966, *44*, 94-124.

Rosenstock, I. M. "Historical Origins of the Health Belief Model." *Health Education Monographs*, 1974, *2*, 328-335.

Rosenstock, I. M. "Adoption and Maintenance of Lifestyle Modifications." *American Journal of Preventive Medicine*, 1988, *4*, 349-352.

Rosenstock, I. M., and Kirscht, J. P. "The Health Belief Model and Personal Health Behavior." *Health Education Monographs*, 1974, *2*, 470-473.

Rosenstock, I. M., Strecher, V. J., and Becker, M. H. "Social Learning Theory and the Health Belief Model." *Health Education Quarterly*, 1988, *15*, 175-183.

Skinner, B. F. *The Behavior of Organisms*. East Norwalk, Conn.: Appleton & Lange, 1938.

Strecher, V. J., DeVellis, B. M., Becker, M. H., and Rosenstock, I. M. "The Role of Self-Efficacy in Achieving Health Behavior Change." *Health Education Quarterly*, 1986, *13*, 73-92.

Thorndike, E. L. "Animal Intelligence: An Experimental Study of the Associative Processes in Animals." *Psychological Monographs,* 1898, *2* (entire issue 8).

Tolman, E. C. *Purposive Behavior in Animals and Men.* East Norwalk, Conn.: Appleton & Lange, 1932.

Watson, J. B. *Behaviorism.* New York: Norton, 1925.

Chapter 4

William B. Carter

Health Behavior
as a Rational Process:
Theory of Reasoned Action and
Multiattribute Utility Theory

This chapter examines two promising theoretical perspectives: the Theory of Reasoned Action and Multiattribute Utility Theory. These value expectancy theories are based on a well-established body of knowledge in the psychological literature and currently represent state-of-the-art models for predicting a person's intention to perform a specific behavior, as well as personal decisions involved in performing or not performing the behavior in question. They can be applied to a variety of populations and behaviors, they provide a reasonably accurate prediction of voluntary health behavior, and they suggest which decision-related dimensions may be most important to personal health decisions and behavior. The last is particularly pertinent for applications in health education. The effectiveness of interventions to encourage clients to initiate a change in their behavior is determined in large part by being able to identify the major concerns and barriers they confront in making the decision to change. If the intervention emphasizes topics that are not relevant to a client's decision about the behavior in question, it is likely to lead to little behavior change. The models described in this chapter provide methods for systematically identifying those issues that are most important to a person's decision about performing a specific behavior. This information can be readily adapted to behavioral interventions and decision aids in health education.

The first section of the chapter examines some of the historical background issues in modeling the behavior of individuals. The next two sections examine each theory in detail and provide examples of how each has been applied to health-related behaviors. In the next section, the relative strengths and weaknesses of the two theories are discussed. The final section examines how value expectancy theories can be used with other theories of behavior change, the implications of these approaches, and future research topics.

Historical and Theoretical Background

"We seek things which we want, which may be our own or other people's pleasure, or anything else whatever, and our actions are such as we think most likely to realize these goods" Ramey (1964, p. 74).

Value expectancy theory provides a framework for systematically evaluating the issues a person may consider in deciding whether or not to take a specific course of action. Modern expectancy theories have evolved from two areas of research: social-psychological investigations of the relationships between attitudes, beliefs, and behaviors (Cooper and Croyle, 1984; McGuire, 1986) and behavioral decision theory (Edwards, 1954, 1961). In the following sections, the Theory of Reasoned Action (Fishbein, 1967; Fishbein and Ajzen, 1975), from social psychology, and a multiattribute utility model (Beach, Townes, Campbell, and Keating, 1976), from decision theory, are explored in detail with examples of how each has been operationally defined to address specific health issues.

A fundamental proposition of value expectancy theory is the principle of maximization. Formally enunciated by Pascal in 1669, it states that the expected value for any action is the algebraic sum across potential consequences or outcomes of the action, of the values of each outcome, and their respective probabilities of occurrence should the action be performed. Value expectancy theories do not attempt to describe how people make decisions. Rather, they provide a method for operationally defining and systematically assessing the elements of a decision to perform a specific behavior.

These theories have a long history in psychology and are prevalent in the research literature (Lawler, 1971; Ebert and Mitchell, 1975) in areas of learning, attitude formation and decision making (Cooper and Croyle, 1984; McGuire, 1986), leadership, motivation, personality, and social power. Table 4.1 contains examples of psychological theories that employ a value expectancy framework. While these theories operationally define value and probability in somewhat different terms, all are fully functional value expectancy theories.

The value of an outcome can be stated objectively (for example, in terms of dollars) or subjectively (for example, in terms of happiness) on any continuum that permits an estimate of how much the various outcomes contribute to the decision. Subjective judgments of value are called utilities in decision theory and attitudes in the Theory of Reasoned Action. Attitudes are subjective judgments of value stated on a continuum that reflects the favorableness or unfavorableness a person feels toward an object of interest. These evaluative judgments are usually measured on a scale that ranges from good to bad. The construct of attitude is a central theme

Table 4.1. Examples of Psychological Theories That Employ a Value Expectancy Framework.

Theorist	*Determinants of the Intended Course of Action*
Tolman (1952)	Expectancy of goal, Demand for goal
Lewin (1936)	Potency × Valence
Edwards (1954)	Subject probability × Utility
Atkinson (1964)	Expectancy × (Motive × Incentive)
Rotter (1954)	Expectancy, Reinforcement value
Vroom (1964)	Expectancy × Valence
Peak (1958)	Instrumentality × Attitude
Rosenberg (1956)	Instrumentality × Importance
Dulany (1967)	Hypothesis of the distribution of the reinforcers × Value of the reinforcers
Fishbein and Ajzen (1975)	Probability × Attitude

Source: Modified from Lawler, 1971.

in social-psychological research that focuses on understanding and predicting behavior (Cooper and Croyle, 1984; McGuire, 1986).

In value expectancy theories, an attitude or utility can be substituted for "value," and subjective probabilities or beliefs for "objective probabilities." While these variations are indicated by a variety of names in different applications (subjective expected utility, Edwards, 1954, 1961; attitude toward performing the behavior, Fishbein, 1967; Fishbein and Ajzen, 1975), they are for the purpose of this discussion essentially equivalent. The decision rule or maximization principle then says that people choose the behavioral alternative that they believe will provide them with the maximum number of good outcomes and the minimum number of bad outcomes. (Value expectancy theories apply only to behaviors that are under the individual's control. Compulsive behaviors and behaviors that occur in settings where personal choice is restricted are beyond the purview of these theories.)

Collectively, value expectancy theories may be viewed as a chain-of-events model, with substantial variation in the operational detail of each approach (Lawler, 1971). From this perspective, behavior is viewed as the end point of a chain of psychological events that begins with an assessment of the possible consequences or outcomes associated with each behavior under consideration. On the basis of this assessment, the decision maker chooses a course of action that he or she intends to follow. Subsequent events permitting, this intention is carried out by the performance of the chosen behavior. While the specific consequences associated with the target behavior fully specify the interrelationships among behavioral consequences and provide an operational methodology for combining people's evaluations of these consequences to predict behavior or the intention to perform the behavior, for the most part, such consequences or outcomes are not specified by the theoretical framework. Rather, they are derived empirically for each behavior from the target population. The "grounding" of model content for each application gives these approaches considerable flexibility and sensitivity across a wide range of behaviors. In health education, in which behaviors and target populations vary widely, understanding the specific issues that influence a person's decision to undertake each behavior and how those issues vary across subpopulations should provide a powerful tool in the design of more effective intervention strategies.

While value expectancy theories assume the perspective of the individual, they are not limited to a single person. In assembling the content of a model, an attempt is made to represent fairly the diverse issues and concerns of individuals from a target population about a specific behavior. These issues and concerns are then phrased in terms of consequences or outcomes of the behavior under consideration. In a second step, the content of the model is tailored to a specific individual by having each person assign a weight to each consequence or outcome that reflects that person's beliefs and values. The validity of the model is assessed in terms of its accuracy in predicting the behavior of individuals in the target population.

From a health education perspective, the effectiveness of strategies of behavior change depends on (1) understanding the natural history of the target behavior, (2) identifying salient and potentially modifiable cognitive and behavioral "causes" or determinants of the target behavior, and (3) designing and implementing effective strategies to modify those determinants and enhance the practice of health protective behaviors. Value expectancy models provide a methodology for addressing the first and second requirements but not the third. Thus, for health applications, the end product of such efforts is to identify important beliefs and attitudes for subsequent use in behavioral interventions, but the strategies for the design of the intervention must come from other theories (see, for example, McGuire, 1984; Curry and Marlatt, 1987).

Some value expectancy theories also include a variety of other variables (sociodemographic characteristics, personality characteristics, prior behavior) that enhance behavioral prediction. It is important to distinguish the role of these variables from the role of attitude and beliefs in designing interventions. Attitudes and beliefs are mutable and thus are good targets for intervention if their relationship with the target behavior is valid. On the other hand, variables such as prior behavior, age, sex, marital status, and personality characteristics either represent history or stable characteristics of a person that are essentially immutable. While these variables may be of little value in designing behavior interventions, they may be very useful in helping to identify population subgroups at risk for certain behaviors.

Theory of Reasoned Action

The Theory of Reasoned Action (Fishbein, 1967; Fishbein and Ajzen, 1975; Ajzen and Fishbein, 1980; Ajzen, 1985) predicts a person's intention to perform a behavior in a well-defined setting and is graphically summarized in Figure 4.1. The theory can be used to explain virtually any behavior over which an individual has volitional control (Ajzen and Fishbein, 1980; Ajzen, 1985). The model assumes that behavioral intention is the immediate determinant of behavior and that all other factors that influence behavior are mediated through intention. The measurement of intention must closely correspond to the measurement of behavior in terms of the action, target, context, and time in order to accurately predict behavior. For example, if the action of interest is attending a specific diet class for cardiac patients, intention to attend that specific class should be assessed. Measures of intention for a general target, such as attending a diet class, are likely to differ from those obtained from a target that focuses specifically on the class in question. Similarly, the specific time (for example, an evening course) and context (for example, at a clinic) should be included in the measure of intention because other times and settings are likely to influence intention.

The strength of a person's intention to perform a specific behavior is a function of two factors: attitude toward the behavior and the influence of the social environment or general subjective norms on the behavior. Attitudes and subjective norms each have two components. Attitude toward the behavior is determined by an individual's belief that a given outcome will occur if he or she performs the behavior and by an evaluation of the outcome. In health education applications, outcomes may include such things as side effects associated with medication or the time and personal problems that a person might confront in participating in a regular exercise program. Finally, social norm is determined by a person's normative belief about what salient others think he or she should do and by the individual's motivation to comply with those people's wishes.

Figure 4.1. Theory of Reasoned Action.

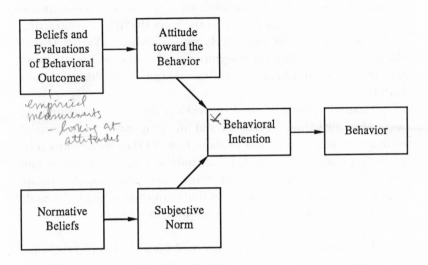

Source: Ajzen and Fishbein, 1980, p. 8.

Outcomes or consequences associated with a specific behavior are obtained empirically through open-ended interviews with individuals in the target population. During such interviews, subjects are asked to list what they perceive to be salient outcomes or consequences of performing the behavior. While it is impossible to determine the point in the list at which beliefs are no longer salient, Fishbein and Ajzen (1975) suggest, as a rule of thumb, that the first five to nine beliefs be considered the salient determinants. When the target group is a large population, Davidson and Morrison (1983) suggest including ten to twelve of the most frequently mentioned beliefs from all the questionnaires administered to a representative sample of the population. To some extent, this procedure controls for the imperfect correspondence in the salient beliefs of different subgroups of the population.

Operationally Defining the Theory of Reasoned Action to Predict Condom Use. Data from a recent study (Baker, 1988) examining the determinants of intention to use condoms by patients in a sexually transmitted disease (STD) clinic are used here to illustrate how the various terms of the Theory of Reasoned Action are operationally defined. The use of barrier methods such as condoms is instrumental in the primary prevention of STDs. Since the risk for contracting STDs depends almost exclusively on an individual's behavioral choices, understanding the determinants of sexual decision making has important implications for the design of health education interventions.

Salient outcomes used to develop the study questionnaire were identified from interviews and an open-ended questionnaire with a representative sample of about forty STD clinic patients. The model's variables, for example, attitude toward the behavior and subjective norms, were measured on seven-point bipolar rating scales and appropriate wording modifications were made for male and female patients. Examples of the measures follow.

1. *Behavioral intention* was measured on a likely-unlikely scale. For men, the question was stated, "I would use a condom during sexual intercourse with a new or infrequent partner to prevent infection," and for women, "I would ask a new or infrequent partner to use a condom during sexual intercourse to prevent infections." The same questions were repeated for steady sexual partners.

2. *Attitude toward the act* was obtained by summing the responses to a number of semantic differential evaluative scales (for example, foolish-wise, bad-good) attached to the question "Using a condom with new or infrequent sexual partners to prevent infections is" for men, and for women, "Asking a new or infrequent partner to use a condom to prevent infection is."

3. *General subjective norm* was defined as follows: "Most people who are important to me think that if I have sex with a new or infrequent partner I (definitely should–definitely should not) use condoms to prevent infections."

4. *Belief about the behavior:* Each belief outcome (for example, "Using a condom is an effective way for me to prevent getting or spreading sexually transmitted infections"; "Sometimes condoms can slip off or break when I use them"; "Having sex is not as pleasurable for me when I use them"; "Using a condom interrupts sex or makes it less spontaneous") was rated on a

likely-unlikely scale in statements such as "Using condoms is an effective way for me to prevent getting and spreading VD."

5. *Evaluation of the consequences:* Each belief outcome was rated on a good-bad scale in statements such as "For me preventing VD is."

6. *Normative belief* was defined by including each of specific normative beliefs (for example, "My health care provider thinks I should use condoms with new or infrequent partners to prevent infections"; "My steady partner thinks we should use condoms to prevent infections") in statements such as "My health care provider thinks that with new and infrequent partners I (definitely should–definitely should not) use condoms to prevent infections."

7. *Motivation to comply* used the same content as above in statements such as "Generally speaking, I try to do what my health care provider wants me to do" (likely-unlikely).

In this study, both attitude toward condoms and general subjective norm significantly predicted intention to use condoms for both steady and new or infrequent partners (Baker, 1988). The total variance accounted for in behavioral intention was 36 percent for steady partners and 8 percent for new and infrequent partners. While the explanatory power of the Theory of Reasoned Action for steady partners is comparable to other applications, it is very modest for new and infrequent partners. The latter is likely the result of a methodological problem that has important implications for the application of all value expectancy theories. In the initial elicitation of salient beliefs, an open-ended question asked about the factors that influence the use of condoms, following the recommendations of Davidson and Morrison (1983). Responses from the forty STD clinic patients did not uncover a single comment that indicated that the issues may differ with a steady partner versus new or infrequent partners. Later, in an attempt to understand why the explanatory power was not higher for new or infrequent partners, a few in-depth exploratory interviews were conducted with a new sample of STD clinic patients. Subjects mentioned a number of factors that suggested that behavioral outcomes may be quite different with new or infrequent partners.

This problem is presented here because it has two important implications for the application of all value expectancy theories. First, the predictive power of these theories is dependent upon the identification of all or most of the outcomes that are salient to the target population. Since the salient outcomes provide the content of these theories, the process of eliciting information from the target population is extremely important. Second, many health education applications are complex, and the elicitation of salient outcomes may require a more rigorous data collection process than indicated previously. At the very least, it appears that probes or questions about specific aspects of the behavior in question should be added to the elicitation process.

Further analyses in the Baker (1988) study suggested also that salient beliefs differ across subgroups of the clinic population. This may provide practical information for the design of behavior change interventions. The analyses examined the contribution of individual belief/evaluation products for individual outcomes to the attitude toward the act and general subjective norm. That is, belief/evaluation products for individual outcomes were used as independent variables in multiple regression analyses, with attitude toward the act, general subjective norm, or behavioral intention as the dependent variable. Outcomes that explain a significant proportion of the variance in the dependent variable may provide some insight into the determinants of attitudes, norms, or behavioral intention. For example, belief/evaluation products of two outcomes, the belief that one's health care provider thinks that one should use condoms with a steady partner and the partner's opinons, were among the most important predictors of intention to use condoms for all groups. For gay men, another important predictor of intention to use condoms with a steady partner was the belief that using condoms will decrease the individual's and partner's sexual pleasure. For heterosexual males, the risk of a condom slipping or breaking, the interruption of sex, not having a condom, and making sex last longer were all important predictors of the intention to use condoms with a steady partner. For women, important predictors of intention to use condoms with a steady partner were preventing pregnancy, a decrease in the individual's and partner's pleasure, interruption of sex, and embarrassment in purchasing condoms.

The variation in the most salient beliefs illustrates how the examination of the outcome and normative beliefs of various subsets of this clinic population can provide useful information for the design of interventions that address the most critical beliefs of each group.

Other Applications of the Theory of Reasoned Action to Sexual Decision Making. A number of other applications of the Theory of Reasoned Action relate to sexual decision making, including decisions about abortion (Smetana and Adler, 1979, 1986), birth planning intentions (Davidson and Beach, 1981; Crawford and Boyer, 1985; Davidson and Jaccard, 1975), Lamaze childbirth intentions (Lowe and Frey, 1983), and contraceptive decision making (Adler and Kegeles, 1987; Cohen, Severy, and Ahtola, 1978; Davidson and Morrison, 1983; Jaccard and Davidson, 1972; Jorgensen and Sosnstegard, 1984; McCarty, 1981; Werner and Middlestadt, 1979). The proportion of variance in intentions to use contraceptive methods accounted for by attitudes and norms is typically very high. For example, the attitudes and norms of college students accounted for 79 percent of the variance in intention to use birth control pills (Jaccard and Davidson, 1972) and 74 percent of the variance for married women (Davidson and Jaccard, 1975). Moreover, further analyses of salient beliefs across subgroups of the former study population provided practical information for the design of behavior change interventions. The subgroups of interest in these studies were women who did and did not intend to use birth control pills. Among college students, for example, both intended birth control pill users and nonusers agreed that birth control pills were inexpensive and convenient and would enable them to regulate birth intervals and family size. Women who did not intend to use birth control pills held a number of negative beliefs about them not held by women who intended to use them. These beliefs included concerns about major side effects, birth defects, and detrimental effects on sexual morals (for example, conflict with religious beliefs, promiscuity).

Multiattribute Utility Theory

Multiattribute Utility (MAU) Theory predicts behavior directly from an individual's evaluation of the consequences or outcomes associated with both performing and not perfoming the behavior in question. The strength of MAU Theory is that it provides (1) a methodology for breaking down a complex decision into individual attributes (consequences or outcomes) that may influence a decision, (2) a methodology for having the decision maker evaluate each attribute, and (3) a methodology for combining these evaluations into a single overall score that should predict the course of action each decision maker is likely to take. If the MAU model* for the decision in question is valid, that is, if it accurately predicts the choice of action, it also provides (4) a methodology for identifying which attributes were most influential in the decision maker's choice of action. These characteristics make MAU models particularly helpful for health education applications. Unlike the Theory of Reasoned Action, it is possible to predict behavioral performance for a single person directly from his or her evaluations of consequences or outcomes. It is also possible to identify which consequences were most influential in that person's probable course of action. Both of these factors make an MAU approach a potentially valuable counseling tool.

MAU Theory is operationally defined in a variety of forms (Keeney, 1982). One form that is particularly successful is the hierarchical multiattribute utility model developed by Sayeki (1972). The purpose of the hierarchical form is to break a complex, multiconsideration decision problem into smaller units of similar considerations so that the decision maker can manage them more easily and so that he or she need not compare dissimilar considerations (apples and oranges, so to speak). This form of MAU Theory has been applied to important health-related decisions (Beach, Townes, Campbell, and Keating, 1976; Carter and others, 1986) to achieve either or both of two goals: to facilitate the development of intervention designed to influence personal decisions and/or to provide decision makers with a decision aid, a simplified version of an MAU model that is designed to help an individual think through the most important considerations of a decision. While MAU Theory is opera-

---

*The term *model* is used here to indicate a specific operational form or a specific behavioral application of a theory.

tionally defined in a variety of formats, all are variants of the general subjective expected utility (SEU) theories (Edwards, 1954).

In MAU models, behavioral consequences or outcomes are obtained empirically from extensive exploratory interviews with a representative sample of the target population. The content of the theory is totally dependent on issues and concerns related to the behavior that are elicited from these interviews. Information from the interviews is subjected to a detailed content analysis that yields a taxonomy of issues and concerns (see Carter and others, 1986). Once the taxonomy of behavioral consequences or outcomes is established, individuals are asked to evaluate the subjective probability that a given consequence will occur if the behavior is performed and the subjective value or utility of that consequence should it occur. (The interested reader is referred to Sayeki, 1972, and Beach, Townes, Campbell, and Keating, 1976, for a more detailed treatment of the mathematical formulations of a hierarchical MAU model.)

Formal measures of subjective probability and utility must meet a number of stringent mathematical criteria that are not easily achieved by human judges (experts or lay people) without considerable training. Although a high level of mathematical precision is critical in MAU applications designed to advise expert decision making—for example, for physicians making a differential medical diagnosis—this level of precision is much less important in most applications that are designed to evaluate personal decisions (such as deciding to follow the dietary recommendations given to you by your doctor).

A common approach in adapting MAU schemes to personal decisions is to relax the formal measurement constraints for utility assessment and to substitute another, more understandable continuum for subjective probability, for example, the extent to which a person believes that a consequence or outcome related to the behavior would argue for or against performing the behavior in question. These approaches, which utilize a continuum for subjective probability, are often called net-weighted utility models. They are similar in all other respects to an SEU formulation. The validity of a net-weighted utility model, however, must be assessed empirically to determine the extent to which it accurately predicts the target behavior.

SEU and net-weighted utility (NWU) scores range from +1.0 to -1.0. The decision rule for predicting whether a person will perform the behavior under consideration is usually based on a simple maximization of SEU or NWU. A score greater than zero indicates that the decision maker favors the behavior under consideration (for example, you favor following the dietary advice of your physician). Conversely, a negative score indicates that the cons outweigh the pros and the decision maker is unlikely to perform the behavior. The larger the score, either by positive or negative, the stronger the disposition to either perform or not perform the action.

Operationally Defining an MAU Theory to Predict Influenza Vaccination. Influenza and related complications constitute the fifth leading cause of death for older people in the United States (*Health Statistics on Older Persons, 1987*). Despite long-standing medical recommendations and the wide availability of effective vaccines, national surveys indicate that only 20 percent of the population at risk for influenza complications (people over the age of sixty-five and people with certain chronic conditions) obtain flu shots in any given year. MAU Theory is described here in the context of a series of studies conducted in the outpatient clinics of a Veterans Administration medical center to determine the validity of a utility maximizing approach (a weighted hierarchical utility model) to modeling patients' flu shot decisions and behavior and to determine whether this approach led to more effective clinical management of noncompliance (Carter and others, 1986).

The content for the hierarchical utility model was based on concerns about flu and flu shots expressed by a stratified (age, diagnosis, and prior year flu shot status) random sample (N = 63) of high-risk clinic patients during hour-long exploratory interviews. The interviews began with an open-ended segment in which patients were asked to discuss the issues and concerns they considered in making a decision about whether or not to obtain a flu shot. Next, a number of issues from the literature on flu shots (for example, knowledge about the risks of influenza, side effects of the injection) and comments from previously interviewed patients were discussed in terms of whether these were relevant issues for the subject. Patient comments were recorded verbatim, transcribed on cards, and sorted independently by two investigators into categories of similar content. This process resulted in the identification of fifteen categories of perceived consequences of getting the flu and of getting a flu shot that formed the basis for the hierarchical scheme illustrated in Figure 4.2. Since most participants were old and ill, large "worksheets" that corresponded to the two major components (flu and flu shot) were developed. The lowest-level categories contained brief paragraphs that were obtained from patient comments that described both pro and con consequences. An example of the first two categories on the flu worksheet is shown in Figure 4.3.

Another sample of 517 high-risk patients participated in MAU interviews. An interviewer led each patient through the worksheets step-by-step. For each of the fifteen consequences shown in Figure 4.2, the interviewer read the descriptive paragraph, and patients distributed ten "weights" in the pans of the "balance scales" (see left side of Figure 4.3) to indicate the extent to which that category of consequence argued for or against getting a flu shot.

After the for and against weights were assigned for each branch of the hierarchy (for example, the pair of consequences labeled Discomfort and Complications, which constitute the Health branch shown in Figure 4.2), patients were asked to divide ten weights (on the right side of Figure 4.3) between the consequences to indicate the relative importance of each to their decision. The same procedure was followed for the three branches on each worksheet (for example, the branches labeled Health, Activities, and Other People in Figure 4.2) and for the flu versus flu shot worksheet, to indicate their relative importance to the decision.

Following the procedures outlined by Beach and others (1976), the relative-importance weights were combined with the for and against weights to yield a net relative importance weight for each consequence. This weight indicated the relative extent to which each consequence had a pro or con influence on a patient's thinking about getting a flu shot. Net relative importance weights were then summed to give an overall score that was used to predict behavioral intention and vaccination behavior. Behavioral intention was measured in a manner similar to that described for the

Figure 4.2. Summary of Content Categories for Hierarchical Weighted Utility Model of Patients' Decisions Regarding Influenza Vaccination.

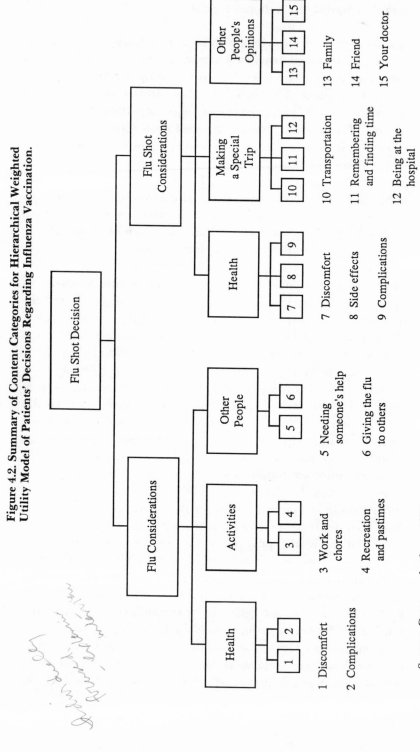

Source: Carter and others, 1986.

**Figure 4.3. Two Examples from the Flu Decision Model Worksheets
for Influenza-Related Outcomes.**

A. Possible Effects of the Flu on Your Health

1. Discomfort

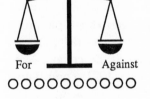

For ▬▬▬ Against

OOOOOOOOOO

Examples: Some people think that having the flu is not too bad, a lot like having a cold; they may be uncomfortable and have a mild fever and aching muscles, but it will go away in a few days. Other people think that they will be miserable if they get the flu (fever, congestion, nausea, vomiting, diarrhea) and that it might last a week or even a month or longer.

O
O
O
O
O
O
O
O
O
O

2. Complications

For ▬▬▬ Against

OOOOOOOOOO

Examples: Some people are healthy or they feel that they could get over the flu without much trouble. Others think they are in pretty good shape, but because of age or lowered resistance, having the flu might lead to other problems, such as pneumonia. Still others already have health problems (asthma, arthritis, diabetes, heart problems, or lung problems), and they worry about the flu making these problems worse, or even killing them.

Source: Carter and others, 1986.

Theory of Reasoned Action, and vaccination behavior was assessed from clinic records and patient reports of vaccination status (Carter and others, 1986).

The results of this study (Carter and others, 1986), indicated that the decision model correctly predicted behavioral intention for

87 percent and vaccination behavior for 82 percent of the patients who participated in the study. More importantly, the model differentiated "flu shot takers" and "nontakers" along several consequences that suggested specific content areas for intervention strategies. Each of these salient consequences or misconceptions was addressed directly in a "flu quiz" that formed the content of a new intervention. This intervention was effective in improving vaccination rates for patients who were refractory to other intervention materials (Carter, Beach, and Inui, 1986). In addition, 64 percent of patients who received the intervention for the first time obtained flu shots compared to only 34 percent of the control group. When the intervention was repeated annually for several years, vaccination rates increased to 80 percent (Carter and others, 1989a). The intervention also was effective in other patient populations in other VA and HMO settings (Carter and others, 1989a; Westbrook, Carter, and Wagner, 1987). In an extensive evaluation in other VA settings, this vaccination-enhancing program was also found to be cost-effective, saving both money and lives (Carter and others, 1989b).

Other Health Applications of MAU Theory. MAU schemes similar to the one used in the flu study have been applied to birth-planning decisions (Beach, Townes, Campbell, and Keating, 1976; Beach, Campbell, and Townes, 1979; Townes, Campbell, Beach, and Martin, 1976; Townes, Beach, Campbell, and Martin, 1977); compliance behavior in women with abnormal Pap smears (Paskett, Carter, Chu, and White, submitted), and decisions to abstain from high-risk sexual practices for gay and bisexual men at risk for AIDS (Gayle, Carter, and Inui, submitted). In each application, the MAU model accurately predicted behavior or behavioral intention and identified important dimensions of the decision that can be used in the design of intervention strategies.

The first health application of the MAU scheme was designed to provide a decision aid for couples considering having a child (Beach, Campbell, and Townes, 1979). The MAU model structured the components of a relatively complex and infrequent decision. The initial validation study of the MAU model predicted with 73 percent accuracy whether or not a couple had a child within a two-year period. A simplified self-administered version of the original MAU model was developed as a decision aid to help prospective parents work through their own concerns about having a child. This helpful decision aid was adopted by Planned Parenthood for inclusion in its self-help counseling materials.

A second application of MAU theory predicted with 68 percent accuracy whether women complied with follow-up medical recommendations for an abnormal Pap smear (Paskett, Carter, Chu, and White, submitted). In addition, elements of the decision model were used to develop an interactive patient teaching brochure to be mailed to patients along with reminders for follow-up treatment. The effectiveness of the new intervention materials is being assessed in a randomized trial. Preliminary data suggest that the new intervention is improving compliance rates by approximately 15 percentage points over rates achieved with the usual clinic intervention alone.

A final study, which is also currently in progress (Gayle, Carter, and Inui, submitted) examines whether an MAU model is useful for predicting whether gay and bisexual men at risk for AIDS abstain from high-risk sexual practices. Exploratory interviews yielded sixteen outcome categories that fall within two general areas: personal sex/sexuality issues (for example, sexual release, physical/sensory pleasure, health) and interpersonal issues (for example, intimacy, rejection, need to satisfy partners, concern for health of partners). The MAU questionnaire was completed by sixty men, and preliminary analyses suggest that the model predicts with approximately 70 percent accuracy the subjects' intention to abstain from the risk behavior over the subsequent three months.

Comparison of Theories

"If it is our serious purpose to understand the thoughts of a people, the whole analysis of experience must be based upon their concepts, not ours" Boaz (1943).

The Theory of Reasoned Action and Multiattribute Utility Theory have many more common characteristics than differences (Davidson and Beach, 1981), and both approaches provide strong and valid behavioral prediction in a variety of settings. The importance of grounding our attempts to understand the determinants of behavior to the concerns of the target population is the cornerstone of modern value expectancy theories. Grounded theories such as MAU Theory and the Theory of Reasoned Action have an overwhelming advantage over theories that have a fixed content.

There are, however, important differences in how the grounding process is operationalized in the Theory of Reasoned Action and Multiattribute Utility Theories. As discussed earlier, content for the Theory of Reasoned Action is obtained from relatively brief interviews with members of the target population, and the frequency with which different consequences are mentioned is the basis upon which items are selected. In contrast, the content of MAU Theory is based on extensive interviews, and an attempt is made to represent fairly all the behavioral consequences mentioned.

Recent data from two studies suggest that the more rigorous MAU methodology may have a number of advantages (Baker, 1988; Carter and others, 1989c) over methods used in the Theory of Reasoned Action. First, Baker (1988) found that brief interviews and questionnaires failed to uncover important differences in the consequences associated with using a condom with a steady partner versus a new or infrequent partner. Second, in an MAU application for understanding how patients value the humanistic skills of their physicians (Carter and others, 1989c), the frequency with which consequence categories were mentioned in the exploratory interviews was systematically compared with the categories that had the greatest relative importance to the decision. About a fourth of these key determinants would have been omitted had the rule of thumb suggested by Fishbein and Ajzen (1975) been used. More importantly, the most frequently mentioned outcome would not have been included as a key determinant had the Theory of Reasoned Action been used.

Unfortunately, no data are available to assess the relative impact of these two value expectancy theories on predictive validity. While at least two studies have made direct comparisons by administering both theories to the same subjects (Carter, 1983; Pagel and Davidson, 1984), in both cases, a common set of consequences or outcomes was used for the evaluation. Thus, the major contrast evaluated in these studies was in differences in scaling methods, and in both cases the theories were comparable.

Each approach, however, has relative advantages in different settings and applications. The focus of prediction in the Theory of Reasoned Action is the group, instruments can be self-administered, and the theory is best suited for survey research applications. In contrast, the focus of MAU prediction is on the individual, and it is ideally suited as a decision aid to help individuals resolve complex health decisions. MAU models, however, should be administered by an interviewer.

There are some differences in theory content regarding normative beliefs in the two theories. The Theory of Reasoned Action routinely includes normative beliefs, whereas in MAU theory, inclusion of normative beliefs occurs only if they are mentioned by the subjects in exploratory interviews. Currently, there is no empirical evidence to evaluate the predictive importance of these differences.

Finally, both of these theoretical approaches are relatively complicated and require a substantial commitment of resources to apply to behavioral problems in health education. While a full implementation of these theories will yield the best results for identifying important interventions, this may not be feasible in many settings. For both theories, the most important issues or barriers to behavioral performance are identified from the people who are to perform the behavior. Thus, a careful and thorough survey of the target population is an essential prerequisite to designing any health education intervention. A second critical step is to determine which of the noted behavioral consequences or outcomes are most important to the target population. Currently, there are no published studies that suggest appropriate shortcuts. Thus, when resources are limited, the best strategy may be to conduct a small pilot study of one of these theories with a random sample (stratified by past behavior when possible) from the target population.

Implications and Future Directions

Selecting Target Behaviors and Populations. The development of any predictive model of health behavior should determine behaviors that need intervention and identify the appropriate target population. The target groups should be identified on the basis of clinical evidence or data.

The cornerstone of most health behaviors is the inability to maintain positive behavior over the long run. Value expectancy theories capture only a snapshot of a personal decision, which represents only one point in time. Decisions, however, are dynamic, and values are likely to change over time. It is useful to introduce this dynamic process as we broaden our perspective of individual decision making (Prochaska and DiClemente, 1983).

Value expectancy theories are also diagnostic in that they describe the issues and concerns that differentiate people who have successfully accomplished a behavior change from those who have not. In addition, this approach may be used to evaluate changes in the issues that are important to people as they move from contemplating behavior change to actually attempting to change their behavior over time. Value expectancy theories are constructed to represent a target population. Therefore, content relevant to all stages of behavior change should be represented in the theory. The weights assigned to specific issues related to behavior change, however, may vary as the individual gains more experience with changing the behavior. Subgroup analyses based on individuals at each stage of the behavior change process can provide insight into issues and concerns at different points along the behavior change continuum.

Integrating Value Expectancy and Relapse Prevention Models. Addressing specific behavior-related issues and concerns of the target population is an effective strategy for encouraging behavior change via the mass media or communications distributed to specific target populations (McGuire, 1984). As discussed in Chapter Eight on Social Learning Theory, information about the perceived consequences of behavior change is also instrumental throughout the stages of intensive behavior change programs such as relapse prevention (Curry and Marlatt, 1987; Marlatt, 1985; Marlatt and Gordon, 1980). This information, however, is only rarely collected in any systematic fashion. Systematic identification of the instrumental concerns underlying a specific behavior with value expectancy theories may improve our capacity to help individuals change complex or addictive behaviors.

Decision Aids for Health Education Settings. One practical implication of the information presented in this chapter is the need to be very specific and candid about the target behavior when discussing guidelines for risk reduction. Using a decision balance sheet approach such as that developed by Janis and Mann (1977) or the decision aids mentioned previously could be potentially useful during the course of a health education counseling session. A balance sheet or decision aid may help the health educator systematically explore and clarify the client's personal values and beliefs about a target behavior and identify important personal consequences of changing that behavior. Such an exercise may identify the beliefs that are most salient in hindering or maintaining change. Moreover, it could be used as a powerful instrument of self-discovery because it tends to gauge the level of current motivation or commitment to change in a manner that is more graphic for the client as well as the health professional. Aside from its obvious utility during the initial stage of change, the decision balance sheet can also be a personal reminder of an individual's values and beliefs surrounding his or her original decisions to change when facing challenges and setbacks.

In other settings, information derived from modeling beliefs can be used to develop teaching aides and client handouts. Because such handouts and aids address specific misconceptions and misunderstandings of the target population, they may be effective educational materials in a variety of settings. The "flu quiz" is an example of this type of application. This quiz addresses specific misconceptions about the flu and flu vaccine (for example, the belief that influenza is not a serious health risk, concern that flu vaccine interferes with other medications) that were found to be instrumental in high-risk patients' decisions not to get vaccinated. The flu quiz and a letter from the clinic are mailed to high-risk patients at regular intervals when flu vaccine becomes available, inviting patients to get a flu shot. This type of intervention provides an inexpensive, yet effective intervention for a large target population.

Summary

The Theory of Reasoned Action and Multiattribute Utility Theory currently represent state-of-the-art models for predicting whether a person will perform specific health behaviors. Theory content is derived empirically for each behavior from a specific target population. The objective is to represent fully important consequences or outcomes associated with the performance of the behavior in question and care is taken to query the target population adequately. The grounding of model content gives these approaches considerable flexibility and sensitivity across a wide range of behaviors. Both theories fully specify the interrelationships among behavioral consequences and provide an operational methodology for combining peoples' evaluations of these consequences to predict behavior or the intention to perform the behavior. The Theory of Reasoned Action and Multiattribute Utility Theory have many more common characteristics than differences, and both approaches have provided strong and valid behavioral prediction in a variety of settings.

References

Adler, N. E., and Kegeles, S. M. "Understanding Adolescent Contraceptive Choice: An Empirical Test." Paper presented at the annual meeting of the American Psychological Association, New York, 1987.

Ajzen, I. "Attribution of Dispositions to an Actor: Effects of Perceived Decision Freedom and Behavioral Utilities." *Journal of Personality and Social Psychology*, 1971, *18*, 144-156.

Ajzen, I. "From Intentions to Actions: A Theory of Planned Behavior." In J. Kuhl and J. Beckman (eds.), *Action Control: From Cognition to Behavior*. New York: Springer-Verlag, 1985, pp. 11-39.

Ajzen, I., and Fishbein, M. "The Prediction of Behavior from Attitudinal and Normative Variables." *Journal of Experimental Social Psychology*, 1970, *6*, 466-487.

Ajzen, I., and Fishbein, M. "Attitude-Behavior Relations: A Theoretical Analysis and Review of Empirical Research." *Psychological Bulletin*, 1977, *84*, 888-918.

Ajzen, I., and Fishbein, M. *Understanding Attitudes and Predicting Social Behavior*. Englewood Cliffs, N.J., Prentice-Hall, 1980.

Atkinson, J. W. *An Introduction to Motivation*. New York: D. Van Nostrand, 1964.

Baker, S. A. "An Application of the Fishbein Model for Predicting Behavioral Intentions to Use Condoms in a Sexually Transmitted Disease Clinic Population." Unpublished doctoral dissertation, University of Washington, 1988.

Beach, L. R., Campbell, F. L., and Townes, B. O. "Subjective Expected Utility and the Prediction of Birth-Planning Decisions." *Organizational Behavior and Human Performance*, 1979, *24*, 18–28.

Beach, L. R., Townes, B. O., Campbell, F. L., and Keating, G. W. "Developing and Testing a Decision Aid for Birth-Planning Decisions." *Organizational Behavior and Human Performance*, 1976, *24*, 19-28.

Boaz, F. "Recent Anthropology." *Science*, 1943, *98*, 311-314, 334-337.

Carter, W. B. *Decision Making and Preventive Health Behavior: Prospective Modeling and Prediction of Influenza Vaccination.* Final report for Health Services Research and Development Grant No. IIR 80-569. Washington, D.C.: Health Services Research and Development, Veterans Administration, 1983.

Carter, W. B. *A Test of Influenza Vaccination Program Effectiveness in VA Settings.* Final report for Health Services and Research Development Grant no. IIR 82-091. Washington, D.C.: Health Services Research and Development, Veterans Administration, 1987.

Carter, W. B., Beach, L. R., and Inui, T. S. "The Flu Shot Study: Using Multiattribute Utility Theory to Design a Vaccination Intervention." *Organizational Behavior and Human Decision Making*, 1986, *38*, 378-391.

Carter, W. B., and others. "Developing and Testing a Decision Model for Predicting Influenza Vaccination Compliance." *Health Services Research*, 1986, *20*, 897-932.

Carter, W. B., and others. "A Patient-Centered Organizational Program to Improve Influenza Vaccination Rates: I. Effectiveness in a VA Multi-Center Randomized Trial." Submitted for publication, 1989a.

Carter, W. B., and others. "A Patient-Centered Organizational Program to Improve Influenza Vaccination Rates: II. Cost- Effectiveness Analysis." Submitted for publication, 1989b.

Carter, W. B., and others. "How Patients Judge the Humanistic Skills of Their Physicians." Submitted for publication, 1989c.

Cohen, J., Severy, L., and Ahtola, O. "An Extended Expectancy-Value Approach to Contraceptive Alternatives." *Journal of Population*, 1978, *1*, 22–41.

Cooper, J., and Croyle, R. T. "Attitudes and Attitude Change." *Annual Review of Psychology*, 1984, *35*, 395–426.

Crawford, T. J., and Boyer, R. "Salient Consequences, Cultural Values, and Childbearing Intentions." *Journal of Applied Social Psychology*, *1985*, *15*, 16–30.

Curry, S. G., and Marlatt, G. A. "Building Self-Confidence, Self-Efficacy and Self-Control." In W. M. Cox (ed.), *Treatment and Prevention of Alcohol Problems: A Resource Manual*. Orlando, Fla.: Academic Press, 1987.

Davidson, A. R., and Beach, L. R. "Error Patterns in the Prediction of Fertility Behavior." *Journal of Applied Social Psychology*, 1981, *37*, 1364–1376.

Davidson, A. R., and Jaccard, J. J. "Population Psychology: A New Look at an Old Problem." *Journal of Personality and Social Psychology*, 1975, *37*, 1073–1082.

Davidson, A. R., and Morrison, D. M. "Predicting Contraceptive Behavior from Attitudes: A Comparison of Within- Versus Across-Subjects Procedures." *Journal of Personality and Social Psychology*, 1983, *45*, 997–1009.

Dulany, D. E. "Awareness, Rules, and Propositional Control: A Confrontation with S-R Behavior Theory." In D. Horton and T. Dixon (eds.), *Verbal Behavior and General Behavior Theory*. Englewood Cliffs, N.J.: Prentice-Hall, 1967.

Ebert, R. J., and Mitchell, T. R. *Organizational Decision Processes*. New York: Crane, Russak, 1975.

Edwards, W. "The Theory of Decision Making." *Psychological Bulletin*, 1954, *51*, 380–417.

Edwards, W. "Behavioral Decision Theory." *Annual Review of Psychology*, 1961, *12*, 473–498.

Fishbein, M. "Attitude and the Prediction of Behavior: Results of a Survey Sample." In M. Fishbein (ed.), *Readings in Attitude Theory and Measurement*. New York: Wiley, 1967.

Fishbein, M., and Ajzen, I. *Beliefs, Attitudes, Intention, and Behav-

ior: An Introduction to Theory and Research. Reading, Mass.: Addison-Wesley, 1975.

Gayle, T. C., Carter, W. B., and Inui, T. S. "A Decision Model to Predict Whether Gay and Bisexual Men Will Abstain from Unsafe Anal and Oral Sex." Submitted for publication.

Health Statistics on Older Persons: United States. Public Health Service Publication no. 87-1409, 1987.

Jaccard, J. J., and Davidson, A. R. "Toward an Understanding of Family Planning Behaviors: An Initial Investigation." *Journal of Applied Social Psychology,* 1972, *2,* 228-235.

Janis, I. L., and Mann, L. *Decision Making.* New York: Free Press, 1977.

Jorgensen, S. R., and Sosnstegard, J. S. "Predicting Adolescent Sexual and Contraceptive Behavior: An Application and Test of the Fishbein Model." *Journal of Marriage and the Family,* 1984, *46,* 43-55.

Keeney, R. L. "Decision Analysis: State of the Field." *Operations Research,* 1982, *30,* 803-838.

Lawler, E. E. *Pay and Organizational Effectiveness: A Psychological View.* New York: McGraw-Hill, 1971.

Lewin, K. *Principles of Topological Psychology.* New York: McGraw-Hill, 1936.

Lowe, R. H., and Frey, J. D. "Predicting Lamaze Childbirth Intentions and Outcomes: An Extension of the Theory of Reasoned Action to a Joint Outcome." *Basic and Applied Social Psychology,* 1983, *4,* 353-372.

McCarty, D. "Changing Contraceptive Usage Intention: A Test of the Fishbein Model of Intention." *Journal of Applied Social Psychology,* 1981, *11,* 192-211.

McGuire, W. J. "Public Communication as a Strategy for Inducing Health-Promoting Behavior Change." *Preventive Medicine,* 1984, *13,* 299-319.

McGuire, W. J. "The Vicissitudes of Attitudes and Similar Representational Constructs in Twentieth-Century Psychology." *European Journal of Social Psychology,* 1986, *16,* 89-130.

Marlatt, G. A. "Cognitive Assessment and Intervention Procedures for Relapse Prevention." In G. A. Marlatt and J. R. Gordon (eds.), *Relapse Prevention.* New York: Guilford Press, 1985.

Marlatt, G. A., and Gordon, J. R. *Relapse Prevention: Maintenance Strategies in the Treatment of Addictive Behaviors.* New York: Guilford Press, 1980.

Pagel, M. D., and Davidson, A. R. "A Comparison of Three Social-Psychological Models of Attitude and Behavioral Plan: Prediction of Contraceptive Behavior." *Journal of Personality and Social Psychology,* 1984, *47,* 517–533.

Paskett, E. D., Carter, W. B., Chu, J., and White, E. "Compliance Behavior in Women with Abnormal Pap Smears: Development and Testing a Decision Model." Submitted for publication.

Peak, H. "Psychological Structure and Psychological Activity." *Psychological Review,* 1958, *58,* 325–347.

Prochaska, J. O., and DiClemente, C. C. "Stages and Processes of Self-Change of Smoking: Toward an Integrative Model of Change." *Journal of Consulting and Clinical Psychology,* 1983, *51,* 390–395.

Ramey, F. P. "Truth and Probability." In H. E. Kyburg, Jr., and H. E. Smokler (eds.), *Studies in Subjective Probability.* New York: Wiley, 1964.

Rosenberg, M. J. "Cognitive Structure and Attitudinal Affect." *Journal of Abnormal and Social Psychology,* 1956, *53,* 367–372.

Rotter, J. B. *Social Learning and Clinical Psychology.* Englewood Cliffs, N.J.: Prentice-Hall, 1954.

Sayeki, Y. "Allocation of Importance: An Axiom System" *Journal of Mathematical Psychology,* 1972, *9,* 55–65.

Smetana, J., and Adler, N. "Understanding the Abortion Decision: A Test of Fishbein's Value Expectancy Model." *Journal of Population,* 1979, *2,* 338–357.

Smetana, J., and Adler, N. "Fishbein's Value x Expectancy Model: An Examination of Some Assumptions." *Personality and Social Psychology Bulletin,* 1986, *6,* 89–96.

Tolman, E. C. "A Cognition Motivation Model." *Psychological Review,* 1952, *59,* 389–400.

Townes, B. O., Beach, L. R., Campbell, F. L., and Martin, D. C. "Birth-Planning Values and Decisions: The Prediction of Fertility." *Journal of Applied Social Psychology,* 1977, *7,* 73–88.

Townes, B. O., Campbell, F. L., Beach, L. R., and Martin, D. C. "Birth-Planning Values and Decisions: Preliminary Findings."

In S. Newman and V. Thompson (eds.), *Population Psychology: Research and Educational Issues.* Washington, D.C.: U.S. Government Printing Office, 1976.

Vroom, V. H. *Work and Motivation.* New York: Wiley, 1964.

Werner, P. D., and Middlestadt, S. E. "Factors in the Use of Oral Contraceptives by Young Women." *Journal of Applied Social Psychology,* 1979, *9,* 537–547.

Westbrook, L. J., Carter, W. B., and Wagner, E. H. "An Evaluation of Strategies to Increase Influenza Vaccination Rates Among High-Risk Elderly at Olive Way Medical Center." Final project report, Center for Heath Studies, Group Health Cooperative of Puget Sound, Seattle, Washington, 1987.

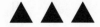

Chapter 5

Frances Marcus Lewis
Lawren H. Daltroy

How Causal Explanations Influence Health Behavior: Attribution Theory

Health professionals are concerned with the ways in which people explain health-related events in their lives. Such explanations affect how people respond both to health threats and to opportunities for health enhancement. *Attributions* are the causes individuals generate to make sense of their world. Attribution Theory describes the processes of explaining events and the behavioral and emotional consequences of those explanations.*

Central to Attribution Theory is the assumption that people spontaneously engage in attributional activities; they ask "Why?" (Bulman and Wortman, 1977; Wong and Weiner, 1981). Ascribing causes is especially relevant when one's health is threatened, when symptoms or tension is heightened, or when a catastrophic event takes place. The assignment of causes makes effective management possible and provides a guide for future action (Weiner, 1985; DuCette and Keane, 1984). Attributions can predict behavior, feelings, and expectancies and are useful in maintaining self-esteem and reducing anxiety (Abramson, Seligman and Teasdale, 1978;

*Work on this chapter was partly supported by the following grants from the National Institutes of Health: National Cancer Institute (P01-CA-38552); Institute of Arthritis, Musculoskeletal, and Skin Diseases (AR 36308); and the Center for Nursing Research (R01-NR-01000-06).

92

Lewis, 1982, 1989; Weiner, 1979). They also contribute to feelings of hopelessness (Weiner, 1979), depression (Peterson, 1988), and motivational and cognitive deficits (Abramson, Seligman, and Teasdale, 1978; Wortman and Dintzer, 1978). Attributions have also been successful predictors of change in achievement programs (Weiner, 1979).

The purpose of this chapter is to analyze Attribution Theory and to present two applications of the theory that are relevant to health behavior and health education. The chapter contains four sections: a brief historical overview of the theory, an analysis of the essential concepts, applications to health education and future directions.

Historical Development of Attribution Theory

Attribution theory emerged from the "naive" or "lay psychology" of Heider (1958) and the subsequent reformulations by Jones and Davis (1965) and Kelley (1967). Heider posited a set of rules of inference by which the ordinary person might attribute responsibility to another person (an "actor") for an action. Heider distinguished between internal and external attributions, arguing that both personal forces and environmental factors operate on the actor, and the balance of these determines the attribution of responsibility (Heider, 1958).

Kelley (1967) significantly advanced Heider's earlier formulations by adding hypotheses about the factors that affect the formation of attributions: consistency, distinctiveness, and consensus. Consistency is the degree to which the actor performs the same behavior toward an object on different occasions. Distinctiveness is the degree to which the actor performs different behaviors with different objects. Consensus is the degree to which other actors perform the same behavior with the same object. Both Heider's and Kelley's analyses influenced the later formulations by Weiner, which are discussed in the next section (Heibsch, Brandstatter, and Kelley, 1982).

Attribution Theory: An Analysis

Antecedents, Processes and Consequents. Generating attributions is an inferential activity, and most attribution researchers have favored an information-processing model (Harvey and Weary, 1985, p. 5). (Information processing is discussed further in Chapter Six.) The individual responds to environmental cues and information and draws inferences or conclusions.

Attributions have been studied in terms of process, content, and consequents (Olson and Ross, 1985). *Process* involves the way in which individuals construct their causal beliefs. Such processes were the initial emphasis on both Heider's and Kelley's works. The study of process is the same as the study of the antecedents of attribution.

Content is the "stuff" or material of the attributions, that is, the categories of response people offer when explaining their worlds in lay terms. The *consequents* of attributions are the outcomes or effects of people's explanations on their own behavior. Some studies focus on the effects of attributions on the person generating them. Studies of the consequents of attributions link the arenas of motivation and personality psychology (Kelley, 1973).

Attribution Theory assumes that people are motivated to explain, interpret, and understand their causal environments. They are information seekers who attempt to decrease ambiguity. A search for explanation ultimately is connected with the broader concept of personal or cognitive control. Attributions render the world predictable and controllable (Pittman and D'Agnostino, 1985; Thompson, 1981, Miller, 1979; Lewis, 1987; Wortman, 1974).

Although causal attributions are the major emphasis in Attribution Theory, not all explanations deal with causes. People also can explain by giving reasons rather than causes and by describing, excusing, or justifying (Antaki, 1982). The larger context of explanation, which goes beyond the scope of this chapter, deals with the derivation of meaning by an individual, only a portion of which is comprised of causal attributions (Lewis, 1987, 1989; Lewis, Haberman, and Wallhagen, 1986; Thompson, 1981; Yalom, 1980).

People are motivated particularly to conduct attributional searches in ambiguous, extraordinary, unpredictable, or uncontrollable situations (Pittman and D'Agnostino, 1985). Such situations include the diagnosis or exacerbation of chronic illness (Gotay, 1985; Baider and Sarell, 1983; Felton and Revenson, 1984), accidental injuries, personal crises, or relief or cure of a symptom or illness.

Under such conditions, the person asks the question "Why me?" and then attempts to explain why something did or did not happen (Bulman and Wortman, 1977; Jaspars, Hewstone, and Fincham, 1983; Lowery, Jacobsen, and Murphy, 1983; Lowery and Jacobsen, 1985).

The Content of Attributions. Attribution processes may be conscious, deliberate, and reportable, or preconscious, below a level of immediate awareness and therefore inaccessible to direct report (Weiner, 1979). The types of attributions people use to explain their worlds can be classified along four broad dimensions: locus of causation, globality, controllability, and stability (Weiner, 1979, 1985; Forsyth and McMillan, 1981; Abramson, Seligman, and Teasdale, 1978). The first dimension, *locus of causation*, locates the source of the cause as internal or external to the person. This dimension derives from Weiner's review of both Heider's (1958) and Rotter's (1966) work. Weiner distinguishes between the dimension of locus of causation and the concept of controllability. Examples of external locus of causation attributions include luck and chance, test difficulty, clarity of directions, family, physicians and health care workers, and environmental pollutants.

The second dimension, *controllability*, describes the extent to which causes are believed to be controllable or uncontrollable (Weiner, 1979). Innate ability and task difficulty are examples of uncontrollable causes. Level of effort and physician or observer bias are examples of controllable causes (Weiner, 1979). Weiner does not distinguish between control by self and control by other; the issue for him is whether the cause is controllable (Brewin and Antaki, 1982).

The third dimension of causal attributions, *stability*, is a person's location of causes on a continuum of stable (invariant) to unstable (variant) (Weiner, 1979). Personal ability and family are examples of relatively stable causes; attention span and mood are examples of relatively unstable causes.

Globality is the fourth dimension of causal attribution (Abramson, Seligman, and Teasdale, 1978). Causes are global if they affect a wide variety of outcomes; causes are specific if they affect a limited set of outcomes. An example of a global cause is lack of innate intelligence. An example of a specific cause is anxiety when taking standardized tests.

Consequents of Attributions. The types of attributions people generate have major implications for their subsequent thoughts, expectancies, feelings, and actions. Table 5.1 summarizes several types of causal explanations and their hypothesized consequences. More research is still needed to establish the conditions under which these hypotheses are true, what factors affect them, and how illness or wellness states might alter them.

Consequents of the Stability Dimension. Attributions about the stability of the cause affect how much a person expects further situations to have similar results. They are an important determinant of goal expectations (Weiner, 1979) and predict cognitive and motivational deficits (Abramson, Seligman, and Teasdale, 1978). Failure that is ascribed to a stable cause, for example, low innate ability ("I wasn't smart enough to do this") or task difficulty ("The treadmill was an impossible test") decreases the expectation of future success more than when failure is ascribed to unstable causes, for example, bad luck, mood, or a lack of immediate effort ("I didn't give it my best try") or transient environmental conditions ("The room was too hot"). Generally, when a cause is ascribed to stable factors, there is a greater shift in expectancy than when it is ascribed to unstable factors. Thus, the person who thinks success is possible will persist. The person who thinks that outcomes were due to unstable causes will give up. Seligman's Theory of Learned Helplessness relates to this process of giving up and has been reformulated in terms of Attribution Theory (Abramson, Seligman and Teasdale, 1978).

Consequents of the Locus of Causation Dimension. The locus of causation dimension affects self-esteem and affect (Weiner, 1979). When failure occurs under conditions of internal ascriptions, self-esteem decreases. When success occurs under conditions of internal ascriptions, self-esteem is raised. Attributions of internal locus of causation in chronic illness are associated both with depression and with taking responsibility for one's treatment. Attributions of blame for others in chronic illness and disability are associated with

Table 5.1. Hypotheses About Causal Explanations and Their
Behavioral Consequences.

Hypothesis 1	Attributions for failure made to *stable* factors result in expectations for failure in future related situations.
	Attributions for success made to *stable* factors result in expectations for success in future related situations.
Hypothesis 2	*Internal* attributions for failure result in deficits in self-esteem.
	External attributions for failure result in the enhancement or protection of self-esteem.
Hypothesis 3	Attributions for failure made to *controllable* factors result in heightened effort.
	Attributions for failure made to *noncontrollable* factors result in decreased effort.
Hypothesis 4	Attributions for failure made to *global* causes result in decreased effort.
	Attributions for failure made to *specific* causes do not affect subsequent effort in other areas.

either poorer long-term morbidity (Affleck, Tennen, Croog, and Levine, 1987; Taylor, Lichtman, and Wood, 1984) or with better coping and adjustment (Bulman and Wortman, 1977).

Consequents of the Controllability Dimension. The development of the dimension of controllability is somewhat primitive in both Weiner's (1979, 1985) and Seligman's (1975) theories. In contrast, Wortman and Dintzer (1978) argue that controllability of the causal factor is of utmost importance in predicting subsequent performance. Causes that are perceived as under one's own control result in heightened efforts (Wortman and Dintzer, 1978). When a person perceives the cause as uncontrollable, future performance deficits will be large; the person thinks that there is little hope of affecting future outcomes. When the cause is perceived as under the control of the individual, subsequent performances will be enhanced.

Consequents of the Globality Dimension. Globality is the fourth dimension of causal attributions (Abramson, Selgiman, and Teasdale, 1978). Global factors affect a wide variety of outcomes, whereas specific factors affect performance in only the original situation. Attributions of failure to global causes result in subsequent performance deficits across a variety of situations. Performance deficits, both motivational and cognitive, will be far-reaching. Global attributions of failure imply that when people confront new situations, the outcome will not be related to any of their responses. If, in contrast, they make specific attributions, performance deficits will not necessarily occur.

Optimum Explanatory Style

There is probably some optimum or ideal set of attributions that best predict a person's exercise of health-enhancing behaviors. Under conditions of success, stable, global, and internal causal attributions for desirable outcomes are to be reinforced. Under conditions of failure, unstable, specific, uncontrollable, and external causes are to be reinforced (Peterson and Seligman, 1984; Sweeney, Anderson, and Bailey, 1986; Seligman and Schulman, 1986). However, research in this area is limited. There is early but strongly suggestive evidence that a pessimistic explanatory style is not health enhancing and may indeed have deleterious effects on one's health. Recent work by Peterson, Seligman, and Vaillant (1988) indicates that pessimistic attributions in early adulthood (age twenty-five) appear to predict poor health in middle and late adulthood (ages thirty to sixty), even when initial physical and emotional health are controlled. There is also some preliminary evidence that pessimistic people have more physician visits than do optimistic people (Peterson, 1988). Such people also show more severe helplessness than people who explain bad events with unstable, specific, and external causes (Seligman, 1975).

Attributions and Health Education Interventions

Attribution Theory can be applied to health education in six ways: (1) in the development of therapeutic relationships between the health care professional and the client, (2) in the development of correct attributions, (3) in the alteration of incorrect attributions,

(4) in altering the focus of attributions, (5) in attributing character-istics to the individual, and (6) in the maintenance of perceived personal effectiveness. Although research is still needed in each ap-plication area, a number of implications can be drawn for health behavior and health education from accumulated knowledge.

Development of Therapeutic Relationships. Determining a per-son's causal explanations for the state of his or her current health is often a first step in aligning the health professional with the client (Stoeckle and Barsky, 1980). It promotes empathy, or the ability to state in the client's terms his or her explanation of his or her health or illness. By obtaining information on the client's attributions, the health professional begins to understand what motivates the client's behavior. Knowledge of the client's perception of his or her health or illness allows the health professional to tailor the treatment regi-men and to use the client's language in discussing compliance or self-care management.

The importance of knowing a client's attributions is illus-trated in the following example. A patient in rural Kentucky who had an eye irritation was given a medical explanation and an eye ointment for the condition. Because it was clear to the physician that her patient could not understand her explanation, she added, "Some folks would call it weed poisoning." This physician as-sumed soundly that an agreed-on explanation would increase the probability that the patient would use the ointment correctly (Watts, 1982, p. 136). In checking back with the patient, the physi-cian learned that it was the "weed poisoning" explanation that the patient remembered.

Assessing attributions also helps the health professional act as an interpreter and client advocate within the larger arena of health care. Interpreting the client's explanations to others can mean that the client becomes less of a "problem patient" and more someone with whom all health professionals can work effectively.

Creation of Correct Attributions. It now appears that some explana-tions for a person's condition, even if biomedically erroneous and based partly or totally on illusion, may have positive effects on that person's psychosocial adjustment (Taylor, Lichtman, and Wood,

1984; Taylor and Brown, 1988). The role of the health professional is to assist patients to formulate informed explanations of their conditions. This means fostering the creation of causal explanations for illness. Although the transmission of information is part of this process, it is probably not sufficient. Research is still needed to evaluate different methods of creating attributions.

Alteration of Incorrect Attributions. Two types of interventions focus on altering attributions. One type alters the inaccurate or incomplete information that causes a misattribution; the other type alters the dimensional structure of an already existing attribution. The first type involves the acquisition of new or additional information. For example, groups of patients undergoing chemotherapy for cancer might attribute their fatigue to treatment failure rather than to a side effect of the therapy. This incorrect attribution should be replaced with a correct conception of the cause of the fatigue, perhaps forestalling despondency and treatment noncompliance. There are many examples in the counseling literature that illustrate the professional's ability to change people's attributions (Brewin and Antaki, 1982).

The second type of alteration of an attribution assumes the health educator's ability to discern an attribution whose dimensions need correcting. It involves a comparison of the dimensions of a client's attributions with an alternative "ideal" set of attributions. Two types of attributions appear to be especially important to modify: attributions of failure that are based on internal, global, stable, or controllable causes and attributions of success that are based on external, specific, unstable, or uncontrollable causes. These sets of attributions constitute the pessimistic explanatory style described earlier. The goal of the health professional is to help people replace these attributions with alternative ones. In general, the goal is to encourage attribution of failure (for example, failure to lose weight or failure to stop smoking) to uncontrollable, external, specific, and unstable causes. Uncontrollable and unstable causes are important in these cases because a person can act on the belief that the health behavior or health outcome was not potentially achievable at that point in time. Thus, things need to be modified to make the health behavior and its outcome possible, and it was not the person's deficiencies or lack of ability that resulted in an earlier unsuccessful outcome. External locus of causation is important because the person can act on the belief that the failure was not inherently related to any personal shortcoming. Specificity is important because the person can view the failure as circumscribed to a particular situation and not generalizable to future attempts to change the health behavior.

Alteration of the Focus of the Attribution. Sometimes the areas over which a person makes attributions need to be shifted. This seems particularly important in chronic or life-threatening illness in which the disease is medically unstable and only partially controllable. Sometimes people erroneously attribute controllability and stability to such medical conditions. These ideas, which are often inaccurate, may serve a temporary purpose of making the condition seem less threatening. Interventions focused on shifting the person's attributions from an area over which he or she actually has little or no control to an area over which he or she can maintain control may facilitate the person's adjustment. A study of late-stage cancer patients revealed that psychosocial adjustment (measured by both self-esteem and anxiety) was unrelated to the locus of causation over their own health but was significantly related to other areas over which the patients attributed control (Lewis, 1982, 1989). Further, patients readily identified areas over which they could maintain control despite the unpredictability and uncontrollability of their disease, for example, their attitudes and how they allocated their time for activities (Lewis, Haberman, and Wallhagen, 1986).

Attribution of Characteristics of the Individual. In addition to altering a person's attributions directly, the health professional can make direct statements of attribution about the person's characteristics in order to affect his or her behavior. This is accomplished by attributing certain characteristics to the person in the person's presence. In an experimental study, Miller, Brickman, and Bolen (1975) taught fifth-graders not to litter and to clean up after others. Members of an attribution group were repeatedly told that they were neat and tidy; members of a persuasion group were repeatedly told that they should be neat and tidy; and members of a control group received no intervention. The attribution manipulation was considerably more effective in modifying behavior than was the persuasion manipulation. Extending this work, it may be possible to design health education interventions similarly to make health-related attributions to children and to adults.

Maintenance of Perceived Personal Effectiveness. People make attributions about their own success and competencies at initiating or maintaining healthy behavior. Attribution Theory argues the importance of a person's attributions of his or her own efficacy in carrying out the necessary behaviors to get or stay well. (This is consistent with Bandura's Social Learning Theory, 1977, 1986, which is discussed in Chapter Eight.) What is critical is that clients attribute potential effectiveness to their own behavior. Under these conditions, health-related skills will not be abandoned in the face of failure (Brewin and Antaki, 1982), difficult tasks will be initiated, and task persistence will occur even in the face of obstacles.

The two applications that follow provide examples of Attribution Theory that address psychosocial adjustment to chronic illness, and symptom attribution and medication compliance.

Causality and Control in Chronic Illness

The first application of Attribution Theory focuses on attributions in chronic disease. It highlights the importance of attributions in affecting patients' psychosocial adjustment to chronic illness. Recent research in cancer, arthritis, and heart disease has shown that attributions can have powerful effects on psychological adjustment, behavior, and morbidity. The most potent attributions center around controllability and locus of causation of disease (Weiner, 1979).

One million people survive heart attacks each year in the United States. Rehabilitation and the return to productive, fulfilling roles are paramount goals that may be helped or impeded by patients' attributions.

In a study by Bar-On and Cristal (1987), eighty-two male, first-time myocardial infarction patients admitted to an intensive coronary care unit (ICCU) were interviewed three times: within forty-eight hours after admission to the ICCU, after two to three weeks and before being released from the hospital, and at a regular checkup at the clinic four to six months after the myocardial infarction. Sixty wives of the patients were interviewed at the second and third measurement times, and forty-five physicians were interviewed on all three occasions.

Two central questions were asked of respondents in the three groups: "Why did the MI [myocardial infarction] happen?" and "What will help you [or the patient] to cope with it?" They were asked to select their answers to each question separately from a list of twenty possible answers. Two dimensions were used to construct a four-category scale: internal-external and controllable-uncontrollable. At the first interview, patients were also rated on an anxiety and depression scale and a denial scale.

Subjects' choices for both questions were factor analyzed. Five main factors organized the type of causal attributions about why the MI happened and the types of activities respondents said helped them cope with the MI. (1) The "Fate-and-Luck" factor included items that attributed the MI and coping with it to external causes such as fate, luck, lack of attention from others, pressure of life in this country. (2) The "Denial" cluster included responses such as "Nothing happened to me; it is just a matter of chance. I will do exactly what I have done until now." (3) In terms of the "Control and Future" factor, no causes for MI were mentioned, only internal locus of causation for coping: for example, "I will build up my body." (4) The "Limits and Strength" factor included such statements as "My anger, not fate, caused the attack." (5) In terms of the last cluster, "the Physical Model of Man," the typical response was "It happened to me because I smoked, ate too much, because of heredity—medication will help."

According to Bar-On and Cristal (1987), the Fate-and-Luck factor is similar to external locus of causation attributions. The Control and Future cluster implies internal, controllable causation. The Limits and Strength factor, though basically internal, also includes external elements (especially in predicting coping); the Physical Model of Man cluster and the Denial cluster are specific to the setting of the illness.

Several results are important. First, all patients in the study made attributions; the motivation seems to exist. Second, although locus of causation and controllability are important, other clusters also are important, and they seem to be disease-specific. Third, actors (patients) are more consistent and use a wider variety of "facts" to make attributions about their diseases than do observers (wives and physicians).

In the study, two instruments were created to measure outcomes. A subjective rehabilitation instrument, Return-to-Work-and-Functioning (RWF), combined physical, sexual, and work-load functioning with degree of return to work. An objective rehabilitation instrument included the number of subsequent rehospitalizations, MIs, and "false alarms" (patients being sent home from the hospital within two hours).

Depression was the only variable significantly associated with objective rehabilitation. Educational level, severity of MI, depression, and the attributions of both the patients and their wives significantly predicted subjective rehabilitation (RWF). Patients who attributed the MI to Fate-and-Luck returned to work more slowly and functioned at a significantly lower level than patients who attributed the MI to Limits and Strength. A similar pattern, though slightly weaker, was found among patients' wives and added to the impact of the patients' attributions.

Patients who attributed the MI to external causes planned and practiced fewer changes overall, relied less on the help of the wife and physician, and returned to work and normal functioning at lower levels. At the other extreme, patients who attributed the MI to Limits and Strength did significantly better in terms of RWF. The results suggest that a multidimensional attributional style in which internal and external attributions are interwoven might be more effective in complex real-life situations than the more unidimensional types of attributions (Denial, Fate-and-Luck, Control and Future).

Internality-training interventions could be developed for Fate-and-Luck patients and their spouses, who could be identified easily with an interview or card-sort exercise such as the one used in this study. Results from the study suggest that it is especially useful to focus on changing Fate-and-Luck attributions (unstable, uncontrollable, external) to controllable, stable, and internal attributions when developing an intervention. Patients and spouses may thereby be encouraged to plan and undertake productive life-style changes. Physicians may also benefit from exploring patients' attributions. A physician who attributes a patient's heart attack solely to the Physical Model of Man cluster, as most did in this study, is unlikely to be effective in uncovering the meaning of the disease to the patient, in explaining the diagnosis and treatment in the patient's language, and in motivating the patient and spouse to assume responsibility for self-management.

Symptom Attributions and Medication Compliance

People develop theories of disease on the basis of their knowledge, information, and symptom experience (Pennebaker, 1982; Rodin, 1978). They make attributions about disease severity and treatment efficacy and use these ideas to regulate self-management (Arluke, 1980; Leventhal, Safer, and Panagis, 1983).

Symptoms abound in daily life, and reorganization of one's attributional (interpretive) theory, based on the knowledge that one has a chronic disease, can considerably alter attention to and interpretation of symptoms that may be random or unrelated to the disease. Patients may become needlessly hypochondriacal, anxious, and self-limited (for example, the cardiac invalid) by constant misattribution of symptoms to a chronic disease or its worsening (Gulledge, 1979).

Medication taking may be strongly affected by attributions if patients make judgments about the activity and effectiveness of their medications on the basis of inaccurate models (Leventhal, Safer, and Panagis, 1983; Arluke, 1980). There is evidence that the placebo effect is enhanced by medication side effects, or at least attribution of random symptoms to a medication, which is then interpreted as evidence of the medication's activity or potency (Pennebaker, 1982). Experimental evidence indicates that information about medication side effects, while not increasing the likelihood of perceived side effects, can increase the chances that both true side effects and random, unrelated symptoms will be attributed to the medication (Morris and Kanouse, 1982).

Psychologically induced side effects often occur because people are highly suggestible (Morris and Kanouse, 1982). Thus, forewarning patients about possible side effects might be expected to produce those effects through suggestion. For this reason, some clinicians hesitate to warn patients about possible side effects. However, because such warnings may help patients respond more appropriately to symptoms, one could argue that patients have the right to know this information.

Morris and Kanouse (1982) randomly assigned 249 newly diagnosed hypertensive patients who were prescribed an antihypertensive medication to one of three groups. The first group received information about the uses and side effects of thiazide in a written pamphlet (patient package insert or PPI), and was interviewed immediately after reading it (at the diagnostic visit) and at the next two clinic visits. The second group was not given the PPI but was interviewed at the diagnostic visit and the next two visits. The third group received the PPI but was not interviewed until the revisits. Of the 249 patients who participated in the initial interviews, 216 returned for at least one visit. The patients were predominately black and Spanish-American. The median age was 51.5 years, and 54 percent were male. Only 39 percent were high school graduates.

A knowledge test showed that the PPI successfully communicated information about side effects. At the initial interview, 76 percent of subjects in the first group (PPI plus interview) but only 33 percent of those in the second group (interview only) correctly named the drug's side effects.

At the first and second revisits, subjects were given a list of seventeen health problems and asked which, if any, they had experienced and which they attributed to the thiazide. Ten of the problems were those mentioned in the PPI and seven were plausible but not listed in the PPI. There were no significant differences when groups were compared on the number of health problems reported or the number still being experienced. Thus, PPIs probably have little effect on the number of side effects that patients report.

In contrast, patients who received the PPI were more likely at the first revisit to attribute any problems they had experienced to the drug. This difference was significant for all seventeen health problems they were asked about at the first revisit *and* for the ten problems listed in the PPI. There were no significant differences in the attribution of problems not listed in the brochure; nor were there any significant differences at the second revisit. Patients receiving the PPI attributed a greater percentage of the health problems they experienced to the drug. In general, the percentage of health problems attributed to the drug was small—usually less than 33 percent. Patients in all three groups reported fewer side effects and less attribution to the medication at the later visits.

Results showed that patients who were informed about possible drug side effects had significantly greater knowledge of these effects. This greater knowledge did not, however, lead to significantly greater reporting of the side effects. Since both PPI-listed and other nonlisted problems tended to be attributed to the drug, it appears that patients forgot the specific side effects over time and retained only a general impression of the kinds of side effects that the drug could cause. When asked to decide whether a given reaction was caused by the drug, subjects may have drawn on this general impression rather than trying to recall whether that specific reaction was mentioned in the PPI. The tendency to attribute a reaction to a drug is probably also influenced by the availability of plausible, alternative nondrug-related explanations. Patients recognized quite rightly that many of the other problems (for example, loss of appetite) could be caused by other factors and made attributions (at least two-thirds of the time) to some nondrug factor. Potential negative effects of information provision did not occur, as informed and uninformed patients did not differ in their likelihood to drop out of therapy, be on time for appointments, comply with medications, or have controlled blood pressure levels.

This documentation of the attribution effect suggests that informing patients about their medications does not stimulate untoward effects. Attribution-based health education interventions could focus on the elicitation of existing attributions about the experienced symptoms and on correcting erroneous attributions. For example, patients on medications could be questioned in an open-ended manner at follow-up medical visits about symptoms they experienced after starting a medication. The health professional could then elicit patient attributions about those symptoms. Incorrect attributions could be targets for educational intervention with the goal of preventing possible noncompliance. Side effects could be investigated by the physician or primary care provider, and the regimen could be adjusted accordingly. To query the patient only about those side effects that are most likely would fail to detect erroneous attributions that could lead patients to stop therapy needlessly.

Directions for Research

The evidence of Attribution Theory is not conclusive. Weiner (1979) as well as his critics (Shaver and Drown, 1986; Lowery, 1981; Lewis, 1982) questions the adequacy with which the dimensions of attributions have been mapped. Health-related work by Lowery's and Lewis's teams as well as others aims to extend and refine the dimensions of attributions and their effects on adjustment to illness.

Counter to the basic assumption of Attribution Theory, there is increasing evidence that some individuals, though a minority, do not engage in causal searches or attempt to generate attributions (Lowery, Jacobsen, and McCauley, 1987). We need to know the conditions under which this occurs and its consequences for the individual. Also, some people generate multiple attributions, some of them mechanistic and some of them philosophical (Bulman and Wortman, 1977; Wortman and Dintzer, 1978). There may also be preliminary attributions as well as final ones (Wortman and Dintzer, 1978). These activities and their consequences deserve further attention.

Under certain conditions, some individuals may prefer causal ambiguity over causal certainty. This seems particularly relevant when the event or outcome is objectively uncontrollable by either the self or others (Wortman and Dintzer, 1978; Haberman, 1987). Further research is needed about causal ambiguity and its importance to the individual.

The utility and impact of attributions may vary over time from onset of disease, across diseases, and by age and educational level (Taylor, Lichtman, and Wood, 1984; Marks, Richardson, Graham, and Levine, 1986). Further research is needed on the role of illusion as a type of incorrect attribution. Health education focuses on the provision of accurate information that individuals may use responsibly and voluntarily to guide their health behavior. If, however, under some conditions inaccurate causal explanations are linked to better psychosocial adjustment (see, for example, Taylor, Lichtman, and Wood, 1984), what are the implications for health education? Is our role to correct the misattributions? If it is, then we should examine the potential deleterious as well as positive effects of such actions.

We have highlighted the importance of the controllability dimension of causal attributions. Three fundamental questions still remain unanswered: When does a perceived lack of controllability result in motivational and cognitive deficits? When does it result in more intense effort? When does it result in active relinquishing of control or a shift to areas over which control can be maintained?

Health education is an intervention-oriented discipline. Despite the firmness with which hypotheses about the consequences of different types of attributions have been stated, caution is in order. No reported experimental study has systematically manipulated the various dimensions or types of attributions. Additional research is needed. There is enough evidence now to claim that attributions are potent, but we do not know if we can manipulate various dimensions of attributions. If so, which ones? By what methods can the attributions be manipulated? If we assume that stable, internal, global, and controllable causes for failure have the most deleterious effects on an individual's behavior and self-appraisal, do altered attributions in these areas positively affect health behavior or health outcomes? Clearly more evaluation of attribution-based interventions is needed.

References

Abramson, L. Y., Seligman, M.E.P., and Teasdale, J. D. "Learned Helplessness in Humans: Critique and Reformulation." *Journal of Abnormal Psychology*, 1978, *87*, 49–74.

Affleck, G., Tennen, H., Croog, S., and Levine, S. "Causal Attribution, Perceived Benefits, and Morbidity After a Heart Attack: An 8-year Study." *Journal of Consulting and Clinical Psychology*, 1987, *55*, 29–35.

Antaki, C. "A Brief Introduction to Attribution and Attributional

Theories." In C. Antaki and C. Brewin (eds.), *Attributions and Psychological Change*. London: Academic Press, 1982.

Arluke, A. "Judging Drugs: Patients' Conceptions of Therapeutic Efficacy in the Treatment of Arthritis." *Human Organization*, 1980, *39*, 84–88.

Baider, L., and Sarell, M. "Perceptions and Causal Attributions of Israeli Women with Breast Cancer Concerning Their Illness: The Effects of Ethnicity and Religiosity." *Psychotherapy and Psychosomatics*, 1983, *39*, 136–143.

Bandura, A. "Self-Efficacy: Toward a Unifying Theory of Behavioral Change." *Psychological Review*, 1977, *84*, 191–215.

Bandura, A. *Social Foundations of Thought and Action: A Social Cognitive Theory*. Englewood Cliffs, N. J.: Prentice-Hall, 1986.

Bar-On, D., and Cristal, N. "Causal Attributions of Patients, Their Spouses and Physicians, and the Rehabilitation of the Patients After Their First Myocardial Infarction." *Journal of Cardiopulmonary Rehabilitation*, 1987, *7*, 285–298.

Brewin, C., and Antaki, C. "The Role of Attributions in Psychological Treatment." In C. Antaki and C. Brewin (eds.), *Attributions and Psychological Change*. London: Academic Press, 1982.

Bulman, R. J., and Wortman, C. B. "Attributions of Blame and Coping in the 'Real World': Severe Accident Victims React to Their Lot." *Journal of Personality and Social Psychology*, 1977, *35*, 351–363.

DuCette, J., and Keane, A. " 'Why Me': An Attributional Analysis of a Major Illness." *Research in Nursing and Health*, 1984, *7*, 257–264.

Felton, B. J., and Revenson, T. A. "Coping with Chronic Illness: A Study of Illness Controllability and the Influence of Coping Strategies on Psychological Adjustment." *Journal of Consulting and Clinical Psychology*, 1984, *52*, 343–353.

Forsyth, D. R., and McMillan, J. H. "Attributions, Affect, and Expectations: A Test of Weiner's Three-Dimensional Model." *Journal of Educational Psychology*, 1981, *73*, 393–403.

Gotay, C. C. "Why Me? Attributions and Adjustment by Cancer Patients and Their Mates at Two Stages in the Disease Process." *Social Science and Medicine*, 1985, *20*, 825–831.

Gulledge, A. D. "Psychological Aftermaths of Myocardial Infarction." In W. D. Gentry and R. B. Williams, Jr. (eds.), *Psychological Aspects of Myocardial Infarction and Coronary Care*. (2nd ed.) St. Louis, Mo.: Mosby, 1979.

Haberman, M. R. "Living with Leukemia: The Personal Meaning Attributed to Illness and Treatment by Adults Undergoing a Bone Marrow Transplantation." Unpublished doctoral dissertation, University of Washington, 1987.

Harvey, J. H., and Weary, G. *Attribution, Basic Issues and Applications*. Orlando, Fla.: Academic Press, 1985.

Heibsch, H., Brandstatter, H., and Kelley, H. H. (eds.). *Social Psychology*. Proceedings of 22nd International Congress of Psychology. New York: North-Holland, 1982.

Heider, F. *The Psychology of Interpersonal Relations*. New York: Wiley, 1958.

Jaspars, J., Hewstone, M., and Fincham, F. D. "Attribution Theory and Research: The State of the Art." In J. Jaspars, F. D. Fincham, and M. Hewstone (eds.), *Attribution Theory and Research: Conceptual, Developmental and Social Dimensions*. London: Academic Press, 1983.

Jones, E. E., and Davis, K. E. "From Acts to Dispositions: The Attribution Process in Person Perception." In L. Berkowitz (ed.), *Advances in Experimental Social Psychology*. Vol. 2. Orlando, Fla.: Academic Press, 1965.

Kelley, H. H. "Attribution in Social Psychology." *Nebraska Symposium on Motivation*, 1967, *15*, 192–238.

Kelley, H. H. "The Processes of Causal Attribution." *American Psychologist*, 1973, *28*, 107–128.

Leventhal, H., Safer, M. A., and Panagis, D. M. "The Impact of Communications on the Self-Regulation of Health Beliefs, Decisions, and Behavior." *Health Education Quarterly*, 1983, *10*, 3–29.

Lewis, F. M. "Experienced Personal Control and Quality of Life in Late-Stage Cancer Patients." *Nursing Research*, 1982, *31*, 113–119.

Lewis, F. M. "The Concept of Control: A Typology and Health-Related Variables." *Advances in Health Education and Promotion*, 1987, *2*, 277–309.

Lewis, F. M. "Attributions of Control, Experienced Meaning, and

Psychosocial Well-Being in Advanced Cancer Patients." *Journal of Psychosocial Oncology*, 1989, 7, 105-119.

Lewis, F. M., Haberman, M. R., and Wallhagen, M. I. "How Adults with Late-Stage Cancer Experience Personal Control." *Journal of Pathosocial Oncology*, 1986, 4, 27- 42.

Lowery, B. J. "Misconceptions and Limitations of Locus of Control and the I-E Scale." *Nursing Research*, 1981, 32, 294-298.

Lowery, B. J., and Jacobsen, B. S. "Attributional Analysis of Chronic Illness Outcomes." *Nursing Research*, 1985, 34, 82-88.

Lowery, B. J., Jacobsen, B. S., and McCauley, K. "On the Prevalence of Causal Search in Illness Situations." *Nursing Research*, 1987, 36, 88-93.

Lowery, B. J., Jacobsen, B. S., and Murphy, B. B. "An Exploratory Investigation of Causal Thinking of Arthritics." *Nursing Research*, 1983, 32, 157-162.

Marks, G., Richardson, J. L., Graham, J. W., and Levine, S. "Role of Health Locus of Control Beliefs and Expectation of Treatment Efficacy in Adjustment to Cancer." *Journal of Personality and Social Psychology*, 1986, 51, 443-450.

Miller, R., Brickman, P., and Bolen, D. "Attribution Versus Persuasion as a Means for Modifying Behavior." *Journal of Personality and Social Psychology*, 1975, 31, 430-441.

Miller S. M. "Controllability and Human Stress: Method, Evidence, and Theory." *Behavioral Research and Therapy*, 1979, 17, 287-304.

Morris, L. A., and Kanouse, D. E. "Informing Patients About Drug Side Effects." *Journal of Behavioral Medicine*, 1982, 5, 363-373.

Olson, J. M., and Ross, M. "Attribution Research: Past Contributions, Current Trends, and Future Prospects." In J. H. Harvey and G. Weary (eds.), *Attribution, Basic Issues and Applications*. Orlando, Fla.: Academic Press, 1985.

Pennebaker, J. W. *The Psychology of Physical Symptoms*. New York: Springer-Verlag, 1982.

Peterson, C. "Explanatory Style as a Risk Factor for Illness." *Cognitive Therapy and Research*, 1988, 12, 119-132.

Peterson, C., and Seligman, M.E.P. "Causal Explanations as a Risk Factor for Depression: Theory and Evidence." *Psychological Bulletin*, 1984, 91, 347-374.

Peterson, C., Seligman, M.E.P., and Vaillant, G. E. "Pessimistic Explanatory Style Is a Risk Factor for Physical Illness." *Journal of Personality and Social Psychology*, 1988, *55*, 23–27.

Pittman, T. S., and D'Agnostino, P. R. "Motivation and Attribution: The Effects of Control Deprivation on Subsequent Information Processing." In J. H. Harvey and G. Weary (eds.), *Attribution, Basic Issues and Applications*. Orlando, Fla.: Academic Press, 1985.

Rodin, J. "Somatopsychics and Attribution." *Personality and Social Psychology Bulletin*, 1978, *4*, 531–540.

Rodin, J. "Aging and Health: Effects of the Sense of Control." *Science*, 1986, *19*, 1273–1275.

Rotter, J. B. "Generalized Expectancies of Internal vs. External Control of Reinforcement." *Psychological Monographs*, 1966, *80*, 1–28.

Seligman, M.E.P. *Helplessness: On Depression, Development, and Death*. New York: W. H. Freeman, 1975.

Seligman, M.E.P., and Schulman, P. "Explanatory Style as a Predictor of Productivity and Quitting Among Life Insurance Sales Agents." *Journal of Personality and Social Psychology*, 1986, *50*, 832–838.

Shaver, K. G., and Drown, D. "On Causality, Responsibility, and Self-Blame: A Theoretical Note." *Journal of Personality and Social Psychology*, 1986, *50*, 697–702.

Stoeckle, J. D., and Barsky, A. J. "Attributions: Uses of Social Science Knowledge in the 'Doctoring' of Primary Care." In L. Eisenberg and A. Kleinman (eds.), *The Relevance of Social Science for Medicine*. Boston: Reidel, 1980.

Sweeney, P. D., Anderson, K., and Bailey, S. "Attributional Style in Depression: A Meta-Analytic Review." *Journal of Personality and Social Psychology*, 1986, *50*, 974–991.

Taylor, S. E., and Brown, J. D. "Illusion and Well-Being: A Social Psychological Perspective on Mental Health." *Psychological Bulletin*, 1988, *103*, 193–210.

Taylor, S. E., Lichtman, R. R., and Wood, J. V. "Attributions, Beliefs About Control, and Adjustment to Breast Cancer." *Journal of Personality and Social Psychology*, 1984, *46*, 489–502.

Thompson, S. C. "Will It Hurt Less If I Can Control It? A Complex

Answer to a Simple Question." *Psychological Bulletin*, 1981, *90*, 89–101.

Watts, F. N. "Attributional Aspects of Medicine." In C. Antaki and C. Brewin (eds.), *Attributions and Psychological Change*. London: Academic Press, 1982.

Weiner, B. "A Theory of Motivation for Some Classroom Experiences." *Journal of Educational Psychology*, 1979, *71*, 3–25.

Weiner, B. "A Theory of Motivation for Some Classroom Experiences." In D. Gorlitz (ed.), *Perspectives on Attribution Research and Theory, The Bielefeld Symposium*. Cambridge, Mass.: Ballinger, 1980.

Weiner, B. "An Attributional Theory of Achievement Motivation and Emotion." *Psychological Review*, 1985, *92*, 548–573.

Wong, P.T.P., and Weiner, B. "When People Ask 'Why' Questions, and the Heuristics of Attributional Search." *Journal of Personality and Social Psychology*, 1981, *40*, 650–663.

Wortman, C. B. "Causal Attributions and Personal Control." In J. Harvey, W. Ickes, and R. Kidd (eds.), *New Directions in Attribution Research*. Vol. 1. New York: Wiley, 1974.

Wortman, C. B., and Dintzer, L. "Is Attributional Analysis of the Learned Helplessness Phenomenon Viable? A Critique of the Abramson-Seligman-Teasdale Reformulation." *Journal of Abnormal Psychology*, 1978, *87*, 75–90.

Yalom, I. D. "Meaninglessness." In I. D. Yalom, *Existential Psychotherapy*. New York: Basic Books, 1980.

Chapter 6

Joel Rudd
Karen Glanz

▲ ▲ ▲

How Individuals Use Information for Health Action: Consumer Information Processing

The Role of Information in Health-Related Decisions

Information is critical to sound health-related decisions. Consumers and patients desire information about health-related products, services, and therapeutic regimens (Glanz and Mullis, 1988; Glanz and Rudd, 1989; Ley, 1987). Though accurate knowledge is generally considered necessary but not sufficient to stimulate appropriate health behavior, it plays a central role in life-style choices, health care interactions, and compliance with therapeutic advice. An understanding of how people acquire and use health information can help professionals and educators influence the quality of consumer and patient health actions.

Information processing affects health behavior when consumers choose health services, providers, and health-related products and when patients or consumers receive health information and advice for avoidance or management of illness. This is particularly evident when communications contain information regarding what, how, where, and when to perform actions to preserve or promote health. If consumers lack knowledge regarding optimal preventive practices, their actions are not likely to help maintain or promote good health.

Background of Consumer Information Processing Theory

Consumer Information Processing (CIP) Theory rose to prominence in the study of consumer behavior in the late 1970s. It owes its principal intellectual debt to human problem solving and information processing and to the domain of cognitive psychology. Interest in cognitive processes such as problem solving and information processing dates from the time of Aristotle. Recently, these and related topics have come to be addressed under the rubric of cognitive science (Stillings, Feinstein, and Garfield, 1987). Cognitive science blends traditional interests in human cognition with computer science efforts to create artificial intelligence. Before CIP theory is discussed, relevant material on human problem solving and information processing is reviewed briefly.

Human Problem Solving and Information Processing

Two areas in the literature on human problem solving and information processing are of particular interest. One is theoretical: How do individuals process large amounts of information in a task involving decisions? The second is methodological: How can researchers accurately measure information-processing and decision-making activities?

Theoretical Premise: Individuals as Limited Information-Processing Systems. The human problem-solving and information-processing tradition views individual decision making as search activity within a problem space (Newell and Simon, 1972). A problem space consists of a series of information points relevant to the decision task. Individuals processing information within a problem space are thus seen as limited information-processing systems. Information processing occurs in a short-term memory having a limited holding capacity and a limited ability to transfer information to long-term memory.

 Memory is used to refer to almost any way that current behavior reflects sensitivity to past experience. Short-term memory refers to retrieval from what can be thought of as working memory. Rehearsal is one of the most effective means of retaining information within working memory. Often the retrieval situation occurs some time later. By then, the information may have been transferred to long-term memory. It only will be recalled if it survives in the network of declarative knowledge (Stillings, Feinstein, and Garfield, 1987).

A major implication of the limited nature of human information processing is that the amount of information acquired in a decision task will be limited and that cognitive techniques will be used to increase the utility of the limited information acquired. For example, the technique of chunking may be used to integrate a number of relatively simple and related information bits into higher-order, more meaningful information chunks. Information chunks are familiar configurations of information that greatly increase the capacity of short-term memory (Newell and Simon, 1972). One of the predictions of human problem solving and information processing is that individuals prefer and tend to seek out or infer chunk information from a problem space.

Methodology and Measurement of Information Processing. Accurate measurement of individual information processing and decision making presents difficulties for the researcher, who cannot "get inside the mind" of the person being studied. Two measurement techniques that were developed and widely used in the early problem-solving and information-processing tradition are the gathering of verbal protocols, in which the subject is asked to think aloud as decision making occurs (Ericsson and Simon, 1980), and eye fixation measures, in which the subject's line of sight is tracked by sophisticated instruments during an information-processing task (Simon, 1979). A third technique to measure information processing and decision making was developed within the more recent CIP perspective: matrix display methodology, in which the subject is asked to acquire information from a multidimensional matrix display device (Jacoby, Syzbillo, and Busato-Schach, 1977).

Matrix display methodology is an experimental laboratory procedure in which subjects are asked to engage in prepurchase information acquisition using a multidimensional matrix display (either on a physical board or a computer screen) typically containing a large amount of information about a particular project (Hoyer and Jacoby, 1983). The matrix might consist of the names of product attributes, brand name alternatives, and sources of attribute information. The actual information values for these categories are hidden but easily accessible to the subject. Subjects freely choose (acquire) these information values, and their choices are recorded for later analysis. Matrix display methodology makes it possible for researchers to study the information-processing experience through observation of a simulated situation and thus allows insights that are not available through verbal protocols. Further, this methodology may be quite useful for formative evaluation of health information programs.

Consumer Information Processing Theory in Perspective

This chapter focuses on CIP theory, which has a strong *individualistic*, or intraindividual, orientation. It attempts to illuminate the "black box" of what is going on in the consumer's mind. The CIP conceptual framework stresses *processes* rather than static states and is intended to help us understand fluid cognitive development. An important overarching theme is that *learning occurs through information processing* and that learning is a cumulative experience that affects future information seeking, acquisition, and use.

CIP complements other approaches to understanding and influencing health-related behavior, particularly the large body of communication theories (for example, Hovland, Janis, and Kelley, 1953). Clearly, information provision is only part of the health education mix. The intent of this chapter is to provide examples of situations where CIP has a good fit, and to encourage others to apply CIP to whole problems or parts of problems, where it can guide understanding, prediction, and intervention strategies in health education.

There is currently some dissatisfaction with CIP theory and its strong rationalistic and individualistic bias. At present, two types of frameworks seem to be attracting interest: (1) those focusing on the role of affect in consumer behavior and (2) more holistic, environmental, or "systems" approaches. The interest in affect, defined as feeling, emotions, and the experiential dimension of consumer choice, is distinct from earlier attitude models. A number of scholars have proposed movement in this direction, though such thinking currently lacks clearly developed research models.

Characteristics of the Consumer Choice Environment

From the CIP perspective, the most important characteristics of the consumer choice environment are the quantity and quality of information available. Both of these characteristics of information are critical determinants of its *processability*, the extent to which consumers can and do use the information in making choices. The mere availability of information does not ensure that it is processable or, if it is processable, that it will be used in decision making (Bettman, 1979).

With a few notable exceptions, the consumer choice environment is information rich. That is, there is a large amount of information available to be brought to bear on a decision process. Some characterize the situation as one in which there is often too much information available, exacerbating the consumer's ability to make decisions. The information environment includes such prevalent information sources as advertising, product labeling, word-of-mouth, news reports, and entertainment.

Emphasis on Information Search and Acquisition

Probably more research has been performed on information search and acquisition than on all other aspects of consumer information use combined. These stages in the decision-making process are of direct interest to product marketers, who have generated much of the research on consumer behavior. In addition, information search and acquisition present fewer data gathering barriers than do other stages in the decision-making process.

In applying CIP to health behavior, several types of information warrant attention, including information for "life-style" health practices such as eating and exercise. An additional focus area is information as a basis for choosing providers and sources of health care. Within medical care, most attention has centered on the provision of information by doctors and other patient educators. An evolving health care "consumer" orientation has more recently addressed ways to stimulate consumer or patient questioning of health professionals (Haug and Lavin, 1983).

Components of Consumer Information Processing Theory

Overview of Stages and Variables

The information-processing approach to consumer decision making is not a unified theory but rather a conceptual framework to guide researchers, program planners, and policy makers in understanding consumer behavior. CIP draws on theories of cognition, decision making, and behavior change. Scholars identified with the CIP perspective posit that consumer decision making is essentially a multistage process in which information is acquired and processed (search), a decision is made and acted upon (choice and purchase), and the quality of the decision is evaluated (use).

Major Concepts and Definitions

The most thorough conceptual and empirical exposition of consumer behavior from a CIP perspective is set forth by Bettman (1979). The basic elements of consumer choice proposed are consumer information processing capacity, motivation, attention and perception, information acquisition and evaluation, decision rules and processes, and consumption and learning (see Figure 6.1). As depicted in Figure 6.1, the CIP framework assumes a continuous and reciprocal interaction among elements, resulting in feedback loops in the decision-making process. When the CIP framework is used as a basis for research, processes within a given element and/or relationships between a subset of selected elements are tested empirically.

Consumer Information Processing Capacity. The fact that consumer information processing capacity is limited affects several of the other elements of consumer choice, most notably attention and perception, information acquisition and evaluation, and decision rules and processes. Consumers are often deterred from engaging in extended information processing because processing capacity is

Figure 6.1. Consumer Information Processing Model of Choice.

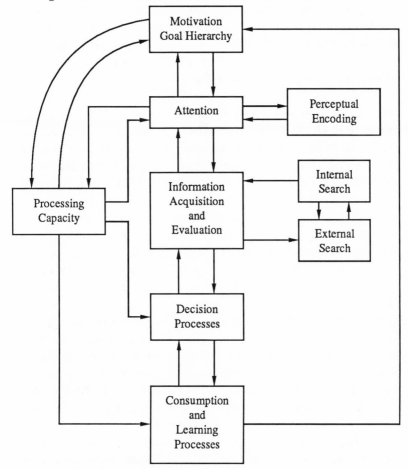

Source: Excerpted from Bettman, 1979.

limited. Further, processing information requires the expenditure of finite resources, primarily effort and time (Bettman, 1979).

Motivation. Motivation is a set of mechanisms for controlling movement from a beginning state (such as recognition of a need) to a desired state (such as purchase or use of a product). One mechanism Bettman proposes to characterize this process is a hierarchy of goals and subgoals. Goals and subgoals are viewed as continually being constructed and reconstructed as motivation levels change and environmental factors, including new information, intervene. Such continual construction and reconstruction provides consumers with the opportunity to decide how much information-processing capacity, time, and other resources to devote to the task of making a choice (Bettman, 1979).

Attention and Perception. In Bettman's (1979) model, attention and perception refer to those activities used by consumers to attend to an information stimulus and to interpret it. Attention may be voluntary, that is, relevant to current goals, or involuntary, that is, not directly related to current goals (Bettman, 1979; Kahneman, 1973).

Information Acquisition and Evaluation. The central processes in Bettman's (1979) model are information acquisition and evaluation. These processes, clearly affected by motivation, attention, and perception, are at the core of consumer decision making. People acquire information through both an internal search (from memory) and an external search (from the environment). Bettman suggests that in the normal course of events, consumers first engage in an internal search. Next, they use what they find there to guide the degree and direction of an external information search. Information derived from an internal search is generally based on past experience and attention to advertising (Bettman, 1979). Lack of sufficient information from an internal search may trigger an external search.

Information processing is an active process in which consumers generate cognitive responses to information from either internal or external sources. Consumers make judgments about the "quality" or veracity of information they have acquired and processed. These judgments may result in a perceived need for additional external information. The direction of an external information search may be influenced by factors such as degree of prior knowledge held by consumers about the product class and the relative availability of information (Bettman, 1979). Moreover, the amount of external information searching is often influenced by the consumer's internal cost-benefit analysis and by environmental factors such as the availability of the information, the difficulty of the choice task, and time pressure (Bettman, 1979; Russo, 1988). In addition, individual differences such as information-processing ability (often a function of educational level) and consumer concern about making a good choice may affect the amount of external searching.

Consumers frequently use a "satisficing" rather than an "optimizing" criterion in determining when to discontinue an information search. That is, they stop acquiring information after locating a satisfactory alternative rather than searching until they have located the best alternative. This is consistent with what Haines (1974) calls the "principle of information processing parsimony." Consumers seek to process as little information as possible in order to make rational decisions quickly.

One of the important implications of the parsimony principle is that consumers are unlikely, under most circumstances, to engage in extended information searching and processing when making health-related decisions. Even when the consequences of suboptimal decisions may be grave, the drive to make decisions quickly is strong. Consumers take many information-processing and decision-making shortcuts. Many such shortcuts involve the development and use of decision rules.

Decision Rules and Processes. In Bettman's (1979) model, decision processes are the heuristics or rules of thumb that consumers develop and use to help them select from among alternatives within the constraints of limited processing capacity. Heuristics, which may be called up from memory or constructed on the spot, provide consumers with a way to simplify and shorten the choice task and perhaps even to routinize it. An example of a simple heuristic is select the cheapest (or closest, most familiar, most accessible) alternative. Bettman describes many more complicated heuristics, most of which are placed into one of two basic information-processing forms: those that involves choice by processing brands (each alternative is evaluated as a whole) and choice by processing attributes (all alternatives are evaluated on a single attribute, then on a second attribute, and so on).

Clearly, the nature of the information environment affects the ease of applying either of these two basic processing forms. For example, package label information in the supermarket and appliance energy-efficiency rating label information are arranged by brand, "forcing" consumers to use choice by processing specific brands. On the other hand, when information is summarized in tabular form for several brands, such as in some supermarket point-of-purchase displays and in *Consumer Reports* magazine, the ease-of-processing differences between the two processing forms disappear.

Consumption and Learning. The consumption and learning processes component of Bettman's model provides both the raison d'être for the stages already discussed and the major feedback mechanism in consumer decision making (Bettman, 1979). This component focuses on the temporal nature of consumer choice, emphasizing the effect of intraindividual feedback from prior decisions and consumption behaviors on current choice. The notion that decision and consumption outcomes are evaluated is basic to this process, and the evaluation process results in cumulative consumer learning. Bettman notes that consumers often develop attributions of causality when evaluating choice outcomes. That is, they evaluate the outcome (positive, negative, or neutral) and then attempt to assign a cause to that outcome (for example, something about the product, their use of it, the conditions under which they used it, and so on).

One mechanism by which past choice outcomes affect consumer choice is through changes in heuristics. Positive, expected outcomes may result in simplification of the heuristic used; negative, unexpected outcomes may result in its elaboration (Bettman, 1979). Thus, when consumers are satisfied with the results of a previous choice, they are likely to take a simplistic view of future choice decisions in the same product category. When consumers are not satisfied or experience undesirable outcomes, they may introduce new decision rules into the heuristic used to make related choices in the future.

Critical CIP Assumptions and Hypotheses
Relevant to Health Behavior

Because Consumer Information Processing theory was developed to explain and predict a broad range of consumer decisions, it is helpful to examine several key issues related to the application of CIP models to health behavior. We will comment briefly on these concerns about correlates of information acquisition and use, minimum requirements for use of health information, and policy issues in health information provision.

Correlates of Information Acquisition and Use

The most revealing findings from studies based on CIP models are those illuminating the process by which individuals learn a particular type of information under a given set of circumstances. However, population-level differences are useful for identifying predispositions to acquire and process information. Key demographic factors that may prove useful include socioeconomic status (education and income levels) and age (John and Cole, 1986). Another important identifier of interest level or involvement might be the extent to which individuals possess a special health interest because of past experience of known risk status (for example, homosexual men's interest in AIDS, family members of Alzheimer's disease patients seeking information about the course of the disease).

Minimum Requirements for Use of Health Information

There are several minimum necessary conditions for consumers to make use of health information in their health actions. First, it must be available. Some types of product information (for example, the chemical makeup of a prescription medication, the chemicals used in some manufacturing processes, the ingredients in a restaurant menu item) and health services information (for example, whether and how often a physician has performed a specific surgical procedure) may be considered proprietary and thus be either unavailable or difficult to obtain. Next, the information must be considered to be useful; it must yield new insights about the characteristics of a product, service, or behavior that the consumer *wants* to gain or believes to be helpful. The information must be *processable* within the time, energy, and comprehension level of the consumer. Further, it must be "format friendly" to processing, that is, strategi-

cally placed for the decision-making situation and time frame, easy
for sensory acquisition, and not confusing.

Policy Issues in Health Information Provision

Probably the most important policy issue that CIP researchers have
addressed is how much and what kind of information should be
provided to improve the quality of consumer decision making.
Early research by Jacoby and colleagues (for example, Jacoby,
Speller, and Berning, 1974) seemed to indicate that at higher information input levels, consumers suffered from "overload" and decision quality declined. However, conceptual and statistical
reanalyses of the Jacoby data and later research have indicated that
increased information loads either improve consumer decision making or have no effect at all (Rudd, 1983).

   While it appears that increased information quantity does
not, in itself, inhibit consumer decision making, the effect of information quality has received less research attention. It is self-evident
that very high quality and very low quality information will have
an impact on the effectiveness of decision making. However, evidence of the effect on decision making of information whose quality
is not at the extremes awaits systematic empirical investigation.

   Private firms, consumer organizations, scientists, and government agencies each have a stake in the amount, type, and channels through which health information is provided. For example,
automobile manufacturers may oppose attempts to require reporting of safety records, and medical device manufacturers may prefer
to conceal health problems resulting from use of their products.
Consumer organizations strive for more information disclosure but
may object to the cost of such information being passed on to consumers. Scientists may insist that for repeated actions (for example,
annual or biennial use of screening tests such as Pap smears and
mammograms) the information must not only be provided but provided repeatedly over time. And the government may be reluctant to
press for information provision requirements because of private-
and public-sector demands or its own assessment of their cost-
effectiveness.

Applications of CIP Theory in Health Education

The major elements of CIP Theory are illustrated here as they apply to two areas of growing concern in health education: consumers' use of nutrition information in food choices, and patients' use of quality of care information in selecting health care providers. These two areas provide contrasts with respect to the amount of available research and the most important CIP factors in the effective use of information. They also differ in the degree of government involvement in the provision of health information. Government intervention in the marketplace to require or encourage information provision is now well established in the area of nutrition information. On the other hand, the government has only recently been involved in similar processes to provide or require disclosure of information to help consumers select high-quality health care providers.

Consumer Use of Nutrition Information in Food Choices

Public interest in nutrition is widespread, and most consumers now recognize the connection between diet and health (Levy, Ostrove, Guthrie, and Heimbach, 1988). Moreover, a growing number of people are making food choices, at least in part, on the basis of nutritional concerns.

While the amount of nutrition information available to consumers has been increasing, its quality varies widely. For example, nutrition labeling on food packages provides a fairly reliable and consistent source of information, largely because the Food and Drug Administration (FDA) mandates the format and monitors the content of nutrition labeling. However, nutrition labels have been heavily criticized, both for the type of information they provide (content) and for the way in which that information is presented (format) (Glaser, 1988). In addition, supermarket shelf tags and other point-of-purchase nutrition information sources are considered nutrition labeling by the FDA, and these appear to be much less consistent in their content and format than packaged food nutrition labels (Pennington and others, 1988).

Three types of research have been used to determine consumer desire for, understanding of, and use of nutrition information on food package labels and in point-of-choice nutrition information programs: consumer surveys, laboratory experiments, and field experiments in naturalistic settings. Consumer surveys and controlled experiments have been most common for studying label use, and field experiments in grocery stores and dining establishments have dominated evaluations of response to point-of-choice nutrition information. We first review some of what is known from research on consumer response to nutrition labeling and then address the effectiveness of point-of-choice interventions.

Effectiveness of Nutrition Information on Food Labels. Liefeld (1983) reviewed the research evidence concerning nutrition labeling and consumer behavior, drawing his conclusions from 100 published articles and reports from 1973 to 1983. Close to half of all consumers said that they would like nutritional information on food packages and labels, but significantly fewer consumers said that they would or did use such information in making food selections. Consumers most often wanted information about salt, sugar, additives, cholesterol, and calories. Both the public in general and those trying to follow special diets focused their information needs on substances to avoid, such as sodium, sugar, and cholesterol, rather than on micronutrient needs to assure dietary adequacy. Consumers preferred simplified information and limited the amount of information they would attend to, acquire, and use.

Some experimental research suggests that when nutrient information on food labels is used, it helps consumers decide which *brand* of a product to buy. Consumers rarely use such information to choose generally nutritious types of foods for more "balanced" diets, however.

Effectiveness of Point-of-Choice Nutrition Information. Point-of-choice (or "point-of-purchase") nutrition information functions as an intermediate cue or source of information between the many stimuli of the grocery store (or restaurant) and a detailed nutrition label on a single food package. It further provides nutrition guidance for items not carrying full nutrition labels. A recent review of more than twenty reports of programs in supermarkets, restaurants, cafeterias, and vending machines found that the research varies along several dimensions: specific goals of programs, brand versus generic food endorsement, placement and complexity of information, length of the intervention, and design and timing of the evaluation study (Glanz and Mullis, 1988).

In general, point-of-choice information programs in supermarkets have been more successful in affecting improvements in nutrition knowledge and attitudes than in changing consumers' purchasing behaviors (for example, Ernst and others, 1986). In studies that have found significant changes toward purchase of "more nutritious" foods, an emphasis on brand-specific choices appears to have been influential (Levy and others, 1985). Russo and others (1986) conducted two experiments testing the use of simplified information formats, one with lists of "desirable" nutritional characteristics (that is, vitamins and minerals) and the other with information about a "negative" component to be avoided (that is, added sugar). These studies, conducted in fourteen supermarkets in the Chicago area, showed that the simplified format was effective in changing behavior only when it focused on nutritional qualities to be limited or avoided.

Several studies of supermarket point-of-choice programs have included questions asking whether shoppers saw or were aware of the nutrition information (for example, Achabal, Bell, McIntyre, and Tucker, 1987; Russo and others, 1986). These studies conclude that only a minority of shoppers are even aware of in-store nutrition information programs, and even fewer probably use them to choose foods.

The literature on point-of-choice nutrition programs includes both apparent failures and encouraging successes. The findings are inadequate either to support or to discredit the value of these programs for improving health. The literature will impress any health education practitioner or researcher with the complexity and difficulty of implementing and maintaining a quality program while simultaneously studying a range of intervening variables and outcomes, as well as controlling for competing explanations for the findings.

Use of Quality of Care Information to Select
Health Care Providers

The increasingly competitive health care market has strengthened the need for patients to make informed choices about the quality and costs of their health care. In order to consider quality of care when choosing among health care providers, people must either have information about the quality of care available in a form that they can understand or be able to acquire such information easily (Glanz and Rudd, 1989). Until recently, little information on the quality of care provided by hospitals, physicians, and other providers was available to consumers. Currently, quality of care information is increasingly generated by government agencies, consumer organizations, the popular press, and health care organizations.

Quality of care information (QCI) is defined as information about the presence or absence or the worth (from poor to excellent) of different dimensions of health care—technical, interpersonal, and amenities of care. QCI involves comparison with a standard of acceptable quality of facilities or performance.

At present, empirical study of the question of whether the availability of quality of care information influences consumers' choices of physicians or hospitals is insufficient to conclude that such information does or does not have a significant impact. However, the answer is most likely neither yes nor no but rather, how much effect can be attributed to what kind of information for what audiences, under what circumstances. To examine these issues, we will use the CIP framework to analyze the question of the effects of quality of care information on consumer choice of physicians and hospitals.

The likely effects of QCI on consumer choices can be discussed in terms of three major areas: audience characteristics, characteristics of QCI, and the literature on reasons for choosing and changing doctors.

Audience Characteristics. While employers, physicians, and consumers and their families all play important roles in the choice and purchase of physician and hospital services, individual consumers (potential patients) and their families make most of the decisions about which physician will provide their health care. About half of all nonhospital physician visits are made by people who know in advance that they need to see a physician and thus may be reasonably well informed. Such visits include pediatric care, general checkups, pre- and postnatal care, and visits for chronic conditions (Pauly, 1982).

Two elements of the CIP model are important in understanding audience characteristics: motivation and consumer information processing capacity (Bettman, 1979). The likelihood that people will seek information about the quality of care depends in part on their propensity to adopt an active consumer stance in health care decisions. Consumer assertiveness in medicine is inconsistent with traditional authority relationships between physicians and patients; it implies "buyer's challenge of seller's claims" (Haug and Lavin, 1983) and willingness to seek information from a variety of sources (Hibbard and Weeks, 1987). A review of studies of consumer information seeking in health provider choice indicates that an estimated 60 to 80 percent of health care consumers conduct only a limited information search because of low motivation (Glanz and Rudd, 1989). The information search may increase as the public learns that quality of care information is available. However, it is likely that extensive consumer education will be necessary even if QCI becomes readily available.

Even if consumers desire information about the quality of care, they will be unlikely to use it correctly unless they understand it. Yet fewer than 30 percent of Americans say that they are well informed about good medical care, and most of those who feel they are well informed are of middle to upper socioeconomic status (General Mills, 1979). However, most consumers (79.3 percent) correctly believe that hospitals vary in terms of the quality of care they offer (Inguanzo and Harju, 1985).

Little research has examined consumer knowledge about the medical care system. Newhouse, Ware, and Donald (1981) studied nearly 5,000 adults and found that educational level was significantly correlated with an eight-item scale of sophistication and that more sophisticated consumers viewed health services more critically, that is, had a more active "consumer orientation." More research on the level of knowledge about the health care system in various population segments is needed to anticipate the effects of quality of care information. For some consumers, it appears that improved knowledge about existing differences in the quality of medical care may act as a stimulus to increased effort to acquire and process quality of care information.

Characteristics of Quality of Care Information. Quality of care information includes indicators of the structure (accreditation status, staff size and type, scope of services, facilities), process (volume of services, tests provided, interpersonal quality of care), and outcome (treatment effectiveness, morbidity and mortality rates), as well as "global" assessments of reputation (U.S. Congress, 1988).

Even simple information, such as the educational background of private practice physicians, is often difficult or impossible for consumers to obtain (Glassman and Glassman, 1981). Furthermore, even when information is available it may be too technical or too complicated for most consumers to use. Information that consumers may perceive to be "simple" (for example, mortality data, volume of surgery) represents complex phenomena. For example, a high-risk patient facing surgery might avoid a certain hospital because of its high absolute mortality rate. But an operation at a less well equipped hospital might result in complications, disability, and even death. Likewise, a consumer obtaining elective surgery at a hospital with a high volume of that surgery may in fact receive *unnecessary* surgery with its concomitant risks. To avoid misleading consumers, quality of care information should only be presented in conjunction with clear interpretation of its meaning.

The extent of an external information search depends, in part, on the consumer's perceptions of the relative costs and benefits of seeking additional information. In addition to the significant environmental barriers currently preventing consumers from acquiring quality of care information, there is an information-processing factor related to degree of search: consumers' confidence in their ability to use the information (Wilkie, 1986). Consumers are likely to feel most confident about using consumer-based indicators (satisfaction with care, interpersonal quality of care, reputation) and structural indicators (particularly facilities/amenities, convenience, and provider background). Consumer interest in quality of care information is likely to increase only through access to information and guidance on how to interpret and use it.

Reasons for Choosing and Changing Health Providers. Two well-researched aspects of consumer prepurchase behavior in the choice of health care providers are reasons for the choice of health services and decisions to change health care providers ("doctor shopping"). Research on these two aspects of consumer health choice behavior is particularly useful for understanding the likely effects of QCI on the heuristics, or decision rules and processes, that consumers develop and use.

Studies indicate that consumers often rely on lay referral (the recommendations of friends and relatives) in choosing health care services. Consumers use lay referral as a simple choice heuristic because they lack quality of care information, have difficulty evaluating such information when it is available, and believe that lay opinion is an adequate substitute for expert opinion. These studies demonstrate that "quality" is important to consumers even in the absence of objective quality of care indicators. Consumers routinely seek informal "quality of care" assessments from friends and family. Because consumers frequently rely on the opinions of friends and family, providing quality of care information in settings where existing friendship and family groups gather might enhance its impact. In sum, the research indicates that simple, accessible QCI may facilitate consumer decision processes.

To the extent that perceptions of quality of care are important in consumer choice of health care, they should also play an important role in the decision to change doctors or to use outside services when covered by a prepaid health plan. The prevailing idea that continuity of care is valuable mitigates against doctor shopping, suggesting that a willingness to change physicians is driven by strong motivations (except when a doctor retires or relocates or when a consumer relocates or changes medical plans).

Research on doctor shopping indicates that consumers change health care providers on much the same bases that they make initial health care choices: lay referral, a desire for better interpersonal quality care, or a lack of confidence in the current provider's technical competence. These findings lend considerable support to the contention that social networks, affective qualities of the physician, and perceived technical quality of care are among the most important factors in consumer health care decisions.

An estimated 20 to 30 percent of consumers choose a new physician each year (Glanz and Rudd, 1989). This suggests that opportunities to acquire and process quality of care information for making health care choices are fairly common. Those who are most likely to engage in doctor shopping are high socioeconomic status, white consumers. The simple, subjective, external search heuristics (for example, rely on advice of family and friends) and experiential decision criteria underscore the low effort expended to obtain objective or expert-generated QCI in most consumer decisions about health care.

Quality of Care Information and Consumer Choice. This review of theory and data leads to a number of conclusions regarding consumer information about health services. First, it appears that most individuals do not actively seek out health care information. The cost of seeking information may deter information-seeking behavior. Strong promotional efforts to encourage medical consumerism may increase the potential effects of QCI on choice of health care. Both information seeking and information processing for *use* will not only require knowledge but also motivation, skills, and peer or social support.

Second, studies of consumers' reasons for choosing and changing health providers indicate that consumers often rely on the recommendations of friends and relatives because of the lack of information about quality of care, the difficulty of evaluating such information when it is available, and/or the belief that lay opinion is an adequate substitute for expertly developed indicators. However, experts' and consumers' notions of quality are often quite different (U.S. Congress, 1988).

In order to promote effective consumer use of quality of care information, (a) QCI should be made widely and readily available; (b) it should be presented so that it is not too technical or complicated for most consumers to use; (c) it should include physician- and hospital-specific information; (d) existing information sources about quality of care should be coordinated and widely disseminated by the government, the private sector and nonprofit groups; and (e) more research needs to be conducted in this area. Research is necessary at both the micro and macro levels to assess information acquisition, understanding, and use in various populations and for various purposes. Health education practitioners and researchers can be important leaders in carrying out or facilitating these advances in consumer education about medical care choice.

Conclusion

The role of information in health-related behavior is widely recognized. However, knowledge is considered necessary but not sufficient to inform those desiring information to guide their health actions and to stimulate health-enhancing behaviors in patient and public health education. Even though efforts to improve health communication through the use of concepts related to Consumer Information Processing theory are not intended to stand alone as health education and promotion strategies, written information plays an important role in both interpersonal and self-managed health decision making. There is much room for improving such communications (Ley, 1987). If health information materials are constructed according to principles based on CIP theory, they can maximally enhance understanding and the probability of recall. For example, hospital mortality information organized to allow consumers quick and easy access to brief, summary data on local hospitals will be more likely to be accessed and processed than venues presenting detailed information on large numbers of hospitals. Acquisition of mortality information will be increased if access is available to consumers via computer or telephone and if such access is free of monetary costs.

McGuire (1984) and Winett (1986) have articulated environmental systems approaches to the understanding of communication and information effects. McGuire (1984) has described an expansion of his earlier information-processing work and proposed two broad types of strategies to improve the public's health: institutional strategies to engineer or establish the context for behavior change, and information and persuasion to convince individuals to alter their life-styles to reduce health risks. These ideas are viewed as complementary and were expressed earlier in other contexts for their potential in health education interventions (Glanz, 1981; Sims and Smiciklas-Wright, 1978; Glanz and Seewald-Klein, 1986). Winett (1986) has presented a comprehensive behavioral systems framework to analyze and predict how information is formed, used, channeled, and delivered in different systems and contexts with different impacts. His framework subsumes CIP theory and amalgamates social learning, communication, and behavioral analysis principles. Its scope is broader than CIP and therefore may better explain some outcomes. However, the research endeavor concomitantly increases in complexity with the breadth of the model.

These emerging perspectives will most likely stimulate continuing thought related to CIP theory, to incorporate its central cognitive principles, and to help produce relevant research and useful guidance in how health professionals can best provide educational experiences to help individuals maintain, improve, and regain their health.

References

Achabal, D. D., Bell, C. H., McIntyre, S. H., and Tucker, N. "The Effect of Nutrition P-O-P Signs on Consumer Attitudes and Behavior." *Journal of Retailing*, 1987, *63*, 9–24.

Bettman, J. R. *An Information Processing Theory of Consumer Choice*. Reading, Mass.: Addison-Wesley, 1979.

Ericsson, K. A., and Simon, H. A. "Verbal Reports as Data." *Psychological Review*, 1980, *87*, 215–251.

Ernst, N. D., and others. "Nutrition Education at the Point of Purchase: The Foods for Health Project Evaluated." *Preventive Medicine*, 1986, *15*, 60–73.

General Mills, Inc. *Family Health in an Era of Stress: The General Mills Family Report, 1978–1979*. Minneapolis, Minn.: General Mills, 1979.

Glanz, K. "Social Psychological Perspectives and Applications to Nutrition Education." *Journal of Nutrition Education*, 1981, *13*, S66–S69.

Glanz, K., and Mullis, R. M. "Environmental Interventions to Promote Healthy Eating: A Review of Models, Programs, and Evidence." *Health Education Quarterly,* 1988, *15,* 395-415.

Glanz, K., and Rudd, J. "Consumer Information on the Quality of Medical Care: A Health Education and Health Information Policy Review." *Advances in Health Education and Health Promotion,* 1989.

Glanz, K., and Seewald-Klein, T. "Nutrition at the Worksite: An Overview." *Journal of Nutrition Education,* 1986, *16,* S1-S12.

Glaser, S. "How America Eats." *Editorial Research Reports, Congressional Quarterly,* Apr. 29, 1988.

Glassman, M., and Glassman, N. "A Marketing Analysis of Physician Selection and Patient Satisfaction." *Journal of Health Care Marketing,* 1981, *1,* 25-31.

Haines, G. H. "Process Models of Consumer Decision Making." In G. D. Hughes and M. L. Ray (eds.), *Buyer/Consumer Information Processing.* Chapel Hill: University of North Carolina Press, 1974.

Haug, M., and Lavin, B. *Consumerism in Medicine: Challenging Physician Authority.* Newbury Park, Calif.: Sage, 1983.

Hibbard, J. H., and Weeks, E. C. "Consumerism in Health Care: Prevalence and Predictors." *Medical Care,* 1987, *11,* 1019-1032.

Hovland, C. I., Janis, I. L., and Kelley, H. H. *Communication and Persuasion.* New Haven, Conn.: Yale University Press, 1953.

Hoyer, W. D., and Jacoby, J. "Three-Dimensional Information Acquisition: An Application to Contraceptive Decision Making." *Advances in Consumer Research,* 1983, *10,* 618-623.

Inguanzo, J. M., and Harju, M. "What Makes Consumers Select a Hospital." *Hospitals,* 1985, *59,* 90, 92, 94.

Jacoby, J., Speller, D. E., and Berning, C. A. "Brand Choice Behavior as a Function of Information Load: Replication and Extension." *Journal of Consumer Research,* 1974, *1,* 33-42.

Jacoby, J., Syzbillo, G. S., and Busato-Schach, J. "Information Acquisition Behavior and Brand Choice Situations." *Journal of Consumer Research,* 1977, *3,* 209-216.

John, D. R., and Cole, C. A. "Age Differences in Information Processing: Understanding Deficits in Young and Elderly Consumers." *Journal of Consumer Research,* 1986, *13,* 297-315.

Kahneman, D. *Attention and Effort*. Englewood Cliffs, N.J.: Prentice-Hall, 1973.

Levy, A. S., Ostrove, N., Guthrie, T., and Heimbach, J. T. "Recent Trends in Beliefs About Diet/Disease Relationships: Results of the 1979-1988 FDA Health and Diet Surveys." Paper presented at FDA/USDA Food Editor Conference, Washington, D.C., Dec. 1-2, 1988.

Levy, A. S., and others. "The Impact of a Nutrition Information Program on Food Purchases." *Journal of Public Policy and Marketing*, 1985, *4*, 1-13.

Ley, P. "Cognitive Variables and Noncompliance." *Journal of Compliance in Health Care*, 1987, *1*, 171-188.

Liefeld, J. P. *Nutrition Labelling and Consumer Behavior: A Review of the Evidence*. Ottawa: Health and Welfare Canada, 1983.

McGuire, W. J. "Public Communication as a Strategy for Inducing Health-Promoting Behavioral Change." *Preventive Medicine*, 1984, *13*, 299-319.

Newell, A., and Simon, H. A. *Human Problem Solving*. Englewood Cliffs, N.J.: Prentice-Hall, 1972.

Newhouse, J. P., Ware, J. E., and Donald, C. A. "How Sophisticated Are Consumers About the Medical Delivery System?" *Medical Care*, 1981, *19*, 316-328.

Pauly, M. V. "Is Medical Care Different? Competition in the Health Care Sector: Past, Present, Future." *Issues in Health Economics*, 1982.

Pennington, J.A.T., Wisniowski, L. A., and Logan, G. B. "In-Store Nutrition Information Programs." *Journal of Nutrition Education*, 1988, *20*, 5-10.

Rudd, J. "The Consumer Information Overload Controversy and Public Policy." *Policy Studies Review*, 1983, *2*, 465-473.

Russo, J. E. "Information Processing from the Consumer's Perspective." In E. S. Maynes (ed.), *The Frontier of Research in the Consumer Interest*. Columbia, Mo.: American Council on Consumer Interest, 1988.

Russo, J. E., and others. "Nutrition Information in the Supermarket." *Journal of Consumer Research*, 1986, *13*, 48-70.

Simon, H. A. "Information Processing Models of Cognition." *Annual Review of Psychology*, 1979, *30*, 363-396.

Sims, L. S., and Smiciklas-Wright, H. "An Ecological Systems Perspective: Its Application to Nutrition Policy, Program Design, and Evaluation." *Ecology of Food and Nutrition*, 1978, 7, 173–179.

Stillings, N., Feinstein, M., and Garfield, J. *Cognitive Science.* Cambridge, Mass.: MIT Press, 1987.

U.S. Congress, Office of Technology Assessment. *The Quality of Medical Care: Information for Consumers.* Office of Technology Assessment Publication no. H-386, 1988.

Wilkie, W. L. *Consumer Behavior.* New York: Wiley, 1986.

Winett, R. A. *Information and Behavior: Systems of Influence.* Hillsdale, N.J.: Erlbaum, 1986.

Chapter 7

Barbara K. Rimer

Perspectives on
Intrapersonal Theories in
Health Education
and Health Behavior

Part Two presents some of the best-developed theories of individual health behavior. The research base that accompanies them is a rich one. Not only do these theories contribute to a broad and basic understanding of individual health behavior, they also point clearly to methods for changing health behavior. Although all are sufficiently robust to become part of the armamentarium of professionals concerned with understanding and enhancing individual health behavior, each is in a different stage of development. And each has a unique history of health application.

This chapter provides an overview of the theories in Part Two and the strengths and weaknesses of each, how these theories relate to others, and how they can be used in practice, particularly in combination with other theories. Finally, the chapter introduces the reader to other promising theories that deserve further attention.

The Health Belief Model

As indicated in Chapter Three, the Health Belief Model (HBM) is one of the few social-psychological models to be developed expressly to understand health behavior. Health professionals have gained long experience with the Health Belief Model in a variety of health-related contexts, beginning with efforts to explain people's tuberculosis screening behaviors. A critical dimension of the Health Belief Model, the failure to believe in the possibility of having pathology in the absence of symptoms, is as relevant today as it was in helping to explain tuberculosis screening behavior in the 1950s. It is probably a critical variable in explaining participation in cancer screening. We have learned, for example, that women are often reluctant to obtain mammograms when they are feeling healthy, even when they "know" that a mammogram can detect something too small to be found by the woman or her physician in any other way. It appears that it takes a belief in asymptomatology, almost an act of faith, to perform the behavior (Rimer and others, 1989). Health educators who understand the importance of this belief and use it to shape their interventions might elect to combine visual and verbal ways of showing the relative size of cancers detected with and without the aid of mammography. Similar beliefs and corresponding opportunities for shaping interventions undoubtedly apply to testing for fecal occult blood and AIDS infections in the absence of symptoms.

One of the most appealing aspects of the Health Belief Model is its acceptance not only by health educators but by psychologists, physicians, dentists, nurses, and other professionals. It has a sort of intuitive logic, the central tenets are clearly stated, and it can be measured by means of a variety of techniques ranging from clinical interviews to population-based surveys. Mullen, Hersey, and Iverson (1987) show that the Health Belief Model is an economical model in terms of the number of questions needed to assess the key variables.

The Health Belief Model has been thoroughly evaluated, and its limitations have become evident. Critics might argue that according to the strictest definitions of theory, the Health Belief Model is not a theory at all. Certainly it never has had the kind of rigorous quantification that Fishbein and Ajzen (1975) have achieved with the Theory of Reasoned Action. However, as Janz and Becker (1984) show, most of the concepts in the model have received considerable empirical support.

Still, one of the most significant limitations of the Health

Belief Model may be that some of the concepts, as Rosenstock explains in Chapter Three and Janz and Becker (1984) observed earlier, have limited predictive value. Severity, for example, seems to have relatively low utility when applied to some health conditions. In cancer, for example, the perception of severity is a difficult variable to measure or change because many people already think this condition is severe. Thus, it appears that the Health Belief Model, taken as a whole, may not apply equally to all behaviors or all diseases.

The Health Belief Model continues to offer myriad opportunities for further investigation. It will be important to understand even more specifically the conditions under which it applies, as well as to standardize and refine the way in which its concepts are measured.

Some components of the Health Belief Model still are not well understood. As Rosenstock notes, the concept of cue is one of these and deserves further study and experimental manipulation. Rosenstock also points out that we need to know more about the role of fear and how it may foster cognitive and behavior changes. Other theoretical models discussed later in this chapter, such as Protection Motivation Theory (Prentice-Dunn and Rogers, 1986) or Self-Regulation Theory (Leventhal and Cameron, 1987), in combination with the Health Belief Model, may be helpful in this regard.

Mullen, Hersey, and Iverson (1987); Rosenstock, Strecher, and Becker (1988); and Rosenstock in Chapter Three of this book have identified other variables that might be added to the Health Belief Model to improve its predictiveness and utility. The most important of their suggestions are the concepts of self-efficacy (also see Chapter Eight on Social Learning Theory), behavioral intention, and a measure of social network (see Chapter Nine on social support). The inclusion of self-efficacy, in particular, seems especially promising for improving the utility of the Health Belief Model.

The Health Belief Model can best be improved through its continued use in the real world and its application to the development of interventions. It is likely to be most useful when combined with other models. Health educators can start by using a planning model such as PRECEDE (Predisposing, Reinforcing, and Enabling Causes in Educational Diagnosis and Evaluation) (Green, Kreuter, Deeds, and Partridge, 1980) to diagnose the multiple layers and dimensions of a health problem. Then the Health Belief Model can be employed within the PRECEDE model to identify the individual knowledge, attitudes, beliefs, and behaviors that are amenable to change and would likely lead to improvement in the behavior of interest. Next, Social Learning Theory could be used to facilitate the development of interventions; for example, the use of modeling can be powerful. Then, because individuals are not the only important targets of intervention, community organization, organizational change, social marketing, and media advocacy could be used to heighten awareness about the problem, to facilitate community level changes, and to alter important norms that hinder expression of the behavior. Assembling the appropriate combination of theories to guide the development and evaluation of interventions at different levels strengthens the potential for achieving initial and lasting change (Rimer, 1989).

Theory of Reasoned Action and Multiattribute Utility Models

The Theory of Reasoned Action and Multiattribute Utility Theory, like the Health Belief Model, are rooted in the intellectual tradition of value expectancy theories. Value expectancy theories provide a method for defining and assessing the elements of decisions. The Theory of Reasoned Action and Multiattribute Utility Theory also are rooted in Information-Processing Theory. Multiattribute Utility models have much in common with social marketing, especially the collection and use of qualitative data to understand and to alter individual decisions and behaviors. Unlike the Health Belief Model, however, the Theory of Reasoned Action and Multiattribute Utility models were not developed explicitly to understand health behavior, although they are now used for that purpose. Attitudes play a stronger role in the Theory of Reasoned Action than in the Health Belief Model, but both place a strong emphasis on the role of beliefs in understanding health behavior.

Fishbein and Ajzen (Fishbein and Ajzen, 1975; Ajzen and Fishbein, 1980) have devoted much of their research effort to specifying the concepts within the Theory of Reasoned Action. In Chapter

Four, Carter shows how each of the concepts, such as attitude toward the act, subjective norm, and behavioral intention, can be operationalized. Because the components have been so well codified, the Theory of Reasoned Action comes closest of all the theories discussed in Part Two to meeting Kerlinger's strict definition of theory. With increased precision of measurement has come improved precision of prediction. Over time, we have learned that the Theory of Reasoned Action is most predictive when the concepts are defined specifically and are in close temporal order. As Carter shows, the Theory of Reasoned Action provides a method for systematically identifying those issues that are most important to a person's decisions about performing a specific behavior. The end product of these efforts is to identify important mutable beliefs and attitudes for subsequent use in behavioral interventions. But as with the Health Belief Model, the strategies for designing interventions must come from other theories.

For Multiattribute Utility Theory, the focus of prediction is the individual. This approach may be more useful than the Theory of Reasoned Action to practitioners, especially those who counsel patients. In Carter's flu vaccination example, the decisional model correctly predicted behavioral intention and vaccination behavior in more than 80 percent of the cases. Knowledge of salient misconceptions and consequences was then used to design the interventions, and decision aids were used to improve the quality of the decision process.

One of the most important characteristics of the Theory of Reasoned Action and Multiattribute Utility Theory is their grounded nature. Carter illustrates how easy it is to overlook important, salient beliefs and attitudes when one does not use rigorous, comprehensive methods in collecting data prior to developing interventions. A final caveat: As Rosenstock observes in Chapter Eighteen, where good data are available for use in program planning, collecting additional data may be tantamount to reinventing the wheel.

While very appealing, especially from a methodological point of view, the Theory of Reasoned Action and Multiattribute Utility Theory are not without limitations. Mullen, Hersey, and Iverson (1987) criticize the Theory of Reasoned Action as almost entirely rational and not recognizing emotional fear-arousal elements such as perceived susceptibility to illnesses. Thus, to explain behavior better, the Theory of Reasoned Action might need supplementation by the Health Belief Model or another theory, such as that of Protection Motivation (Rogers and Mewborn, 1976) or Self-Regulation (Leventhal and Cameron, 1987).

Further, the measurement of the Theory of Reasoned Action and Multiattribute Utility models, while powerful for prediction, may be cumbersome and time-consuming in practice. Multiattribute Utility Theory relies on extensive interviewer-administered personal interviews. While ultimately useful, this can be a demanding, costly process. Collecting more than pilot data may be beyond the resources of most practitioners and a laborious process when programs must be developed quickly.

Simplification of the theories for practice would make them more accessible to practitioners. Decision aids, which are simplified versions of the Multiattribute Utility model that can be used to help people make decisions about health matters, appear promising and should be refined. The Theory of Reasoned Action and Multiattribute Utility models can help us better understand, predict, and measure health behavior, as well as help people make better choices about health behavior. We only are in the preliminary stages of understanding how to translate these ideas into manageable health programs for practitioners, but they are exciting and promising.

Attribution Theory

Attribution Theory, as applied to health, concerns the important question of how people explain health-related events in their lives. Consciously and unconsciously, we continually ask "why?" and assign causes to things that happen to us. Thus, as Lewis and Daltroy show in Chapter Five, Attribution Theory helps explain what happens as people ask "why?" and helps people use this understanding to enhance health behavior. Ideally, we would like to improve those inferences, thereby improving the quality of decision making (Nisbett, Krantz, Jepson, and Fong, 1982), a goal similar to those who use Multiattribute Utility models.

Ross (1977) suggests that people make a fundamental attributional error when they attach others' (or their own) behaviors to personal characteristics to the exclusion of situational causes or transient environmental influences. This is not merely an abstract concern. People who are trying to change their behaviors tend to lapse occasionally. When people attribute such lapses to personal weakness rather than to some environmental influence, such as exposure to smoking colleagues, relapse is more likely (Marlatt and Gordon, 1985). How people attribute symptoms may also determine whether or not they take appropriate action. A man who attributes his chest pain to the spicy lunch he ate earlier instead of to a potential heart attack may take antacids and continue to work. In his case, picking the wrong cause may be a life and death matter. Attribution Theory can help health professionals understand their patients. It is important not only in explaining health-related behaviors but in guiding the development of interventions to correct faulty attributional processes.

Attribution Theory shares with the Health Belief Model, the Theory of Reasoned Action, and Multiattribute Utility Theory a focus on beliefs in the context of individual behavior. It shares with Consumer Information Processing a concern about how people form cognitions and process health information. Interpersonal Influence (see Chapter Ten), Self-Regulation, and Attribution Theory recognize that patients and providers may have different beliefs about the causes of illness and therefore the way they should be treated. Social Learning Theory and Attribution Theory both include Rotter's concept of locus of control. The concept of self-efficacy is also central to both theories. In the case of Attribution Theory, the primary concern is with the formation of beliefs and the effects of those differential beliefs on the individual health-related behavior.

Attribution Theory can be especially rich in helping professionals understand patients' reactions to their illnesses. The Bar-On and Cristal (1987) study discussed in Chapter Five shows that attributions affect important health outcomes, such as return to work after a heart attack. Patients who attributed their heart attacks to external causes were slower in returning to work and functioning. Easterling and Leventhal's research (forthcoming) suggests that women who have breast cancer are most likely to attribute generic symptoms to relapse if they hold an abstract belief that they are vulnerable to cancer.

Like the other theories presented in this part of the book, Attribution Theory should not stand alone. It helps one to understand behavior but not necessarily how to change it. As Lewis and Daltroy point out, research on health interventions using Attribution Theory is extremely limited. Through its continued use, both researchers and practitioners will be able to advance the understanding of this important theory as it relates to health behavior. Clearly, Attribution Theory can be used by health practitioners to assess and improve clients' attributional processes. Although this theory has been underutilized in the study of preventive health behaviors, it seems very relevant to prevention and early detection beliefs and behaviors. For example, older adults and their physicians tend to overattribute potential cancer symptoms to the effects of aging (Prochaska and DiClemente, 1985; Leventhal, 1989). This may partly explain why many older adults are diagnosed at a later stage of disease (Rimer and others, 1983; Celentano, Klassen, Weisman, and Rosenshein, 1988; Leventhal, 1989). Also, both physicians and older adults may attribute the physiological effects of cigarette smoking to aging. This results in continued smoking among many older adults and the failure of many physicians to advise them to stop (Rimer and others, 1990). Here the attributions of both physicians and older adults require correction.

Changing attributions of failure may be especially important in preventing relapse of health-promoting behaviors, such as stopping smoking and improving diet (Marlatt and Gordon, 1985). Likewise, changing attributions of the causes of illness and side effects is also important in helping patients implement acute and chronic disease regimens. Attribution Theory shows that it is critical to understand patients' meanings. Where patients differ greatly from health professionals, problems may result. Apparent lack of communication and even noncompliance may stem from divergent attributions by patients and physicians.

Researchers should investigate the relationships between attributional style and socioeconomic status and other related variables. Future research should map the dimensions with more specificity while also manipulating the dimensions in an effort to improve attributional processes. Moreover, there should be more examination of people who do not ask "why?" or engage in attributional searches. Lewis and Daltroy also urge researchers to test manipulations of different kinds of attributions. Finally, researchers should examine the relationship between attributional style and informational style. Miller (1987) shows that some people are information monitors, seeking out information, while others are information blunters, utilizing distraction methods rather than engaging in information searches. Further research may very well uncover interactions between informational and attributional styles. It might also explain why some patients prefer causal ambiguity about their diseases to full information. A related concept is mindfulness, as defined by Langer (1989). Being mindful has to do with creation of new categories, openness to new information, and awareness of more than one perspective. People who are mindful may have different attributional styles from those who are not. Understanding such informational styles may help in better matching patients and health education programs.

Consumer Information Processing

Consumer Information Processing is a subset of Information Processing, long one of the dominant paradigms in social psychology. To some extent, each of the other three theories discussed in this chapter has been influenced by Information Processing. That is not surprising. One of the axioms of health education is that knowledge is necessary but not sufficient for behavior change. Information is necessary but not sufficient for knowledge. We are bombarded by information, and on both conscious and unconscious levels, we process this information continually. Some information is never received, some is forgotten quickly, and some is stored in memory for retrieval when it is necessary or useful.

Understanding the nature of information processing is important because it can help health practitioners structure information more effectively. For example, it has been shown that information presented first (primacy) or last (recency) is remembered best (Ley, 1979). So a clinician who wants a patient to remember exactly when to take her insulin will not put this important information in the middle of the discussion (Ley, 1979; Meichenbaum and Turk, 1987). No matter how much educators believe in the power of information, they must be humbled by the limits of information-processing capacity. Just because information is available does not mean that it will be used. There is simply too much information for all of it to be accessed. "Whatever else people are doing, they are always taking in, storing, retrieving, transforming, transmitting and acting on the basis of information" (Stillings and others, 1987, p. 7).

In trying to determine the impact of information on behavior, those interested in the processing of health information have perhaps been most influenced by McGuire (1983), who argues that whether the acquisition of a particular piece of information will lead to some desired behavior is dependent, in part, on whether the information has been appropriately processed by a receiver. According to McGuire (1968), there are five independent variables—source, message, channel, receiver, and destination—and five behavioral steps—attention, comprehension, yielding, retention, and action. Thus, much of the work of health educators and health psychologists has focused on different types of messages delivered by different kinds of sources (such as credible lay people versus physicians) over different media (such as, television versus radio versus in-person). Bettinghaus (1986) states that information processing specifies the conditions under which links between informational messages, persuasive messages, and behavior change will occur. As with the other theories discussed in this chapter, Information Processing and Consumer Information Processing are best regarded as components of an overall behavioral change strategy. Consumer Information Processing could well be supplemented by Social Learning Theory in the development of an intervention using modeling of the recommended behavior or organizational change theories to alter norms and policies, thus enabling people to respond more readily to persuasive messages.

Rudd and Glanz discuss how Consumer Information Processing Theory deals with the acquisition of information necessary to make choices and how information is used to make choices. One of the important lessons from Consumer Information Processing is that, in general, consumers tend not to engage in extended information searches. This has important implications for those who communicate health information. The nutrition application shows just how difficult it is to get the consumer's attention, but once this is done, sometimes positive changes in food choices will occur from exposure to information. The quality of care information example illustrates the kinds of information consumers require to make informed health care decisions. This area is a particularly important one, especially as more information becomes available about health care institutions.

While Consumer Information Processing is still relatively new and has had few health education applications, it is promising and would profit from integration with health models so that it could become more useful to those concerned with health as opposed to more general consumer behavior.

Looking Beyond Part Two: Other Promising Theories

Four theories not in Part Two hold particular promise for health behavior and health education and warrant brief summaries here. They are Protection Motivation Theory, Self-Regulation Theory, the Transtheoretical Model and Relapse Prevention Theory.

Protection Motivation Theory. Protection Motivation Theory shares the Health Belief Model's emphasis on cognitive processes in mediating attitudinal and behavioral change (Prentice-Dunn and Rogers, 1986). Differences in the threat level of a message affect attitudes in the short term. Information about the threat is critical for action and longer-term changes in beliefs. "Threat appraisal" provides the motivation to act, but "coping appraisal" gives direction for how to act (Leventhal, 1989). Like Social Learning Theory, Protection Motivation Theory posits that both internal and external rewards will increase the likelihood of action. Coping refers to judgments about the efficacy of a preventive response ("response efficacy") that will avert the perceived threat. Protection Motivation Theory also includes a self-efficacy component (Beck and Frankel, 1981).

Protection Motivation is maximized when the threat is severe, the individual feels vulnerable, an adaptive response is believed to be an effective means of reducing the threat, the person is confident about completing the response, and the rewards of maladaptive behavior and the costs of the adaptive response are small. These propositions closely parallel the intervention applications that might be derived from the Health Belief Model. Protection Motivation Theory has been used in a variety of areas, including enrollment in exercise programs, smoking cessation, and performance of breast self-examination (Beck and Davis, 1980; Beck and Frankel, 1981).

Self-Regulation Theory. According to Leventhal (1989), Leventhal and Cameron (1987) and Leventhal, Zimmerman and Gutmann (1984), self-regulation models view the person as an active problem solver whose behavior reflects an attempt to close the perceived gap between his or her current status and a goal or ideal state. Behavior depends on the person's cognitive representations of the current state and the goal state, plans for changing the current state, and techniques or rules for appraising progress. Attribution is one of the underlying processes. Leventhal and Cameron (1987) include three stages: cognitive representation of the health threat, the coping stage or action plan, and the appraisal stage, in which the person judges success in reaching the goal. Unlike the Theory of Reasoned Action, the self-regulatory model specifically includes an emotional component, recognizing that emotional responses to threat may well be different from the cognitive responses. The self-regulatory model can be especially helpful in understanding patients' responses to symptoms. Both Protection Motivation Theory and Self-Regulation Theory stress the importance of coping plans.

The development of Self-Regulation Theory is still underway by Leventhal and his colleagues. As yet, there are few outcome data, and the constructs within the theory are not yet fully operationalized (Leventhal and Cameron, 1987). But Self-Regulation Theory has potential and might be particularly relevant for practitioners as they help patients respond appropriately to risk factors and illness.

The Transtheoretical Model. Common processes of change transcend a variety of behavioral changes, including smoking cessation, weight control, substance abuse management, and reduction of psychological distress (Prochaska and others, 1982; Prochaska and DiClemente, 1985). The stages of change are similar. They include contemplation (the interval during which the client moves toward change), determination (the interval during which the client makes a serious commitment to change), action (the initiation of specific change), and maintenance (of the therapeutic gains). The action phase takes about six months, and maintenance can last two to three years. The model is circular rather than linear; a person can enter or exit at any point. The changes appear to be similar whether one seeks professional help or is a self-changer. Likewise, there are consistent processes of change. These include consciousness raising, self-reevaluation, self-liberation, contingency management, helping relationships, counterconditioning and stimulus control. Verbal processes prepare a person for action, whereas behavioral processes become more important once action is initiated. Through their research, Prochaska and DiClemente (1985) have found some differences across problem areas. For example, people who want to lose weight read more articles and books and make more commitments to change than people who stop smoking. But there are remarkable similarities across the change spectrum.

The Transtheoretical Model is directly applicable to practitioners. People in the process of change must have access to interventions that start at their stage in the change process. For example, if a smoker has not started thinking about what smoking is doing to her, there is no point in providing detailed information about behavioral coping processes. It would be far better to raise her consciousness regarding the personal harms associated with smoking and the benefits to be achieved from quitting. This is not very different from the health education principle that Minkler discusses in Chapter Twelve on Community Organization—start where the people are. Once the stage of change has been assessed, people can be provided with therapist-guided or self-initiated interventions that meet their needs.

The Transtheoretical Model is not yet fully developed, and the constructs are not completely operationalized. Moreover, it is not clear how well it applies to such areas as medication compliance and complex self-care regimens. But it is an exciting model for those interested in enhancing behavior change. While it is a theoretical model, it is also highly applied and has been developed through observation of and intervention with people engaged in the process of change. Moreover, the model recognizes that interventions should include a range of options, including self-help individual and group strategies, as well as interventions aimed at environmental, community, and policy levels. Finally, the Transtheoretical Model may provide a larger structure within which other intrapersonal and interpersonal theories of behavior can be integrated. It deserves attention from researchers and practitioners alike.

Relapse Prevention Theory. Many people who begin programs of behavior change, whether formal or informal, self-guided or therapist guided, eventually relapse, that is, return to their previous habits. Most people relapse fairly soon after initial change attempts. Relapse is de rigueur for the addictive disorders—problem drinking, substance abuse, and smoking and eating disorders. Those who seek to help people overcome these problems increasingly recognize that there is a continuum of behavior change, including initiation, modification, cessation, and maintenance of cessation. Different processes operate at each stage, and different strategies for preventing relapse are therefore necessary. According to Marlatt and Gordon (1985), Relapse Prevention Theory is a generic term that refers to a wide range of strategies designed to prevent relapse in the area of addictive behavior change. Following Social Learning Theory, addictive behaviors are regarded as overlearned habit patterns. Thus, Relapse Prevention Theory focuses on changing these patterns through the use of self-management and self-control techniques. Like Attribution Theory, Relapse Prevention Theory emphasizes the role of beliefs, in this case, beliefs about the course of treatment outcome and the causes of lapses. Positive outcome expectancies—a social learning concept—also are important.

Relapse Prevention Theory has already made significant contributions to an understanding of the addictions and how to change them. Especially important is the recognition that the maintenance stage of behavior change requires an analysis and interventions quite different from either initiation or cessation. Relapse Prevention Theory has direct applicability for practitioners who can apply its concepts to the development of programs. Researchers also benefit by adding a Relapse Prevention Theory component to their behavior change programs. As we gain more understanding of individual behavior change, theory-grounded models such as Relapse Prevention can help to enhance our effectiveness. The goal is not only to help people initially change their health behaviors but to maintain them over time.

Conclusion

The theories reviewed in Part Two provide professionals with several viable theoretical choices for designing programs to change health behavior. However, individuals should not be regarded as the only context for intervention. As Winett, King and Altman (1989) argue, individual-focused interventions have the advantage of being tailored to specific population segments. But they lack reach. Moreover, personal change that is not reinforced at other levels is difficult to sustain. McLeroy, Bibeau, Steckler, and Glanz (1988) urge, therefore, that health education programs should include interventions directed at the individual as well as those directed at interpersonal processes, institutional factors, community factors, and public policy. As Green's PRECEDE (Green, Kreuter, Deeds, and Partridge, 1980) and Winett, King, and Altman's (1989) planning model illustrate, personal behavior change must be viewed within a context that also includes interpersonal- and community-level change. In practice, multilevel analysis and intervention should be the rule rather than the exception. The appropriate strategy is that articulated by Simons-Morton, Simons-Morton, Parcel, and Bunker (1988)—that both environmental and personal change are important, and both should be addressed by public health and health promotion efforts. The following chapters in this book will help the reader gain a keener understanding of theories that can be used to achieve health-enhancing changes at the interpersonal level and the community or organization level.

References

Ajzen, I., and Fishbein, M. *Understanding Attitudes and Predicting Social Behavior*. Englewood Cliffs, N.J.: Prentice-Hall, 1980.

Beck, K. H., and Davis, C. M. "Predicting Smoking Intentions and Behaviors from Attitudes, Normative Beliefs, and Emotional Arousal." *Social Behavior and Personality*, 1980, *8*, 185-192.

Beck, K. H., and Frankel, A. "A Conceptualization of Threat Communications and Protective Health Behavior." *Social Psychology Quarterly*, 1981, *44*, 204-217.

Bettinghaus, E. P. "Health Promotion and the Knowledge-Attitude-Behavior Continuum." *Preventive Medicine*, 1986, *15*, 475-491.

Celentano, D. D., Klassen, A. C., Weisman, C. S., and Rosenshein, N. B. "Cervical Cancer Screening Practices Among Older Women: Results from the Maryland Cervical Cancer Case-Control Study." *Journal of Clinical Epidemiology*, 1988, *41*, 531-541.

Easterling, D. V., and Leventhal, H. "The Contribution of Concrete Cognition to Emotion: Judged Risk and Symptoms as Determinants of Worry About Cancer." *Journal of Applied Psychology*, forthcoming.

Fishbein, M., and Ajzen, I. *Belief, Attitude, Intention Behavior: An Introduction to Theory and Research*. Reading, Mass.: Addison-Wesley, 1975.

Green, L. W., Kreuter, M. W., Deeds, S. G., and Partridge, K. D. *Health Education Planning: A Diagnostic Approach*. Mountain View, Calif.: Mayfield, 1980.

Janz, N. K., and Becker, M. H. "The Health Belief Model: A Decade Later." *Health Education Quarterly*, 1984, *11*, 1-47.

Langer, E. J. *Mindfulness*. Reading, Mass.: Addison-Wesley, 1989.

Leventhal, H. "Emotional and Behavioural Processes." In J. Johnston and L. Wallace (eds.), *Stress and Medical Procedures*. Oxford, England: Oxford Science and Medical Publications, 1989.

Leventhal, H., and Cameron, L. "Behavioral Theories and the Problem of Compliance." *Patient Education and Counseling*, 1987, *10*, 117-138.

Leventhal, H., Zimmerman, R., and Gutmann, M. "Compliance: A Self-Regulation Perspective." In W. D. Gentry (ed.), *Handbook of Behavioral Medicine*. New York: Guilford Press, 1984.

Ley, P. "The Psychology of Compliance." In D. J. Oborne, M. M.

Gruneberg, and J. R. Eiser (eds.), *Research in Psychology and Medicine.* London: Academic Press, 1979.

McGuire, W. J. "Personality and Attitude Change: An Information-Processing Theory." In A. G. Greenwald, T. C. Brock, and T. M. Ostrom (eds.), *Psychological Foundations of Attitudes.* Orlando, Fla.: Academic Press, 1968.

McGuire, W. J. "A Contextualist Theory of Knowledge: Its Implications for Innovation and Reform in Psychological Research." *Advances in Experimental Social Psychology,* 1983, *16*, 1-47.

McLeroy, K. R., Bibeau, D., Steckler, A., and Glanz, K. "An Ecological Perspective on Health Promotion Programs." *Health Education Quarterly,* 1988, *15*, 351-377.

Marlatt, G. A., and Gordon, J. R. *Relapse Prevention.* New York: Guilford Press, 1985.

Meichenbaum, D., and Turk, D. C. *Facilitation Treatment Adherence: A Practitioner's Guidebook.* New York: Plenum, 1987.

Miller, S. M. "Monitoring and Blunting: Validation of a Questionnaire to Assess Styles of Information Seeking Under Threat." *Journal of Personality and Social Psychology,* 1987, *52*, 345-353.

Mullen, P. D., Hersey, J. C., and Iverson, D. C. "Health Behavior Models Compared." *Social Science Medicine,* 1987, *24*, 973-981.

Nisbett, R. E., Krantz, D. H., Jepson, C., and Fong, G. T. "Improving Inductive Inference." In D. Kahneman, P. Slovic, and A. Tversky (eds.), *Judgment Under Uncertainty: Heuristics and Biases.* Cambridge, England: Cambridge University Press, 1982.

Prentice-Dunn, S., and Rogers, R. W. "Protection Motivation Theory and Preventive Health: Beyond the Health Belief Model." *Health Education Research,* 1986, *1*, 153-161.

Prochaska, J. O., and DiClemente, C. C. "Common Processes of Self-Change in Smoking, Weight Control, and Psychological Distress." In S. Shiffman and T. Wills (eds.), *Coping and Substance Use.* Orlando, Fla.: Academic Press, 1985, pages 345-364.

Prochaska, J. O., and others. "Self-change Processes, Self-Efficacy and Self-Concept in Relapse and Maintenance of Cessation of Smoking." *Psychological Reports,* 1982, *51*, 983-990.

Rimer, B. "Theory-Driven Health Promotion Interventions for Older Americans." Paper presented at the 1989 SOPHE Midyear Conference, Seattle, Washington, June 1989.

Rimer, B., and others. "Planning a Cancer Control Program for Older Citizens." *Gerontologist,* 1983, *23,* 384–389.

Rimer, B., and others. "Why Women Resist Mammograms: Understanding Patient-Related Barriers to Acceptance of Screening Mammography." *Radiology,* 1989, *172,* 243–246.

Rimer, B. K., and others. "The Older Smoker: Status, Challenges, and Opportunities for Intervention." *Chest,* 1990.

Rogers, R. W., and Mewborn, C. R. "Fear Appeals and Attitude Change: Effects of a Threat's Noxiousness, Probability of Occurrence, and the Efficacy of Coping Responses." *Journal of Personality and Social Psychology,* 1976, *34,* 54–61.

Rosenstock, I. M., Strecher, V. J., and Becker, M. H. "Social Learning Theory and the Health Belief Model." *Health Education Quarterly,* 1988, *15,* 175–183.

Ross, L. "The Intuitive Psychologist and His Shortcomings: Distortions in the Attribution Process." In L. Berkowitz (ed.), *Advances in Experimental Social Psychology.* Volume 10. Orlando, Fla.: Academic Press, 1977.

Simons-Morton, D. G., Simons-Morton, B. G., Parcel, G. S., and Bunker, J. F. "Influencing Personal and Environmental Conditions for Community Health: A Multilevel Intervention Model." *Family Community Health,* 1988, *11,* 25–35.

Stillings, N. A., and others. *Cognitive Science: An Introduction.* Cambridge, Mass.: MIT Press, 1987.

Winett, R. A., King, A. C., and Altman, D. *Health Psychology and Public Health: An Integrative Approach.* Elmsford, New York: Pergamon Press, 1989.

▲ ▲ ▲

PART THREE

▲ ▲ ▲

MODELS OF
INTERPERSONAL HEALTH BEHAVIOR

Interpersonal models of health behavior are the focus of Part Three. Three conceptual perspectives form the basis of this section: Social Learning Theory; Social Support, Control, and the Stress Process; and Health Professionals' Influence on Health Behavior.

Social Learning Theory (SLT) explains human behavior in terms of a triadic, dynamic, and reciprocal model in which behavior, personal factors, and environmental influences all interact. In Chapter Eight, Perry, Baranowski, and Parcel highlight two branches of Social Learning Theory—an operant conditioning branch and a cognitive branch—and offer a creative synthesis of those two branches. The influence of such variables as positive external reinforcements from the operant conditioning branch is coupled with observational learning from the cognitive branch. In two applications, the authors illustrate how the concepts from both branches were used to mold the components of community-based and school-based intervention programs in health promotion.

Chapter Nine, by Israel and Schurman, analyzes a theoretical framework of perceived stress, social support, and control that can explain both short- and long-term health outcomes. Like Chapter Eight, this chapter highlights the importance of reciprocal determinism and the dynamic, multicausal relationships between individuals and their interpersonal environments, including the work setting. The authors use an action research project in a manufacturing setting to analyze how the theoretical framework can be used to guide an intervention to reduce occupational stress among employees.

In Chapter Ten, Joos and Hickam provide an analysis of the main theoretical perspectives that contribute to our understanding of the effects of patient-provider relationships on health behavior and health outcomes. They analyze four perspectives: cognition and information processing, interpersonal interaction, conflict between patients and providers, and social influence. Each of these perspectives has its own research tradition and suggests either specific targets to increase the effectiveness of patient-provider relationships or methods with which to positively affect patient-provider interaction. The applications in this chapter include reviews of observational and intervention studies on patient-provider interaction and patient outcomes.

Chapter 8

Cheryl L. Perry
Tom Baranowski
Guy S. Parcel

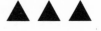

How Individuals, Environments, and Health Behavior Interact: Social Learning Theory

Social Learning Theory (SLT) addresses both the psychosocial dynamics underlying health behavior and the methods of promoting behavior change. The cognitive version of Social Learning Theory emphasizes what people think, that is, their cognitions, and their effect on behavior. Human behavior is explained in SLT in terms of a triadic, dynamic, and reciprocal model in which behavior, personal factors (including cognitions), and environmental influences all interact. An individual's behavior is uniquely determined by these factors. Among the crucial personal factors are the individual's capabilities to symbolize the meanings of behavior, to foresee the outcomes of given behavior patterns, to learn by observing others, to self-determine or self-regulate behavior, and to reflect and analyze experience (Bandura, 1986). These ideas have been particularly valuable in designing effective health education programs.*

Investigators working with SLT have identified procedures or techniques that influence the underlying cognitive variables, thereby increasing the likelihood of behavioral change. Health

*This chapter was funded, in part, by grants from the National Heart, Lung, and Blood Institute (R18 HL-30625, RO1 HL-25523, UO1 HL-39852, RO1 HL-32929, and RO1 HL-35131).

161

behavior programs based on SLT thereby use techniques that emphasize the cognitive mediators of behavior. In this way, the theory not only explains how people acquire and maintain certain behavior patterns but also provides the basis for intervention and learning strategies. This chapter provides a brief history of the development of Social Learning Theory, descriptions of key concepts, and two examples of how the theory has been used to design health education programs.

Brief History of Social Learning Theory

Social learning theory involves a broad conceptual domain that incorporates many theoretical ideas and is employed in many areas of practice. Because an intellectual history of such a broad area would be impossible to review in just one section of a single chapter, publication milestones of SLT in the area of understanding and changing health behaviors are listed in Table 8.1.

Miller and Dollard (1941) originally introduced Social Learning Theory to explain imitation of behavior among animals and humans. The original SLT principles were based on learning principles and the motivational ideas of Hull (1943). Learning theory takes a mechanistic approach to explaining behaviors. The person is seen as a "black box," which emits behaviors called responses to which reinforcements are applied by other people. Reinforcements link the performance of certain responses to particular stimuli and thereby increase the likelihood of those responses. Hull attempted to explain why certain kinds of behavior are more likely to occur than others by considering internal states called drives (not cognitions). Hull believed that organisms (animals and humans) acquired drives, physiological processes that often drive behavior. For example, hunger motivates food search and food consumption. Hull also maintained that one organism's responses provide stimuli for other organisms. Social learning, thereby, is attending to others' responses when motivated by an acquired drive.

Two streams of health-related research flowed from Miller and Dollard's (1941) seminal ideas. Rotter first applied these early social learning principles to clinical psychology (1954), which in turn led to his development of the idea of "generalized expectancies

Table 8.1. Publication Milestones in the Development
of Social Learning Theory.

1941	Miller and Dollard	*Social Learning and Imitation*
1954	Rotter	*Social Learning and Clinical Psychology*
1962	Bandura	*Social Learning Through Imitation*
1963	Bandura and Walters	*Social Learning and Personality Development*
1966	Rotter	"Generalized Expectations for Internal Versus External Control of Reinforcement," *Psychological Monographs*
1969	Bandura	*Principles of Behavior Modification*
1973	W. Mischel	"Toward a Cognitive Social Learning Reconceptualization of Personality," *Psychological Review*
1975	Stokols	"The Reduction of Cardiovascular Risk: An Application of Social Learning Perspectives," *Applying Behavioral Science to Cardiovascular Risk*
	Zifferblatt	"Increasing Patient Compliance Through the Applied Analysis of Behavior," *Preventive Medicine*
1977	Bandura	*Social Learning Theory*
	Bandura	"Self-Efficacy: Toward a Unifying Theory of Behavioral Change," *Psychological Review*
	Farquhar and others	"Community Education for Cardiovascular Health," *Lancet*
1978	Bandura	"The Self System in Reciprocal Determinism," *American Psychologist*
	Wallston and Wallston	"Locus of Control and Health," *Health Education Monographs*
1981	Parcel and Baranowski	"Social Learning Theory and Health Education," *Health Education*
1986	Bandura	*Social Foundations of Thought and Action: A Social Cognitive Theory*
1987	Rodin	"Personal Control Through the Life Course," *Implications of the Life-Span Perspective for Social Psychology*

of reinforcement" (1966). Rotter contends that a person learns or is conditioned operantly on the basis of his or her history of positive or negative reinforcement. The person also develops a sense of internal or external locus of control. Those with an internal locus of control are more likely to self-initiate change, whereas those who are externally controlled are more likely to be influenced by others.

Within a learning theory framework, Zifferblatt (1975) applied behavioral analysis procedures in order to gain an understanding of compliance behavior. Wallston and Wallston (1978) formulated a scale for the assessment of the "health" locus of control. They proposed that their new measure was more useful in health research because an individual's sense of control often varies by domains of experience and action, such as health experiences. The control literature has evolved to a point at which a need or drive for control has been postulated with evidence accruing that giving people control over their lives improves their health outcomes (Rodin, 1987). While this is an important and interesting area of SLT as applied to health, we will emphasize the other stream, which has led to more ideas and techniques for promoting health behavior change.

The other stream of research has progressed far beyond the behavior theory headwaters, employing cognitive concepts to explain behavioral phenomena. Bandura is the leading figure in this stream. In 1962, he first published an article on social learning and imitation. Bandura and Walters (1963) proposed that children learn by watching other children and do not need to be rewarded directly in order to learn a new type of behavior. Instead, a child can learn by observing the behavior of others and the rewards they receive (vicarious reinforcement). Prior to this time, learning theory held that rewards had to be applied directly for learning to occur. In 1969, Bandura provided a conceptual foundation for behavior modification that heavily emphasized traditional learning theory. Mischel (1973) first proposed several cognitive constructs that provided a cognitive basis for Social Learning Theory. Stokols (1975) applied the observational learning concept to the area of cardiovascular disease risk reduction. In 1977, Bandura published his refutation of the adequacy of traditional learning theory principles for understanding learning and provided the first theoretical treatment of his cognitive concept of self-efficacy (Bandura, 1977a). Farquhar and others (1977) reported the first community-wide intervention for heart disease prevention based on SLT. In 1978, Bandura proposed the organizing concept of reciprocal determinism, in which environment, person, and behavior are continually interacting. In 1981, Parcel and Baranowski applied the cognitive formulation of SLT to health education and delineated the stages in the behavior change process at which each concept was most relevant. In 1986, Bandura published a comprehensive framework for understanding human social behavior, using the concepts he helped to develop. In 1986, Bandura renamed SLT a Social Cognitive Theory. This chapter reflects this work but continues to use the long-standing label Social Learning Theory.

Both Mischel and Bandura have introduced a variety of specific constructs in their discussions of the process of human learning. The most pertinent of these constructs to health behavior change are discussed in this chapter. Cognitive Social Learning Theory is particularly relevant to health education programs for three reasons. First, the theory synthesizes previously disparate cognitive, emotional, and behavioristic understandings of behavior change. Second, as demonstrated in this chapter, the constructs and processes identified by SLT suggest many important avenues for new behavioral research in health education. Third, the use of SLT provides an opportunity to apply theoretical models developed in other areas of psychology to new areas of health behavior.

Social Learning Theory Constructs

Mischel (1973) and Bandura (1977a, 1986) have formulated a number of SLT constructs that are important in understanding and intervening in health behavior. Table 8.2 summarizes the constructs that are described in this section as well as their implications for potential intervention strategies in health education.

Reciprocal Determinism. An underlying assumption of SLT is that behavior is dynamic and depends on environmental and personal constructs that influence each other simultaneously. The continuing interaction among a person, the behavior of that person, and the environment within which the behavior is performed is called *reciprocal determinism*. Behavior is not simply the result of the environment and the person, just as the environment is not simply the result of the person and behavior. Instead, these three components are constantly interacting. The interaction is such that a change in one has implications for the others (Bandura, 1978, 1986). According to SLT, the environment provides the social and physical situation

**Table 8.2. Major Concepts in Social Learning Theory
and Implications for Intervention.**

Concept	Definition	Implications
Environment	Factors that are physically external to the person	Provide opportunities and social support
Situation	Person's perception of the environment	Correct misperceptions and promote healthful norms
Behavioral capability	Knowledge and skill to perform a given behavior	Promote mastery learning through skills training
Expectations	Anticipatory outcomes of a behavior	Model positive outcomes of healthful behavior
Expectancies	The values that the person places on a given outcome, incentives	Present outcomes of change that have functional meaning
Self-control	Personal regulation of goal-directed behavior or performance	Provide opportunities for self-monitoring and contracting
Observational learning	Behavioral acquisition that occurs by watching the actions and outcomes of others' behavior	Include credible role models of the targeted behavior
Reinforcements	Responses to a person's behavior that increase or decrease the likelihood of reoccurrence	Promote self-initiated rewards and incentives
Self-efficacy	The person's confidence in performing a particular behavior	Approach behavior change in small steps; seek specificity about the change sought
Emotional coping responses	Strategies or tactics that are used by a person to deal with emotional stimuli	Provide training in problem solving and stress management; include opportunities to practice skills in emotionally arousing situations
Reciprocal determinism	The dynamic interaction of the person, behavior, and the environment in which the behavior is performed	Consider multiple avenues to behavioral change including environmental, skill, and personal change

within which the person must function and thus also provides the incentives and disincentives (expectancies) for the performance of behavior. A person has the behavioral capability to act and the potential for self-control over his or her actions. He or she can also anticipate certain events and outcomes and can respond to them (Argyle, Furnham, and Graham, 1981; Magnusson, 1981). Finally, the behavior, which can be viewed from many levels (Frederiksen, Martin, and Webster, 1979), reflects the environment and the state of the person and can affect the environment, the person, or both.

Behavior may result from characteristics of a particular person or environment, and behavior may be used to change the variable (Bem, 1967). If a variable changes, the situation changes, and the behavior, situation, and person are reevaluated. For example, a man may be so opposed to exercise that his friends come to expect him to maintain a sedentary life-style. The man has strengthened this expectation about exercise by avoiding any physical or social environments in which he might be expected to exercise (for example, gyms or playing fields). At some point, however, a dramatic event may occur in this man's life (for example, the death of a close family member from a heart attack and exposure to the information that heart attacks may in part be caused by a sedentary life-style) that makes him decide to start exercising. The man will now encounter the expectations of his sedentary friends, who may pressure him not to exercise. To avoid these negative pressures, he may seek new friends who value exercise and support his new behavior (reciprocal effect). This change, in turn, may motivate a sedentary friend to begin to exercise as well (a reciprocal effect to that friend), and the friend will then either change the exercise habits of other sedentary friends, or acquire new friends who are interested in exercise.

This kind of behavior change underscores the importance of professionals avoiding the simplicity of "single direction of change" thinking. Reciprocal determinism may be used to advantage in developing programs that do not focus on behavior in isolation but focus instead on changes in the environment and in the individual as well. The following descriptions of environment and person constructs should be considered as part of this dynamic process.

Environments and Situations. The term *environment* refers to an objective notion of all the factors that can affect a person's behavior but that are physically external to that person. Examples of the social environment include family members, friends, and peers at work or in the classroom. The physical environment might include the size of a room, the ambient temperature, or the availability of needed facilities. In SLT, the term *situation* refers to the cognitive or mental representation of the environment (including real, distorted, or imagined factors) that may affect a person's behavior. The situation is a person's perception of the environment, such as place, time, physical features, activity, participants, and his or her own role in the situation. This concept of situation corresponds to Lewin's (1951) notion of the life space or Bronfenbrenner's (1977) idea of microsystem.

The environment can affect behavior without a person's being aware of it (Moos, 1976). For example, if fresh fruits and vegetables are made available in a child's environment, for example, at school, the child will probably learn to include those foods in his or her diet. The situation, on the other hand, guides and limits thinking and behavior. For example, the social and physical situation provides cues about the types of behavior that are acceptable (Rotter, 1955). If a child perceives that all of his or her classmates drink nonfat milk and value its healthfulness, the child may begin to drink it, too. The situation may also pose certain problems that require immediate attention, or it may preclude and limit types of behavior. A person may not be aware of important factors in the environment, thereby limiting the influence of the environment on his or her behavior.

The situation also regulates behavior by providing certain consequences of the behavior. These consequences have positive or negative values called expectancies, which in turn affect what people learn. The environment is the source of social supports, such as friends and family (Baranowski and Nader, 1985a, 1985b; Gottlieb, 1981). From the environmental perspective, social supports in the environment provide cues for reinforcement and discrimination. From the situational perspective, the person generates expectations and expectancies from people in the environment, and these people may be important resources in approaches to emotional coping and self-control (Moos, 1976).

Behavioral Capability. The concept of *behavioral capability* maintains that if a person is to perform a particular type of behavior, he or she must know what the behavior is (knowledge of the behavior) and how to perform the behavior (skill). The concept of behavioral capability leads to a distinction between learning and performance because a task can be learned and not performed, but performance presumes learning. Thus, the purpose of many education programs is to provide the person with the behavioral capability to perform a new type of behavior.

The development of behavioral capability is the result of the individual's training, intellectual capacity, and learning style. The behavioral training technique called mastery learning provides cognitive knowledge of what is to be performed, practice in performing those activities, and feedback about successful performance (Block, 1971).

Expectations. Expectations are the anticipatory aspects of behavior that Bandura (1977a, 1986) calls antecedent determinants of behavior. A person learns that certain events are likely to occur in a particular situation and then expects them to occur when the situation arises again. For behavior that is not performed habitually, people anticipate many aspects of the situation in which the behavior might be performed and develop and test strategies for dealing with the situation. In this way, people develop expectations about a situation before they actually encounter it. In most cases, this reduces their anxiety and increases their skill at being able to handle the situation. According to SLT, expectations learned from previous experiences in similar situations are referred to as performance attainments. When they are learned from observing others in similar situations, this is called vicarious experience. Expectations may also be learned from hearing about these situations from other people or social persuasion. Finally, expectations can result from emotional or physical responses, which are referred to as physiological arousal.

An example of how expectations may develop and be

changed can be seen in the area of adolescent smoking prevention. Generally, an adolescent "learns" that smoking can be fun, exciting, grown-up, or even sexy, from advertising, older peers, or adult role models. In a health education program, peers can be taught to direct discussions on the negative social consequences of smoking and how to handle pressure to smoke from other adolescents. This approach has been successful in deterring smoking onset (Flay, 1985). In essence, this approach succeeds because the expectations around future smoking situations for these young adolescents have been changed.

Expectancies. Expectancies (called incentives by Bandura, 1977a, 1986) are differentiated from expectations in that expectancies are the *values* that a person places on a particular outcome. Expectancies have magnitude: a quantitative value that is usually represented on a continuum from 0 to 1 and that can be positive or negative. Expectancies influence behavior according to the hedonic principle; that is, if all other things are equal, a person will choose to perform an activity that maximizes a positive outcome or minimizes a negative outcome. Mischel (1973) believes that expectancies underlie classical conditioning. For example, in trying to provide weight reduction skills for overweight adults, one may need to help those adults replace the positive outcomes of food consumption with negative outcomes. This can be done by stressing the attractiveness or healthfulness of weight reduction or even more overtly by paying money for weight loss.

A person's positive expectancies should be assessed early in a project that is designed to promote changes in health behavior in order to identify motivators for that behavior. Many researchers have observed, for example, that people are more likely to engage in physical activity to achieve short-term benefits (to become physically attractive, to feel better, or to compete with friends in tennis) than to achieve long-term gains (for example, to avoid a heart attack in thirty years). McAlister and others (1980) show that smoking prevention programs for adolescents are more successful if they emphasize the immediate negative effects of smoking, such as bad breath or unattractiveness, rather than the long-term effects, such as morbidity and mortality from cancer and heart disease. Thus, an emphasis on immediate positive rewards or expectancies may be more likely to influence the initiation of some desired behaviors than an emphasis on long-range benefits.

Self-Control and Performance. The term *performance* refers to the type of human behavior that focuses on achievement of a goal. One of the goals of health education is to bring the performance of health behavior under the control of the individual. Self-control of behavior enhances the learning and maintenance of that behavior (Stuart, 1977; Kanfer, 1975, 1976; Bandura, 1986).

The self-regulation models of Kanfer (1975, 1976) and Bandura (1986) are perhaps the most sophisticated models of *self-control.* According to Kanfer, self-control operates through a set of subfunctions, including self-observations, unambiguous specification of a target behavior, a criterion for performance, a procedure to evaluate performance against the criterion, and self-reward. Kanfer focused primarily on decisions made by people to achieve long-term self-control and found that the setting of a criterion of performance, or goal setting, is the most important factor in the achievement of self-control.

Promotion of self-control requires a focus on a specific type of behavior. In a weight control program, for example, a target of "cutting down on sweets" would be too vague to produce observable results because a person in the program might become confused or could make small changes that conformed to the target but did not lead to weight loss. Instead of trying to "cut down on sweets," therefore, a person might aim to eat eight instead of eleven cookies a day. A specific goal might also help to promote self-motivation (Locke, Bryan, and Kendall, 1968) because if a goal is set too high, a person may become frustrated and give up.

Observational Learning. One reason that SLT considers the environment to be important is that it provides *models* for behavior. A person can learn from other people, not only by receiving reinforcements from them but also through observing them and utilizing his or her symbolic capability. *Observational learning* occurs when an observer watches the actions of another person and observes the reinforcements that the other person receives. This process has also been called vicarious reward or vicarious experience (Bandura, 1986).

Observational learning is a more efficient approach than operant learning for learning complex behaviors. In the operant approach, a person must perform a given behavior that is subsequently reinforced. Through a trial-and-error process, the person continues to perform behaviors that come progressively closer to the desired performance. This is an inefficient process. In observational learning, the observer does not need to go through this time-consuming, trial-and-error process in uncertain circumstances. Instead, the learner discovers rules that account for the behavior of others by observing the reinforcements they receive for their behavior. The person can learn what is appropriate by observing the behaviors, successes, and mistakes of others.

Many types of behavior can be learned through observational learning (Bandura and Walters, 1963; Bandura, 1972, 1986). This process accounts for why people in the same family often have common behavioral patterns. Children observe their parents when they eat, smoke, drink, and use seat belts and see the various rewards or penalties the parents receive for these types of behavior. Some children observe other children smoking at school and notice the rewards and punishments that the smokers receive. If the smokers get reinforcements that the observers consider rewarding (acceptance from peers or a desirable image), the observers are more likely to perform that behavior in the future.

Reinforcement. *Reinforcement* is the primary construct in the operant form, as well as in certain other forms, of learning theory. *Positive reinforcement,* or reward, is a response to a person's behavior that increases the likelihood that the behavior will be repeated. In traditional operant theory, the reinforcement works in an unknown mechanical way to affect behavior. According to cognitive SLT, however, a person behaves in a certain way to achieve an expectancy. Negative reinforcement, or punishment, is not the direct opposite of positive reinforcement in that it does not always decrease the likelihood that a certain type of behavior may be performed. Instead, negative reinforcement may simply reduce the likelihood that a particular behavior will be performed in those situations in which a person expects to receive negative reinforcement but not in other situations.

Cognitive SLT incorporates three types of reinforcement: direct reinforcement (as in operant conditioning), vicarious reinforcement (as in observational learning), and self-reinforcement (as in self-control). These types of reinforcement can be classified further into external (or extrinsic) and internal (or intrinsic) reinforcement. External reinforcement is the occurrence of an event or act that is known to have predictable reinforcement value. Internal reinforcement is a person's own experience, or perception, that an event that has some value for him or her has occurred.

Internal reinforcement (or internal expectancy) accounts for why some people behave in a manner that is not reinforced externally or may even be negatively reinforced externally. For example, a person may choose to return $10 that was given in error as change, because it was the "right" thing to do, even though the $10 would have provided for the fulfillment of some personal desire, an external expectancy.

The difference in reward mechanisms is particularly important in an area that is known as the "overjustification effect." If a person is given an external reward for a task that is intrinsically interesting, he or she may find that task less intrinsically interesting in the future (Lepper and Green, 1978; Bates, 1979). Thus, if a person who usually enjoys jogging is paid to jog for a week, he or she may find that jogging is no longer as enjoyable (valuable) as it was before the payment was provided. Researchers have shown that any external constraint that is imposed on behavior may reduce the level of internal motivation (Lepper and Green, 1978). Health educators, psychologists, and others must therefore be careful not to provide external rewards for all health promotion activities to ensure that the internal appeal of these activities will be maintained. They can, however, use external rewards for behaviors that are part of a behavior change program, for example, maintaining daily diet records, while they emphasize the intrinsic rewards of the behavior change itself (Perry and others, 1988).

Self-Efficacy. Bandura and colleagues (Bandura, 1977b, 1978, 1982, 1986; Bandura and Adams, 1977; Bandura, Adams, and Beyer, 1977) have proposed that one aspect of the notion of self, self-efficacy, is the most important prerequisite for behavior change. Self-efficacy is the confidence a person feels about performing a particular activity. Self-efficacy affects how much effort is invested in a given task and what levels of performance are attained (Ewart, Taylor, Reese, and Debusk, 1983; DiClemente, 1981). In the process of changing behavior, the promotion of self-efficacy becomes a critical concern (Maddux and Rogers, 1983; Condiotte and Lichtenstein, 1981; Strecher, DeVellis, Becker, and Rosenstock, 1986; Rosenstock, Strecher, and Becker, 1988).

Repetition of the performance of a single task builds a person's self-efficacy, which in turn affects task persistence, initiation, and endurance, which promote behavior change. Therefore, health professionals who are training people with diabetes to self-inject insulin may divide the self-injection process into many small steps, each of which they can learn through repetition (for example, filling the syringe with the correct amount of insulin, ensuring that all items remain sterilized, seeing that no bubbles get into the syringe, and being sure that the fluid is at the precise marker on the syringe). Simplifying each step and allowing patients to practice each in isolation with many repetitions, enables them to build self-efficacy about performing each step. When patients are self-confident about each step, they can progressively put the steps together and build self-efficacy about the entire task.

To make use of self-efficacy in promoting self-control of performance, goals should be set in increments that approximate a given behavior and that are each possible to achieve, thereby allowing a person to build self-efficacy about performing the desired behavior. Both observational and enactive (participatory) learning techniques can be used in introducing and promoting each sequence of a targeted behavior (Bandura, 1986).

Managing Emotional Arousal. Bandura (1977a) recognized that excessive emotional arousal inhibits learning and performance and proposed that certain stimuli give rise to fearful thoughts (stimulus-outcome expectancies). These fearful thoughts produce emotional arousal and trigger defensive behaviors. As the defensive behaviors deal effectively with stimuli, the fear, anxiety, hostility, or emotional arousal is reduced.

Categories of behavioral management for emotional and physiological arousal are identified by Moos (1976). One category includes psychological defenses (denial, repression, and sublimation). Another category includes more cognitive techniques, such as problem restructuring. A third category includes stress management techniques (progressive relaxation or exercise) that treat the symptoms of the emotional distress. A fourth category includes methods for solving problems effectively (clarifying a problem and identifying, selecting, and implementing solutions for the causes of the emotional arousal).

Although many programs employ behavioral management strategies, their nature varies across individuals and cultures (Diaz-Guerrero, 1979). For example, severely overweight people may find it difficult to deny or repress their condition. People often react negatively to overweight people, and these reactions can increase anxiety about being overweight (Hudson and Williams, 1981). For some obese people, this anxiety causes overeating (Leon and Roth, 1977; Slochower and Kaplan, 1980; Slochower, Kaplan, and Mann, 1981). Heightened anxiety also makes it difficult to attend to the health messages coming from health professionals (Ley and Spelman, 1965). Therefore, health educators must learn methods to aid people in their ability to minimize emotional arousal, before they can help them to change their behavior, or these educators should postpone educational efforts until anxiety has subsided.

The following sections provide two concrete examples of the utilization of SLT in health education program design.

The Texas A Su Salud Project

A particularly innovative project based on SLT has focused on smoking cessation and prevention in the community. McAlister and others (submitted) targeted for change the stresses in life that inhibit smoking cessation among lower-income Mexican-American families, thereby enhancing the likelihood of cessation.

As indicated in Table 8.3, many stressful situations either inhibit the initiation of smoking cessation or enhance the recidi-

Table 8.3. Major Concepts in Social Learning Theory and Examples
of Their Application in the Texas A Su Salud Project.

Environment	Neighborhood-based cueing
	Social support for overcoming stressful problems
Situation	Skills to cope with stressful problems (for example, lack of a job) that interfere with health behaviors
Behavioral capability	Skills to stop smoking
	The recognition of stressors that interfere with maintaining nonsmoking
	Individual and family counseling for coping with stressors
Expectancies	The theme of the "six killers" in Maverick County
Observational learning	Mass media role models for stopping smoking, for other positive health behaviors, and for coping with stressors
Reinforcements	874 "lay leaders" providing social reinforcements
Self-efficacy	A target on perceived ability to cope with stressors to help maintain smoking cessation
Reciprocal determinism	Promotion of social support and individual coping skills in dealing with environmental stressors

vism to smoking, after it is stopped. The guiding idea of A Su Salud is that programs should be targeted at creating a supportive environment and enhancing a person's ability to make behavioral changes.

McAlister and others (submitted) used three components in their intervention for stopping smoking. The first technique employed a variety of models who demonstrated smoking cessation activities and examples of behavioral strategies that could be used to respond to the stressors that inhibit those activities. People from the community were recruited to demonstrate practices at which they were proficient, and these were disseminated through newspapers, radio, and television. By means of this technique, behavioral capability (how to stop smoking) and self-efficacy (confidence in ability to stop smoking) are modeled by individuals who have been successful in changing smoking behavior and thereby promote vicarious learning of cessation skills by other community members.

The media campaign builds community participation into the communication through the use of "real-life" stories of community members. Although Social Learning Theory concepts have been employed to actualize modeling in the ideal, the program is dependent on what members of the community have actually done to stop smoking or to change other health-related behaviors.

The second program component involved recruiting several hundred volunteers to establish a community network that is used to facilitate the dissemination of information about the role models in the media and behavioral change. These volunteers, part of the social environment in the target communities, provide the stimuli for paying attention to the role models in the media as well as the social reinforcement for initiated behavior change. The third component provides individual and family counseling for managing life events that make it difficult to attend to and set a priority for changing a health behavior. The primary approach to counseling is referral to the appropriate community agency for mitigating whatever appears to be the participant's primary sources of stress.

The staff has underscored the value of engaging in smoking cessation and the necessary management behaviors by emphasizing the "six killers of Maverick County" (alcohol and drugs, cigarette smoking, obesity and diabetes, absence of regular medical checkups, nonuse of seatbelts, and environmental hazards of the workplace). From work with focus groups, the investigators learned that residents are aware of the major causes of mortality in their community and are interested in engaging in behaviors that will mitigate that burden. In their media and other educational activities, the investigators have linked the targeted behaviors with preventing the effects of the six killers. Repeated practice of the coping skills, such as relaxation techniques, has enhanced self-efficacy over these behaviors. The program has used reciprocal determinism by promoting social support and individual skills in dealing with environmental conditions that increase the likelihood of smoking.

Preliminary results (McAlister and others, submitted) reveal that the media modeling with social reinforcement and support from lay volunteers has been more effective than the media modeling alone in increasing and maintaining the number of nonsmokers. There is also some evidence that the individual and family counseling and referral have been effective in further increasing cessation among women but not among men.

The intervention strategies are targeted at changing behavior (smoking) as well as responding to obstacles that inhibit behavior change. The media messages and role models increase behavioral capability and influence outcome and efficacy expectations for the behavior. The community volunteers serve as a means to reinforce the media messages and to give reinforcement to individuals for making a behavior change. The volunteer component is a critical part of the program because it creates a positive expectancy for behavior change from the social environment. A Su Salud is a good example of how Social Learning Theory intervention strategies can address the interaction between individual cognitive factors, behavior, and the environment. The use of a community-based approach (in contrast to most clinic-based programs) that does not rely on self-monitoring or other intensive therapeutic techniques, appears promising for enhancing health behaviors.

Minnesota Home Team Study

Social Learning Theory was used in the development of a parent involvement program for families of third-graders (ages eight and nine) in an attempt to change the children's eating patterns. The research study has been described in detail elsewhere (Perry and others, 1988). The design and results are summarized here, with primary attention being given to the content of the intervention program. The challenge was to translate the concepts described in Social Learning Theory into a creative and situation-appropriate educational package.

The Home Team program is a correspondence course for third-graders. Each week for five weeks the students receive a Home Team packet in the mail. Each packet provides the instructions and materials for two to three hours of activities to be carried out by each student and his or her parent(s). Each packet includes a Hearty Heart and Friends adventure book that tells the story of four characters (Hearty Heart, Dynamite Diet, Salt Sleuth, Flash Fitness) from

Planet Strongheart who travel to earth to teach children about how to live healthful lives. The packet also includes a variety of games that provide practice of the basic knowledge and skills that are presented. Students label foods in their home as "everyday" or "sometimes," mix and match foods to rhymes, and look for clue cards of the Hearty Heart characters and messages around the house. Each packet includes a simple snack recipe to prepare, a recipe that the students can subsequently make on their own. The recipes have team-related names such as "Championship Veggies" and "Fruit, Fruit, Fruit for the Home Team." Team Tips, which are refrigerator pin-ups that provide additional nutritional information, are also disseminated weekly. For each activity, points are awarded, recorded on a scorecard, taken to school, and recorded on a scoreboard. Teams that complete the Home Team series are eligible for a grand prize; in the research study this was a family trip to Disneyworld, funded by a local foundation.

Several of the major concepts of SLT guided the development of the Home Team program. These are summarized in Table 8.4. In particular, the use of an overall incentive for parental participation (the "team" concept with a grand prize), age-appropriate role models (the Hearty Heart characters), the experiential nature of the activities (carried out in the home setting), and the option of additional learning and capability development (through the Team Tips) were unique components for a school health education program. These components were necessary, however, from the perspective of SLT.

The Home Team program was evaluated in a study that involved thirty-one schools in Minnesota and North Dakota. The design of the study involved schools assigned randomly to one of four conditions: the Home Team, an equivalent school-based program (Hearty Heart), both the Home Team and Hearty Heart, or a no-program control. At posttest time, students in the Home Team program, regardless of whether they participated in the Hearty Heart school program, had significantly changed their fat and complex carbohydrate consumption (Perry and others, 1988). However, students in the school-based Hearty Heart program had acquired more knowledge. Thus, the application of SLT within the home, a

Table 8.4. Major Concepts in Social Learning Theory and Examples of Their Application in the Minnesota Home Team Program.

Environment and situation	Parental involvement in the program's activities
	Food selection and purchasing changes to prepare the Home Team recipes
Behavioral capability	Team Tips, label reading, and food preparation skills activities
Expectations	Parent-child communication in home-based activities
Expectancies	The possibility of winning the grand prize by completing the Home Team program
Self-control	Goal-setting exercises to increase personal and family consumption of healthful foods
Observational learning	Cartoon role models portraying healthful lives in the *Adventures of Hearty Heart and Friends*
Reinforcements	Small stickers, Salt Sleuth magnifying glasses, points to reward completion of activities
Reciprocal determinism	Targeting eating habit changes in a novel parent-child context through personal skill development

potent environment for learning eating patterns, seemed critical for behavior change.

Caveat

An important caveat is in order. In the development of SLT concepts over the past decades, one concept was often explored while the others were excluded completely. For example, the concept of internal and external locus of control dominated social learning research at one time. Later, the concept of observational learning was used extensively to explain learning among children. In 1982, Bandura stated that self-efficacy may be the single most important factor in promoting behavioral change. This emphasis on a single variable is a reflection of the structure of experimental research, which usually permits analysis of only a few variables at a time; the problems that are selected for analysis; and the tendency for fads to develop in all types of research.

Practitioners who are confronted with real problems often like the simplicity provided by a single-variable explanation. They find, however, that many variables must be addressed in a program to produce behavior change. For example, it makes little sense to help a person with diabetes build self-efficacy at self-injection without providing that person with the behavioral capability to self-inject, ways in which to fit this behavior into his or her life, and suggestions about how to cope emotionally with having diabetes. Although some variables may be more important in certain situations than others, most apply in almost any area of health education. The health professional must therefore explore the ways in which multiple variables are manifested in particular situations and plan interventions that are based on multiple relevant concepts.

Summary

This chapter has focused on Social Learning Theory and its relevance in the design of health education programs. By incorporating a concern for environment, people, and behavior, SLT provides a framework for designing and implementing comprehensive behavior change programs.

Social Learning Theory is an attractive theory to apply to health education and health promotion programs because it not only illuminates the dynamics of individual behavior but also gives direction to the design of intervention strategies to influence behavior change. A large number of intervention studies that provide support for the effectiveness of SLT as a theoretical base for promoting health behavior change have been conducted.

In the development of health promotion programs, great emphasis is placed currently on the importance of multicomponent interventions. Recent approaches are including interventions that address not only behavioral change at the individual level but also change within the environment to support behavioral change (Simons-Morton, Simons-Morton, Parcel, and Bunker, 1988; Parcel, Simons-Morton, and Kolbe, 1988). SLT can be applied to the multi-level change strategy because of the inclusion of environmental, personal, and behavioral constructs. The ability of SLT to address all three domains can contribute to the design of multicomponent health promotion interventions.

As reviewed in this chapter, SLT is a robust theoretical framework that can be applied to health education and health promotion activities with as much diversity as individual counseling, community-based interventions, and the diffusion of innovative programs. However, inappropriate applications of SLT sometimes occur because of an oversimplification of the intervention methods. To guard against inappropriate applications, designers of intervention strategies should first specify the desired behavioral outcome and identify the SLT variables most likely to influence changes in the specified behavior. Then SLT intervention methods can be matched with variables targeted for change to influence the desired behavioral outcome. The final step is the creative part of health education: translating the theory into practical and meaningful intervention strategies that can work in the real-life settings of health education programs.

References

Argyle, M., Furnham, A., and Graham, J. A. *Social Situations.* Cambridge England: Cambridge University Press, 1981.

Bandura, A. "Social Learning Through Imitation." In M. R. Jones (ed.), *Nebraska Symposium on Motivation,* Vol. 10. Lincoln: University of Nebraska Press, 1962.

Bandura, A. *Principles of Behavior Modification.* New York: Holt, Rinehart & Winston, 1969.

Bandura, A. *Psychological Modeling: Connecting Theories.* Chicago: Aldine/Atherton, 1972.

Bandura, A. *Social Learning Theory.* Englewood Cliffs, N.J.: Prentice-Hall, 1977a.

Bandura, A. "Self-Efficacy: Toward a Unifying Theory of Behavioral Change." *Psychological Review,* 1977b, *84,* 191–215.

Bandura, A. "The Self System in Reciprocal Determinism." *American Psychologist,* 1978, *33,* 344–358.

Bandura, A. "Self-Efficacy Mechanism in Human Agency." *American Psychologist,* 1982, *37,* 121–147.

Bandura, A. *Social Foundations of Thought and Action.* Englewood Cliffs, N.J.: Prentice-Hall, 1986.

Bandura, A., and Adams, N. E. "Analysis of Self-Efficacy Theory of Behavioral Change." *Cognitive Therapy and Research,* 1982, *1,* 287-310.

Bandura, A., Adams, N. E., and Beyer, J. "Cognitive Processes Mediating Behavioral Change." *Journal of Personality and Social Psychology,* 1977, *35,* 125-139.

Bandura, A., and Walters, R. H. *Social Learning and Personality Development.* New York: Holt, Rinehart & Winston, 1963.

Baranowski, T., and Nader, P. R. "Family Health Behaviors." In D. Turk and R. Kerns (eds.), *Health, Illness and Families.* New York: Wiley, 1985a.

Baranowski, T., and Nader, P. R. "Family Involvement in Health Behavior Change Programs." In D. Turk and R. Kerns (eds.), *Health, Illness and Families.* New York: Wiley, 1985b.

Bates, J. A. "External Reward and Intrinsic Motivation: A Review with Implications for the Classroom." *Review of Educational Research,* 1979, *49,* 557-576.

Bem, D. J. "Self-Perception: An Alternative Interpretation of Cognitive Dissonance Phenomena." *Psychological Review,* 1967, *74,* 183-200.

Block, J. H. (ed.). *Mastery Learning: Theory and Practice.* New York: Holt, Rinehart & Winston, 1971.

Bronfenbrenner, U. "Toward an Experimental Ecology of Human Development." *American Psychologist,* 1977, *32,* 513-553.

Condiotte, M., and Lichtenstein, E. "Self-Efficacy and Relapse in Smoking Cessation Programs." *Journal of Consulting Clinical Psychology,* 1981, *49,* 648-658.

Diaz-Guerrero, R. "The Development of Coping Style." *Human Development,* 1979, *322,* 320-331.

DiClemente, C. C. "Self-Efficacy and Smoking Cessation." *Cognitive Therapy and Research,* 1981, *5,* 175-187.

Ewart, C. K., Taylor, C. B., Reese, L. B., and Debusk, R. F. "Effects of Early Post-Myocardial Infarction Exercise Testing on Self-Perception and Subsequent Physical Activity." *American Journal of Cardiology,* 1983, *51,* 1076-1080.

Farquhar, J. W., and others. "Community Education for Cardiovascular Health." *Lancet,* 1977, *1,* 1192–1195.

Flay, B. R. "What We Know About the Social Influences Approach to Smoking Prevention: Review and Recommendations." In C. S. Bell and R. J. Battjes (eds.), *Prevention Research: Deterring Drug Abuse Among Children and Adolescents.* National Institute for Drug Abuse Research Monograph no. 63, 1985.

Frederiksen, L. W., Martin, J. E., and Webster, J. S. "Assessment of Smoking Behavior." *Journal of Applied Behavior Analysis,* 1979, *12,* 653–664.

Gottlieb, B. (ed.) *Social Networks and Social Support.* Newbury Park, Calif.: Sage, 1981.

Hudson, A., and Williams, S. G. "Eating Behavior, Emotions, and Overweight." *Psychological Reports,* 1981, *48,* 669–760.

Hull, C. L. *Principles of Behavior.* East Norwalk, Conn.: Appleton & Lange, 1943.

Kanfer, F. H. "Self-Management Methods." In F. H. Kanfer and A. P. Goldstein (eds.), *Helping People Change.* Elmsford, New York: Pergamon Press, 1975.

Kanfer, F. "The Many Faces of Self-Control, or Behavior Modification Changes Its Focus." Paper presented at the Eighth International Banff Conference on Behavior Modification, Banff, 1976.

Leon, G. R., and Roth, L. "Obesity: Psychological Causes, Correlations, and Speculations." *Psychological Bulletin,* 1977, *84,* 117–139.

Lepper, M. R., and Green, D. (eds.). *The Hidden Costs of Reward: New Perspectives on the Psychology of Human Motivation.* Hillsdale, N. J.: Erlbaum, 1978.

Lewin, K. *Field Theory in Social Science.* New York: Harper & Row, 1951.

Ley, P., and Spelman, M. S. "Communications in an Out-Patient Setting." *British Journal of Social and Clinical Psychology,* 1965, *4,* 114–116.

Locke, E. A., Bryan, J. F., and Kendall, L. M. "Goals and Intentions as Mediators of the Effects of Monetary Incentives on Behavior." *Journal of Applied Psychology,* 1968, *52,* 104–126.

McAlister, A., and others. "Pilot Study of Smoking, Alcohol, and

Drug Abuse Prevention." *American Journal of Public Health,* 1980, *70,* 719-721.

McAlister, A., and others. "Three-Year Panel Study of Health Promotion and Smoking Cessation in Three Southwest Texas Border Communities." (Manuscript submitted for publication.)

Maddux, J. E., and Rogers, R. W. "Protection Motivation and Self-Efficacy: A Revised Theory of Fear Appeals and Attitude Change." *Journal of Experimental Social Psychology,* 1983, *19,* 469-979.

Magnusson, D. (ed.). *Toward a Psychology of Situations, An Interactional Perspective.* Hillsdale, N.J.: Erlbaum, 1981.

Miller, N. E., and Dollard, J. *Social Learning and Imitation.* New Haven, Conn.: Yale University Press, 1941.

Mischel, W. "Toward a Cognitive Social Learning Reconceptualization of Personality." *Psychological Review,* 1973, *80,* 252-283.

Moos, R. H. *The Human Context: Environmental Determinants of Behavior.* New York: Wiley, 1976.

Parcel, G., and Baranowski, T. "Social Learning Theory and Health Education." *Health Education,* 1981, *12,* 14-18.

Parcel, G. S., and Meyer, M. P. "Development of an Instrument to Measure Children's Health Locus of Control." *Health Education Monographs,* 1978, *6,* 149-159.

Parcel, G. S., Simons-Morton, B. G., and Kolbe, L. J. "Health Promotion: Integrating Organizational Change and Student Learning Strategies." *Health Education Quarterly,* 1988, *15,* 435-450.

Patterson, G. R. *A Social Learning Approach.* Vol. 3: *Coercive Family Process.* Eugene, Ore.: Castalia, 1982.

Perry, C. L., and others. "Parent Involvement with Children's Health Promotion: The Minnesota Home Team." *American Journal of Public Health,* 1988, *78,* 1156-1160.

Rodin, J. "Personal Control Through the Life Course." In R. Heise (ed.), *Implications of the Life-Span Perspective for Social Psychology.* Hillsdale, N. J.: Erlbaum, 1987.

Rosenstock, I. M., Strecher, V. J., and Becker, M. H. "Social Learning Theory and the Health Belief Model." *Health Education Quarterly,* 1988, *15,* 175-183.

Rotter, J. B. *Social Learning and Clinical Psychology.* Englewood Cliffs, N.J.: Prentice-Hall, 1954.

Rotter, J. B. "The Role of the Psychological Situation in Determining the Direction of Human Behavior." In M. R. Jones (ed.), *Nebraska Symposium on Motivation.* Lincoln: University of Nebraska Press, 1955.

Rotter, J. B. "Generalized Expectancies for Internal Versus External Control of Reinforcement." *Psychological Monographs,* 1966, *80,* 1-28.

Rotter, J. B. *Social Learning and Clincial Psychology.* New York: Praeger, 1982.

Simons-Morton, D. G., Simons-Morton, B. G., Parcel, G. S., and Bunker, J. F. "Influencing Personal and Environmental Conditions for Community Health: A Multilevel Intervention Model." *Family and Community Health,* 1988, *11,* 25-35.

Slochower, J., and Kaplan, S. P. "Anxiety, Perceived Control, and Eating in Obese and Normal Weight Persons." *Appetite,* 1980, *1,* 75-83.

Slochower, J., Kaplan, S. P., and Mann, L. "The Effects of Life Stress and Weight on Mood and Eating." *Appetite,* 1981, *2,* 115-25.

Stokols, D. "The Reduction of Cardiovascular Risk: An Application of Social Learning Perspectives." In A. J. Enelow and J. B. Henderson (eds.), *Applying Behavioral Science to Cardiovascular Risk.* Dallas, Tex.: American Heart Association, 1975.

Strecher, V. J., DeVellis, B. M., Becker, M. H., and Rosenstock, I. M. "The Role of Self-Efficacy in Achieving Health Behavior Change." *Health Education Quarterly,* 1986, *13,* 73-92.

Stuart, R. B. (ed.). *Behavioral Self-Management: Strategies, Techniques, and Outcomes.* New York: Brunner/Mazel, 1977.

Telch, C. F., and Telch, M. J. "Psychological Approaches for Enhancing Coping Among Cancer Patients: A Review." *Clinical Psychology Review,* 1985, *5,* 325-344.

Wallston, K. A., and Wallston, B. S. "Locus of Control and Health." *Health Education Monographs,* 1978, *6,* 107-117.

Zifferblatt, S. M. "Increasing Patient Compliance Through the Applied Analysis of Behavior." *Preventive Medicine,* 1975, *4,* 173-182.

Chapter 9

Barbara A. Israel
Susan J. Schurman

Social Support, Control, and the Stress Process

A substantial body of research evidence suggests that numerous sources of stress are related to a diverse set of physiological, psychological, and behavioral outcomes (Cohen, Evans, Stokols, and Krantz, 1986; DeLongis and others, 1982; Dohrenwend and Dohrenwend, 1981; Kahn, 1981; Kaplan, 1983; Kasl and Cooper, 1987). This research has found not only an association between stressors and health, but also that numerous psychosocial factors, including social support and control, play a significant role in modifying levels of stress or health or the relationship between stress and health (Cohen, Evans, Stokols, and Krantz, 1986; Cohen and Syme, 1985; House, 1981; House, Umberson, and Landis, 1988; Israel and others, 1989; Karasek, 1979; Lewis, 1987; Sutton and Kahn, 1984). These findings further substantiate a conceptual model of stress that posits stress as a process in which individual and environmental characteristics interact to produce a variety of outcomes. In this conceptual framework, the stress process includes not only the environmental and psychosocial sources of stress and the individual's perception of them but also short-term and long-term physiological, psychological, and behavioral responses and a number of moderating factors that influence the relationships among variables in the stress process (French and Kahn, 1962; House, 1981; Katz and Kahn, 1978; Levi, 1981).

187

This conceptual framework has implications for health education research and practice. In health education practice, the stress model suggests that a comprehensive approach, one that includes interventions aimed at multiple factors in the model, is often necessary. Programs can be more effective if they focus on reducing sources of stress in addition to teaching individuals how to cope with stressful situations. Health education interventions can also be aimed at strengthening the moderating factors of social support and control that may reduce stress and improve health.

The purpose of this chapter is to explicate the stress model and its implications for health behavior.* After providing a general explanation of the entire framework, the chapter describes the relationships among the variables. This is followed by more specific definitions of the three concepts that are the focus of the chapter (stressors, social support, control) and a summary of some of the major hypotheses relating these concepts and health status. Finally, the chapter provides a description and an analysis of a health education action research project within a work setting that is guided by and is a test of the stress model.

Background to the Conceptual Framework

Given the multidisciplinary and multidimensional aspects of the framework, it is not surprising that numerous theories from different disciplines are applicable to the stress model. From sociology and organizational psychology, Systems Theory posits a hierarchical ordering of biological, psychological, and social levels, or systems, each of which has its own resources, needs, and limitations (Katz and Kahn, 1978; von Bertalanffy, 1968). These systems are interrelated in such a way that change at one level inevitably affects behavior at other levels. The relationships between the parts are viewed as

*Preparation of this chapter has been supported by Grant #501 AA06553 from the National Institute on Alcohol Abuse and Alcoholism. We thank James House for his invaluable contribution to our thinking and to the action research project described here. We appreciate the efforts of all members of the research team and the work site Stress and Wellness Committee. A special thanks goes to Sue Andersen for her patience and competence in preparing this chapter.

dynamic, interactive, and frequently reciprocal. The theory is characterized by concepts such as status quo, homeostasis, and equilibrium. Consistent with a systems perspective, the stress model outlined here states that an individual's perception of stress may be the result of as well as contributor to the stressors and changes within the family, work site, neighborhood, nation, and society as a whole.

Drawing from developmental psychology, Bronfenbrenner's (1979) theory of the ecology of human development states that in order to understand human development it is necessary to go beyond the immediate situation of the individual to consider the ecological environment as an expanding series of contexts that surround the individual's immediate setting (that is, microsystem, mesosystem, exosystem, and macrosystem). It is the interrelationships between the environment and behavior and the social processes that mediate these relationships that are important. Similarly, the stress model recognizes the interaction between environmental and individual characteristics and the multilevel moderating factors that affect the association between stress and health.

The historical development of the stress model also reflects the different disciplines that conduct stress research. Two of the early investigators, Cannon (1929) and Selye (1956), developed physiological models of stress that examined the sympathetic nervous system ("fight or flight" response) and pituitary-adrenocortical axis (General Adaptation Syndrome), respectively. Both models focused on the physiological responses of the body to adverse stimuli in which the body moves through a process from homeostasis to disruption to reequilibration.

In the early 1950s, Holmes and his colleagues developed a list of forty-three representative stressful life events (Holmes and Rahe, 1967). The list included items that could be considered desirable as well as undesirable events, and stressfulness was defined in terms of the need for the person to readjust to the event. The items were also assigned a weight or rating of stressfulness that was determined by outside experts, not the people themselves. A rapid increase in the study of stressful life events was stimulated by the availability of the Holmes and Rahe scale (Dohrenwend and Dohrenwend, 1981).

Another early contribution to the stress framework is the work of Lazarus (1966) on the role of cognitive appraisal in assessing objective events as stressful experiences. The important factor here is the recognition that a given objective condition may be perceived positively by one individual and negatively by another and that these subjective factors may play a greater role in the stress process than objective conditions.

In the field of social psychology, early research in this area focused on occupational stress and physical and mental health. In general, these studies used one of three basic conceptual models: an "external" model, which emphasized the role of environmental forces external to the individual (for example, Margolis, Kroes, and Quinn, 1974); an "internal" model, which emphasized characteristics of the individual, such as Type A behavior (for example, Stokols and others, 1978); or an "interaction" model, which assumed that occupational stress was the result of an interaction between individual characteristics of workers and characteristics of their work environment (for example, French and Kahn, 1962; House, 1974). The conceptual framework presented in this chapter draws most closely on the last of these models.

The ideas presented by the epidemiologist Cassel (1976) also provided a historical basis for the current model. In a review of animal and human studies, Cassel argued that there are two sets of psychosocial variables associated with disease susceptibility: stress and social support. He posited that social support can have a direct positive effect on well-being or can serve as a buffer or moderator of the effects of stress on health status.

Conceptual Framework of the Stress Process

Despite the increase in research evidence over the past fifteen years that has shown an association between the experience of stress and the development of a diverse set of physical, psychological, and behavioral disorders (Cohen, Evans, Stokols, and Krantz, 1986; DeLongis and others, 1982; Dohrenwend and Dohrenwend, 1981; Kahn, 1981; Kaplan, 1983; Kasl and Cooper, 1987), there is still considerable debate in the literature on the most fundamental questions, such as how to define the concept of stress. (See Evans and Cohen, 1987, for a review of these problems.) This lack of agreement on the definition of stress is complicated by the multidisciplinary nature of the field and by the fact that research initially focused on stress in different domains (for example, work, family, community), with various conceptualizations and operationalizations in each (for example, chronic role strains, major life events); rarely was the effect of stress examined simultaneously across these domains. Such difficulties led most stress researchers to conceptualize stress as a complex, interactive process that includes not only the environmental sources of stress and the individual's reaction to them but also a number of intervening steps and later consequences that are potentially modified by individual and situational factors (House, 1981). According to this perspective, stress is a relational concept that reflects an imbalance between environmental demands and individual and social resources to cope with those demands (Evans and Cohen, 1987; Lazarus, 1966; McGrath, 1970).

The specific manner in which this process is hypothesized to occur is shown in Figure 9.1. This conceptual framework is based on earlier models of social-environmental determinants of health (French and Kahn, 1962; Katz and Kahn, 1978; Lazarus, 1966; McGrath, 1970), and on the model of relationships among occupational stress, social support, and health (House, 1974, 1981). The model postulates the following set of five elements in the stress process. (1) People may experience a set of objective conditions (for example, death of a loved one, daily hassles with a family member, work overload, poverty status, natural disaster, exposure to toxic wastes) that place them at risk for physical, psychological, and behavioral disorders. These conditions or stressors do not invariably result in long-term negative outcomes; rather, their effects depend on (2) the perceptions and responses to the stressor by the people involved. An individual may perceive a stressor as threatening, exciting, challenging, or stressful. When a stressor is perceived as stressful, individuals may respond in one or more ways, psychologically, behaviorally, and physiologically. The sequences of response to perceived stress are not necessarily bad, and depending on the specific pattern of relationships among stressor, perception, and response, the stress reaction may be helpful and even pleasurable. However, when the demands placed on people by their environment exceed their abilities or when people are not able to meet strong needs, conditions are perceived as stressful (McGrath, 1970).

Figure 9.1. Conceptual Framework of the Stress Process.

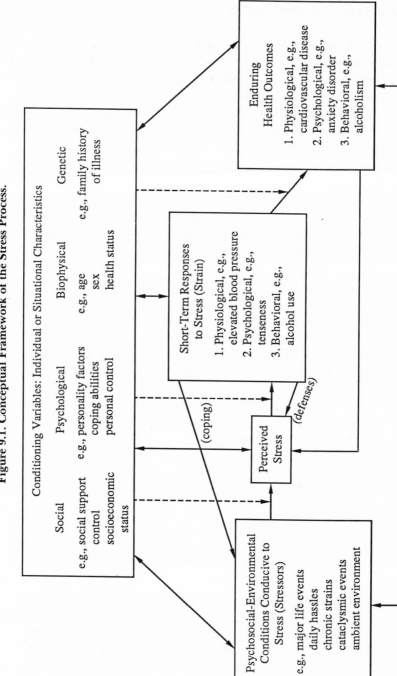

Note: Solid lines between boxes indicate presumed direct relationships among variables. Dotted lines indicate the hypothesized buffering effects of the conditioning variables on the relationship between stressors and perceived stress, between perceived stress

(3) Negative short-term response sequences may occur (for example, elevated blood pressure, tenseness, alcohol use) that may lead over time to (4) enduring poor health outcomes (for example, cardiovascular disease, anxiety disorder, alcoholism). The framework further posits that no objective stressor is likely to produce the same perceptions of stress or resultant short-term responses or enduring outcomes in all people exposed to the stressor. Rather, (5) certain individual and situational factors (presented in Figure 9.1 as four general categories of moderating or conditioning variables) influence how an individual experiences the stress process.

A hypothetical example from an occupational setting illustrates these components of the framework. An individual may experience objective conditions (stressors) at work, for example, too much work to do, conflicting job demands, and uncertainty regarding scope and responsibilities of the job. If this person receives social support from his or her co-workers and supervisor, this support may buffer the effect of the potentially stressful conditions because the individual may appraise the situation as less threatening or stressful. If, however, the stressors are perceived as stressful but the individual is able to exert control over decisions at work, his or her control may reduce the likelihood that the perceived stress will lead to negative short-term consequences. As indicated in Figure 9.1, there are numerous possible short-term responses to perceived stress, some of which may modify the stressor itself (see arrow labeled "coping") or the individual's perception of it (see arrow labeled "defenses"), which in turn may reduce or eliminate the perceived stress and its effect on health and health behavior (House, 1981). Here again, co-workers' support can facilitate efforts at coping and defense and thereby serve as a buffer against the effects of stress. These conditioning variables can also have an impact on whether short-term responses develop into more enduring outcomes. Hence, if an individual is able to exert control over the stressful situation, then the long-term effects may be alleviated. In addition to having these moderating or buffering effects, the conditioning variables may also have a direct or main effect on stress and health (House, 1981). For example, an individual who is supported by co-workers and supervisors and who can exert control over work conditions may experience fewer stressors to begin with. Further explanation of the potential direct and buffering effects of these conditioning variables is presented later in this chapter.

Several additional important aspects of and caveats concerning the conceptual framework shown in Figure 9.1 need to be summarized briefly. As indicated by the two-way arrows and feedback loops, this model reflects a complex and dynamic process. Although social support may have a direct impact on health status, one's health may also affect the extent and nature of social relationships that one is able to develop and maintain. Although social support and control are most frequently identified as a social resource, the lack of social support and the lack of control have also been identified as stressors (Karasek, 1979). The conditioning variables depicted in Figure 9.1 may also mediate the effects of each other and the relationship between stress and health. For example, a sense of personal control may be antecedent to control over decisions at work, which are in turn potential determinants of supportive relationships that may then affect perceptions of job stress and health. The objective conditions conducive to stress encompass different categories of stressors that may occur in different life domains, such as family or work (DeLongis and others, 1982; Evans and Cohen, 1987). There is increased evidence that the effects of some stressors on health, for example, major life events, may be mediated by other stressors, for example, negative daily events (Wagner, Compas, and Howell, 1988). Additionally, stressors that occur in one life domain may have an effect on stressors in another domain and subsequently on health status (Klitzman, House, and Israel, forthcoming). Thus, there are important relationships between and among objective conditions conducive to stress that are not detailed in Figure 9.1. There are other conceptual models that focus more specifically on one of the conditioning variables, for example, social support, and posit the potential determinants of different aspects of social support or social networks and their relationship to health (House, Umberson, and Landis, 1988; Israel, 1982; Kahn and Antonucci, 1980). Hence, social support (as well as each of the other conditioning variables) can be considered an independent, moderating, and dependent variable (House, Umberson, and Landis, 1988). Another dimension of the stress process not reflected in Figure 9.1 is that at numerous points along the model an individual may experience a successful outcome that may lead to no substantive change or to positive effects such as enhanced physical or mental health. The conceptual framework as presented focuses on the effects of stress on individual health status and the role of the individual (as well as the situation) in this process. A parallel approach recognizes that the stress model is applicable to group, organization, community, and societal levels. Thus, the presence of stressors within a community can be assessed along with their effect on such factors as social disintegration and community competence (Cottrell, 1976; Leighton and others, 1963).

The purpose here is to specify further the definitions and hypothesized relationships among three major categories of variables: stressors, social support, and control. These variables were selected for emphasis because research findings substantiate their significance to health and their applicability to health education. (Two additional conditioning variables that will not be elaborated but that play a major role in the stress process are coping abilities and personal control; see for example Cohen, 1987; Cohen, Evans, Stokols, and Krantz, 1986; Evans and Cohen, 1987; Folkman and Lazarus, 1988; Holahan and Wandersman, 1987; Lewis, 1987; Menaghan, 1983).

Definitions of Stressors, Social Support, and Control

Stressors. The psychosocial-environmental conditions conducive to stress, that is, stressors, have been conceptualized and operationalized in different ways by different disciplines (DeLongis and others, 1982; Dohrenwend and Dohrenwend, 1981; Evans and Cohen, 1987; Holt, 1982; House, 1981; Kasl and Cooper, 1987; Thoits, 1983). This diversity has been accompanied by methodological problems, particularly in the measurement of stressor variables. For the purpose of this chapter, stressors are divided into five general categories that represent relatively distinct constructs.

Major life events are discrete events that occur in a person's life and disrupt or threaten to disrupt normal activities and often require adaptive responses (Dohrenwend and Dohrenwend, 1981; Holmes and Rahe, 1967; Thoits, 1983). Examples of major life events include death of a loved one, marriage, divorce, loss of a job, birth of a child, and change in residence. Although studies of major life events have consistently shown an association between events and physical and mental health symptoms, only small portions of the variance are explained by these major events. The dimensions of life events most predictive of poor health outcomes are undesirability, uncontrollability, magnitude, and time clustering (Thoits, 1983). The content of checklists used to measure major life events differs in the extent to which they include, for example, desirable or undesirable events; voluntary or involuntary events; events that are relevant to certain age, gender, race, and income groups; and events that are confounded with physical and mental health outcomes (Thoits, 1983). For a review of the methodological and theoretical problems and research evidence on the role of major life events in health, see, for example, Kasl and Cooper, 1987, and Thoits, 1983.

Daily hassles are the minor events that occur in the day-to-day lives of individuals that may be perceived as frustrating or bothersome (DeLongis and others, 1982). Such events are often assessed by listing a set of items that occur in everyday life and asking an individual to indicate "how much of a hassle" each item was for a given day (DeLongis, Folkman, and Lazarus, 1988). Examples of items include one's spouse; children; fellow workers; work load; meeting deadlines; enough money for necessities, education, extras; physical environment; home repairs; taking care of paperwork; and amount of free time. Daily hassles occur more frequently and are more short term than most major life events. Early studies comparing the effects of daily hassles versus major life events found daily hassles to be a better predictor of health outcomes (DeLongis and others, 1982; Kanner, Coyne, Schaefer, and Lazarus, 1981). More recent research found that the effects of major life events on mental health are mediated by daily hassles; that is, major events lead to daily hassles that in turn influence mental health (Wagner, Compas, and Howell, 1988). Thus, daily hassles have an independent effect on stress and health, as well as an intervening effect between major life events (in addition to other stressors such as chronic strains) and health (Kasl and Cooper, 1987; Wagner, Compas, and Howell, 1988).

Chronic strains are the challenges, hardships, and problems that people experience over time in their daily lives (Pearlin, 1983).

They are most often associated with difficulties experienced in ongoing roles, but they also include broader social and structural contexts (Evans and Cohen, 1987; Pearlin, 1983). Examples of chronic strains include poverty, long-term unemployment, racism, ongoing work overload, interpersonal demands at work, family conflicts, and loss and gain of roles. Chronic strains are not a totally separate category of stressors from daily hassles and are often considered the same concept (Bailey and Bhagat, 1987). The importance of dividing them is due to the distinction between chronic strains as persistent, recurring problems, and daily hassles as often more transient in nature. The extensive research in the area of occupational stress and health defined and measured stressors primarily as chronic strains and found convincing evidence that chronic strains were a significant predictor of health status (Bailey and Bhagat, 1987; Holt, 1982).

Cataclysmic events are sudden disasters that require major adaptive responses from all people who experience them (Evans and Cohen, 1987); thus an individual's perception of the stressor is somewhat less important. Examples of such events include floods, earthquakes, hurricanes, nuclear power plant accidents, war, imprisonment, and discoveries of toxic waste dumps. The last of these (which may subsequently be considered a chronic ambient stressor as described below) has recently gained recognition as an important concern for public health and health education (Edelstein and Wandersman, 1987; Freudenberg, 1984; Gibbs, 1986). For a review of several of these cataclysmic events and their effects, see Fischoff, Svenson, and Slovic, 1987.

Ambient stressors are the more continuous and often unchanging conditions in the physical environment (Evans and Cohen, 1987). Examples of such stressors include chronic air and water pollution and exposure to chronic noise and chemicals within the environment.

In addition to the above types, stressors can be examined along eight dimensions: the degree to which a stressor is easily identifiable, the type of adjustment required, the positive or negative value assigned to the stressor, the degree of controllability over the stressor, the predictability of the stressor, the necessity and importance of the stressor, whether the stressor is linked to human behavior, and the duration and regularity of the stressor (Evans and Cohen, 1987).

Social Support. There is considerable variation and confusion in the literature on how the terms *social support* and *social networks* are defined and operationalized. As reviewed elsewhere (Israel, 1982; Israel and Rounds, 1987), a social network is person-centered and refers to the set of relationships among individuals within a person's web of social ties. Numerous characteristics of social networks have been categorized along three dimensions (Israel, 1982; Mitchell and Trickett, 1980). These dimensions are *structural characteristics,* such as size and density (extent to which people know one another); *interactional characteristics,* such as reciprocity, durability, and frequency of interaction; and *functional characteristics,* such as affective support (caring, love), instrumental support (tangible aid and services), and social outreach (access to new social contacts and roles). Thus, social networks refer to the linkages between people that may or not provide social support. This is an important distinction between social networks and support. For example, there is increased evidence indicating that negative aspects of relationships, such as those characterized by mistrust, hassles, domination, are more strongly related to psychiatric morbidity than that social support is related to mental health (Fiore, Becker and Coppel, 1983; Rook, 1984). Furthermore, these negative aspects of relationships are distinct from, not the opposite of, the lack of social support (Israel and others, 1989). Although the use of a social network approach was suggested previously (Israel, 1982; Israel and Rounds, 1987), the focus in this chapter is on the social support functions of social networks.

The term *social support* has been defined and measured in numerous ways. For a comprehensive review of measurement and methodological issues, see Heitzman and Kaplan, 1988; House, 1981; House and Kahn, 1985; Norbeck, Lindsey, and Carrieri, 1983; Payne and Jones, 1987. According to House (1981), social support is the functional content of relationships that can be categorized along four broad types of supportive behaviors or acts. *Emotional support* involves the provision of empathy, love, trust, and caring and has the strongest, most consistent relationship to health status (House,

1981; Israel and Rounds, 1987). *Instrumental support* involves the provision of tangible aid and services that directly assist a person in need. *Informational support* is the provision of advice, suggestions, and information that a person can use in addressing problems. *Appraisal support* involves the provision of information that is useful for self-evaluation purposes, that is, feedback, affirmation, and social comparison. While these four support functions are differentiated conceptually, they have not always been found empirically to be independent (House and Kahn, 1985; Israel and Rounds, 1987).

In addition to these types of support, it is important to consider the sources of support (such as family, friends, co-workers) and the quantity versus the quality of support (House and Kahn, 1985). In the occupational stress literature, emotional and instrumental support from co-workers and supervisors was more significant in alleviating work stress and buffering its effect on health than was support from friends and relatives (House, 1981). Research evidence suggests that the quality of supportive relationships is a better predictor of health than the quantity of such relationships (House and Kahn, 1985; Israel, 1982). The concept is further differentiated by whether the support provided is general or problem-specific and whether it is perceived (subjective) or actually received (objective) (House, 1981). Thus, there are multiple dimensions of social support that need to be examined in the context of the stress process.

Control. Several different conceptualizations of control are relevant to the stress model. Some of these concepts are distinct and others overlap. They have been variously referred to as personal control, contingency control, cognitive control, behavioral control, existential control, retrospective control, decisional control, processual control, and social control (Cohen, Evans, Stokols, and Krantz, 1986; Evans and Cohen, 1987; Holahan and Wandersman, 1987; Lewis, 1987). The focus in the current chapter is on a more sociological or extrapersonal level, that is, on control aimed at exerting influence (through, for example, participation in decision making) over events and conditions in the environment (Holahan and Wandersman, 1987; Lewis, 1987; Sutton and Kahn, 1984). This definition of control draws on the literature on organizational behavior

(Argyris, 1957; Tannenbaum, 1968; Likert, 1967; Lawler, 1986), workplace democracy (Bernstein, 1976; Spector, 1986; Walker, 1974), group dynamics (Blumberg, Hare, Kent, and Davies, 1983), and citizen participation.

The type of control that is perhaps most familiar to health educators is contingency control, which involves the individual's perception that his or her reactions to a stressor control the outcome (Lewis, 1987). The frameworks and concepts that are relevant to this type of control include Social Learning, locus of control, learned helplessness, and self-efficacy (see Lewis, 1987, for a discussion of their application). This approach to control is primarily psychological and can be considered an intrapersonal moderator of stress (Evans and Cohen, 1987).

A major conceptual problem that has undermined attempts at developing a more general framework of participation and control focuses on whether the most important component is the *act* of participating or the *outcome* of participation in the form of influence or control. A framework developed by Bernstein (1976) clearly emphasizes the outcome of participation in terms of control. He states that each individual case of such participation can be distinguished along three dimensions: (1) the degree of control the individual can exert over any particular decision, (2) the issues over which control may be exercised, and (3) the level of the organization at which control is exercised. In contrast, Walker's (1974) framework, while incorporating many of the same elements, contains a strong emphasis on the act of participating. He focuses more heavily on whether participation takes place formally or informally, directly or indirectly, in an adversarial or cooperative mode.

The concept of control, as defined here, includes both the act of participating in decision making and the effects of that participation in terms of increased influence and control. This approach is consistent with the empirical evidence in the occupational stress field. Studies have found that the degree of participation in decision making (the *act*) is related to job satisfaction, psychological and somatic symptoms, and perceptions of stressors as stressful (Jackson, 1983; Margolis, Kroes, and Quinn, 1974). The ability to control work factors has also been related to cardiovascular and psychosomatic disorders, job dissatisfaction, and depression (Caplan and others, 1975; Frankenhaeuser and Gardell, 1976). The work of Karasek and his colleagues shows that people who experience high levels of stress but also are able to exercise high levels of control are at lower risk for cardiovascular disease (Karasek and others, 1981). Furthermore, the effects of participation on stress and health are mediated through influence (Israel and others, 1989). These components of participation and control are also considered to be key elements of empowerment (see Zimmerman, forthcoming, for a review).

Hypothesized Effects of Social Support and Control on Stressors and Health

This section provides a more specific discussion of the hypothesized effects of social support and control on stress, health, and the stress and health relationship. Figure 9.2 summarizes the potential effects of social support and control on stressors and health.

Figure 9.2 is a somewhat simplified version of the broader conceptual framework depicted in Figure 9.1. The major hypotheses regarding the conditioning variables suggest that social support and control may directly enhance health regardless of stress level (direct or main effects), as well as protect people from negative consequences of stressful situations (buffering effects). Although these two hypothesized relationships were initially posed and investigated as an either-or relationships, more recent evidence suggests that social support and control may have *both* direct and buffering effects on stress and health and that the way in which social support is measured may be what influences the types of effects it has (Cohen, 1987; Cohen and Syme, 1985; Cohen and Wills, 1985; House, Umberson, and Landis, 1988; Israel and Rounds, 1987; Payne and Jones, 1987; Sutton and Kahn, 1984).

According to Figure 9.2, objective conditions conducive to stress (stressors) may have a direct effect on health (arrow c), although much of the effect is mediated through perceived stress (arrows a and b). That is, stressors lead to perceived stress, which in turn leads to negative health consequences. Perceived stress is further hypothesized to have a direct effect on health (arrow b). The primary focus in this chapter is on the arrows numbered 1 through 5

Figure 9.2. Hypothesized Relationships of Social Support and Control on Stressors and Health.

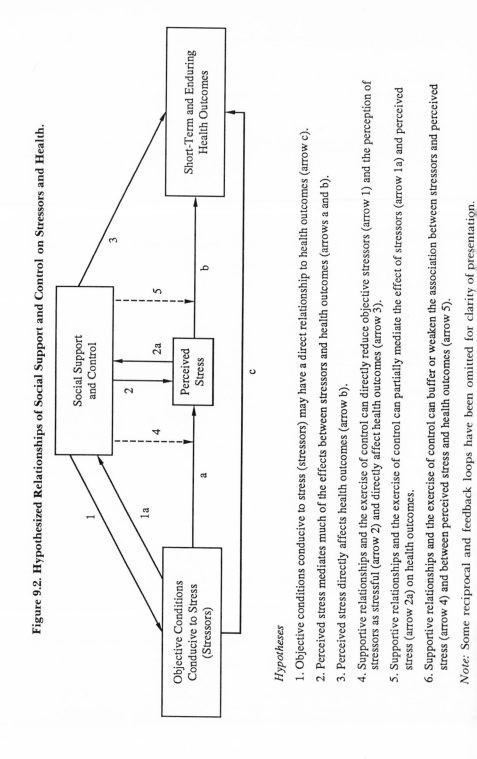

Hypotheses

1. Objective conditions conducive to stress (stressors) may have a direct relationship to health outcomes (arrow c).

2. Perceived stress mediates much of the effects between stressors and health outcomes (arrows a and b).

3. Perceived stress directly affects health outcomes (arrow b).

4. Supportive relationships and the exercise of control can directly reduce objective stressors (arrow 1) and the perception of stressors as stressful (arrow 2) and directly affect health outcomes (arrow 3).

5. Supportive relationships and the exercise of control can partially mediate the effect of stressors (arrow 1a) and perceived stress (arrow 2a) on health outcomes.

6. Supportive relationships and the exercise of control can buffer or weaken the association between stressors and perceived stress (arrow 4) and between perceived stress and health outcomes (arrow 5).

Note: Some reciprocal and feedback loops have been omitted for clarity of presentation.

in Figure 9.2. Social support and control may directly reduce objective stressors (arrow 1) and the perception of stressors as stressful (arrow 2) and have direct effects on health (arrow 3). Also, stressors and perceived stress may be reciprocally causally related to support and control (arrows 1a and 2a). That is, some of the effect of stressors and perceived stress on health will be mediated through the effect of social support and control. Finally, support and control may buffer or weaken the relationship between stressors and perceived stress (arrow 4) as well as the relationship between perceived stress and health (arrow 5).

The direct-effect and buffering-effect hypotheses are somewhat general prescriptions and do not provide the specific mechanisms through which social support and control affect the stress and health relationship. The latter issue has received increased attention conceptually and to a lesser extent empirically (Cohen, 1987; Cohen, Evans, Stokols, and Krantz, 1986; House, Umberson, and Landis, 1988; Payne and Jones, 1987; Pearlin and Anesheusel, 1986). For example, supportive relationships provide an increased probability of having access to useful information and advice that may in turn influence relevant health behaviors or help one to avoid high-risk situations (Cohen, 1987). Also, the presence of supportive relationships may have a tranquilizing effect on the neuroendocrine system that makes people less reactive to perceived stress (House, 1981). In addition, control over stressful situations may enhance self-esteem, which in turn affects health status (Cohen, Evans, Stokols, and Krantz, 1986). The further specification of these mechanisms has important implications for both research and practice in health education.

Guidelines for Applying the Stress Model to Health Education

Drawing from the stress model and accompanying research evidence, a set of general guidelines for health education practice follows. Health education interventions will do well to move away from solely a categorical disease focus and include an examination of the effects of interventions on mental health and alcohol and drug use as well as physical health. Health education can benefit from a comprehensive approach involving multiple interventions aimed at different points in the model. This needs to include greater emphasis on interventions that focus on changing characteristics of the social and physical environment (that is, reducing sources of stress), as compared to changing individual characteristics (for example, teaching individual stress management skills). Health education practice can benefit from the inclusion of collective action aimed at organizational and social change for reducing those stressors that are beyond any one individual's ability to control (for example, unemployment, poverty) and thus achieve lasting and significant change in health status. Health education programs need to be based on an assessment of the specific stressors and psychosocial resources of the target population (individuals, groups, organizations, and communities). Health education interventions may be aimed at strengthening the conditioning factors of social support and control in the general population without reference to specific stressors, thereby having a direct effect on reducing stress or improving health. Health education may also target such programs on identified subgroups who are at risk because of exposure to stressors, thereby buffering the relationship between stress and health. The active involvement and control of participants in planning, implementing, and evaluating health education programs are essential to a potential health-promoting process.

Application of the Stress Model to an Occupational Stress Intervention

The authors of this chapter and their colleagues are presently involved in an action research project in a manufacturing setting that represents both an intervention guided by the conceptual framework of the stress process and an attempt to test and further refine the model. A brief discussion of how this effort has applied the model is presented next. See Israel, Schurman, and House, 1989, for an in-depth description and analysis of the project.

Study Site and Sample. This intervention, now in the fourth year of a six-year project, is being conducted in a component-parts plant of a major manufacturing corporation located in a medium-sized urban area of Michigan. The plant resembles a collection of small businesses (product areas), each made up of several departments and producing a distinct and unrelated product by means of a diverse array of processes, technologies, and managerial practices. The plant is comprised of approximately 1,000 employees, of which 90 percent are hourly (10 percent salaried), 80 percent are white, 95 percent are male, the average age is forty-three, and the average number of years with the corporation is twenty. The hourly work force is represented by a major industrial union.

Research and Intervention Goals. This project involves an action research approach in which professionals and organization members are working collaboratively to increase understanding of the stress process (research objectives) and to meet the immediate needs of the organization (intervention objectives). Thus, the original general objectives were refined and operationalized jointly by the research team and an action research group appointed by the company and the union to implement the project. The three major objectives are (1) to involve employees in planning, implementing, and evaluating interventions for reducing sources of occupational stress and strengthening psychosocial resources (for example, social support and control); (2) to test and evaluate the cumulative effects or impact of an action research strategy on reducing the negative short-term effects and enduring health outcomes of the stress process for employees (for example, job dissatisfaction, overall poor health, depression); and (3) to examine and test the psychosocial predictors and moderators of the stress process in order to gain increased knowledge of (a) the meaning, causes, short-term responses, and enduring outcomes of job stress; (b) the cross-sectional and longitudinal relationships between and among the variables in the stress model; and (c) the processes or mechanisms by which social support and control influence stress and the relationship between stress and health.

Action Research Approach. Several of the key characteristics of the action research approach are being used in this project. (1) It is *participatory;* that is, organization members are involved in all phases of the research and action, and the problems include those identified by organization members and not just the theoretical issues selected by researchers (Elden, 1986a; Elden, 1986b; Peters and Robinson, 1984; Susman and Evered, 1978). (2) The project is *collaborative* in that organization members and researchers are involved in a joint, cooperative process in which both have needs and expertise to contribute (Peters and Robinson, 1984; Susman and Evered, 1978). (3) It is a *co-learning process* in which employees are involved in developing local theory that explains their own situation and is used by employees to change the organization (Elden, 1986a, 1986b). (4) It involves *system development* in that the action research approach develops competencies within the organization to engage in a cyclical problem-solving process to meet identified needs, such as reducing occupational stress (Susman and Evered, 1978). (5) It is an *empowering process* in that through participation, organization members gain increased control over their lives (Elden, 1986a). (See Israel, Schurman, and House, 1989, for a discussion of the rationale for and limitations of using an action research approach.) This emphasis in action research on participation, developing cooperative relationships and problem-solving capacities, and empowerment strongly complements the key elements of the stress model.

Examples of How the Conceptual Framework Guides This Project.
The action research approach is viewed as a cyclical process that involves three overlapping phases: group development, research, and action—with evaluation as an ongoing component in each of the phases (Cunningham, 1976). Several examples of data collection and project implementation show how the conceptual framework of the stress process has been applied in this effort.

First, the framework was the conceptual underpinning of this project, with a particular focus on occupational sources of stress. This led to the selection of the action research method. In accordance with this method, it was essential that the organization members themselves develop their own model of stress to use in guiding data collection and action strategies. The first phase, *group development,* involved taking a series of steps to gain acceptance and support for the project by top union and management personnel and organizing a representative group of employees to participate in the action research. During the first working session of the

Stress and Wellness Committee (the name the group chose to call itself), the authors engaged the group in an experiential activity in which pairs of individuals interviewed each other to discover personal sources of stress at work, perceptions and feelings about the stress, and typical ways of coping with or responding to the perceived stress. During these interviews, the committee generated data that closely fit the model presented here (Figure 9.1) and that included sources of stress specific to the local situation. The committee and the research team were then able to use these data to develop a commonly defined and understood model (referred to in the committee as "the stress connection") to guide the construction of a survey instrument that was administered plantwide.

This initial survey served as a broad-based needs assessment for identifying problems for potential action, as well as a quantitative baseline measure for evaluation and research purposes. Based on the committee's conceptual model, the survey included questions on key variables, such as sources of stress (for example, work load, role demands, lack of information and feedback), social support from co-workers and supervisor, participation and control over decision making, coping strategies, job satisfaction, overall health, and depression. The survey instrument included standardized items with established reliability and validity, as well as questions based on the committee's input that were specifically tailored, in both language and content, to the plant situation.

The committee administered the survey, and the research team analyzed the results. Feedback was given in a report to the Stress and Wellness Committee to use as a basis for intervention. The results of the analyses indicated that job dissatisfaction, negative feelings about work, and physical and mental health were most strongly associated with (1) lack of communication, information, and feedback; (2) hassles with supervisors; (3) job demands related to work overload and demands of other people; (4) lack of job security; and (5) dissatisfaction with participation and influence. It is really apparent that these relationships are similar to previous findings in the literature as presented earlier, thereby supporting the conceptual framework of the stress process. (A major set of regression analyses directly tested components of the model; see Israel and others, 1989.)

On the basis of the findings from the survey, the committee selected four top problem areas for initial stress reduction efforts; problems with supervisors; lack of information, communication, and feedback; lack of participation in and control over decision making; and conflict between producing quality versus quantity of product (considered to be related to job security). Note that the first three major sources of stress are congruent with the psychosocial factors identified in the conceptual framework.

The committee formulated and implemented several action plans on the basis of the results of the survey. An example of one intervention is the development of a pilot project that is being implemented in one product area of the plant. The goals of this project are to improve product quality and quantity ratings and eliminate waste, to increase participation in and control over decisions on the job, and to increase trust and improve relationships between supervisors and supervisees. The project has involved the establishment of a multidisciplinary problem-solving team comprised of a cross section of employees who have received training in areas such as team building, problem solving, communication skills, and statistical quality control. The team has conducted further problem identification and priority setting and is involved in problem resolution. The aim of the project is to expand the use of this team approach to include eventually all members of the product area in such problem-solving teams. The effects of this intervention are presently being evaluated.

Conclusion

The conceptual framework of the stress process described here is a dynamic, multifaceted model that clearly has implications for health behavior and health education research and practice. On the basis of the model, we suggest the importance of taking an ecological, contextual approach in health education interventions that recognizes the social and structural determinants of stressors, health, and the relationship between stress and health. It is essential that our programs strive to eliminate or reduce the social and environmental sources of stress, not just teach individuals how to manage or cope with stressful situations. The effectiveness of such programs can be increased by including strategies for strengthening support-ive relationships and participation and control. In order to accom-plish these tasks, it is necessary to place greater emphasis on the organization, community, and societal levels of practice and the role of the individual, family and small group within these broader contexts.

In doing this work, we believe that multidisciplinary teams—involving researchers, practitioners, and community members—are needed to work collectively and to design and evalu-ate programs jointly. Despite the methodological problems in-volved, we argue that there is a need to consider alternatives to traditional experimental intervention designs in view of the com-plexity of the stress process. Our own experience in an action re-search project suggests that this is a viable strategy for health educators committed both to increasing our knowledge and under-standing of the stress process and to meeting the needs of people in the community. The conduct of action research entails the develop-ment of cooperative, supportive relationships and fosters participa-tion in and control over decision making, two of the conditioning factors that may themselves reduce stress and improve health. This approach has major implications for health educators. Health edu-cators engaged in such action research need to be flexible and able to handle ambiguity and to be comfortable with sharing and transfer-ring the ownership and control of the process to the people with whom they work. This means decreased reliance on "outside ex-pert" models of professional behavior and increased emphasis on collaboration and co-learning as core professional competencies. It is our aim that through the development and evaluation of such collaborative efforts, addressing multiple factors in the stress model and involving different levels of practice, health education research and practice can itself be an empowering process.

References

Argyris, C. *Personality and Organizations: The Conflict Between System and the Individual.* New York: Harper & Row, 1957.

Bailey, J. M., and Bhagat, R. S. "Meaning and Measurement of Stressors in the Work Environment: An Evaluation." In S. Kasl and C. Cooper (eds.), *Stress and Health: Issues in Research Methodology.* New York: Wiley, 1987.

Bernstein, P. "Necessary Elements for Worker Participation." *Journal of Economic Issues,* 1976, *10,* 490–522.

Blumberg, H., Hare, A., Kent, V., and Davies, M. (eds.). *Small Groups and Social Interaction.* Vols. 1 and 2. New York: Wiley, 1983.

Bronfenbrenner, U. *The Ecology of Human Development.* Cambridge, Mass.: Harvard University Press, 1979.

Cannon, W. B. *Bodily Changes in Pain, Hunger, Fear, and Rage.* East Norwalk, Conn.: Appleton & Lange, 1929.

Caplan, R., Cobb, S., French, J.R.P., Harrison, R., and Pinneau, S. *Job Demands and Worker Health.* U.S. Department of Health, Education and Welfare, Publication no. NIOSH, 1975.

Cassel, J. "The Contribution of the Social Environment to Host Resistance." *American Journal of Epidemiology,* 1976, *104,* 107–123.

Cohen, F. "Measurement of Coping." In S. Kasl and C. Cooper (eds.), *Stress and Health: Issues in Research Methodology.* New York: Wiley, 1987.

Cohen, S. "Psychosocial Models of the Role of Social Support in the Etiology of Physical Disease." *Health Psychology,* 1988, *7,* 269–297.

Cohen, S., Evans, G., Stokols, D., and Krantz, D. (eds.). *Behavior, Health, and Environmental Stress.* New York: Plenum, 1986.

Cohen, S., and Syme, S. L. (eds.). *Social Support and Health.* Orlando, Fla.: Academic Press, 1985.

Cohen, S., and Wills, T. "Stress, Social Support, and the Buffering Hypothesis." *Psychological Bulletin,* 1985, *98,* 310–357.

Cottrell, L. S. "The Competent Community." In B. H. Kaplan, R. N. Wilson, and A. H. Leighton (eds.), *Further Explorations in Social Psychiatry.* New York: Basic Books, 1976.

Cunningham, B. "Action Research: Toward a Procedural Model." *Human Relations,* 1976, *29,* 215–238.

DeLongis, A., Folkman, S., and Lazarus, R. "The Impact of Daily Stress on Health and Mood: Psychological and Social Resources as Mediators." *Journal of Personality and Social Psychology,* 1988, *54,* 486–495.

DeLongis, A., and others. "Relationship of Daily Hassles, Uplifts, and Major Life Events to Health Status." *Health Psychology,* 1982, *1,* 119–136.

Dohrenwend, B. S., and Dohrenwend, B. P. (eds.). *Stressful Life Events and Their Contexts.* New York: Prodist, 1981.

Edelstein, M., and Wandersman, A. "Community Dynamics in Coping with Toxic Contaminants." In I. Altman and A. Wandersman (eds.), *Neighborhood and Community Environments.* New York: Plenum, 1987.

Elden, M. "Sociotechnical Systems Ideas as Public Policy in Norway: Empowering Participation Through Worker-Managed Change." *Journal of Applied Behavioral Science,* 1986a, *22,* 239–255.

Elden, M. "Sharing the Research Work: Participative Research and Its Role Demands." In P. Reason and J. Rowan (eds.), *Human Inquiry.* Chichester, England: Wiley, 1986b.

Evans, G., and Cohen, S. "Environmental Stress." In D. Stokols and I. Altman (eds.), *Handbook of Environmental Psychology.* Vol. 1. New York: Wiley, 1987.

Fiore, J., Becker, J., and Coppel, D. "Social Network Interactions: A Buffer or a Stress?" *American Journal of Community Psychology,* 1983, *11,* 423–440.

Fischoff, B., Svenson, O., and Slovic, P. "Environmental Stress: Natural and Technological Disasters." In D. Stokols and I. Altman (eds.), *Handbook of Environmental Psychology.* New York: Wiley, 1987.

Folkman, S., and Lazarus, R. "Coping as a Mediator of Emotion." *Journal of Personality and Social Psychology,* 1988, *54,* 466–475.

Frankenhaeuser, M., and Gardell, B. "Underload and Overload in Working Life: Outline of a Multidisciplinary Approach." *Journal of Human Stress,* 1976, *2,* 35–46.

French, J.R.P., and Kahn, R. L. "A Programmatic Approach to Studying the Industrial Environment and Mental Health." *Journal of Social Issues,* 1962, *18,* 1–47.

Freudenberg, N. *Not in Our Backyards.* New York: Monthly Review Press, 1984.

Gibbs, M. "Psychological Dysfunction as a Consequence of Exposure to Toxins." In A. Lebovits, A. Baum, and J. Singer (eds.),

Health Consequences of Exposure to Toxins. Hillsdale, N.J.: Erlbaum, 1986.

Heitzman, C., and Kaplan, R. "Assessment of Methods for Measuring Social Support." *Health Psychology,* 1988, *7,* 75-109.

Holahan, C., and Wandersman, A. "The Community Psychology Perspective in Environmental Psychology." In D. Stokols and I. Altman (eds.), *Handbook of Environmental Psychology.* Vol. 1. New York: Wiley, 1987.

Holmes, T. H., and Rahe, R. H. "The Social Readjustment Rating Scale." *Journal of Psychosomatic Research,* 1967, *11,* 213-218.

Holt, R. "Occupational Stress." In L. Goldberger and S. Breznitz (eds.), *Handbook of Stress: Theoretical and Clinical Aspects.* New York: Free Press, 1982.

House, J. S. "Occupational Stress and Coronary Heart Disease: A Review and Theoretical Integration." *Journal of Health and Social Behavior,* 1974, *15,* 12-27.

House, J. *Work Stress and Social Support.* Reading, Mass.: Addison-Wesley, 1981.

House, J., and Kahn, R. "Measures and Concepts of Social Support." In S. Cohen and S. Syme (eds.), *Social Support and Health.* Orlando, Fla.: Academic Press, 1985.

House, J., Umberson, D., and Landis, K. "Structures and Processes of Social Support." *Annual Review of Sociology,* 1988, *14,* 293-318.

Israel, B. A. "Social Networks and Health Status: Linking Theory, Research, and Practice." *Patient Counseling and Health Education,* 1982, *4,* 65-79.

Israel, B. A., and Rounds, K. A. "Social Networks and Social Support: A Synthesis for Health Educators." *Advances in Health Education and Promotion,* 1987, *2,* 311-351.

Israel, B. A., Schurman, S. J., and House, J. S. "Action Research on Occupational Stress: Involving Workers as Researchers." *International Journal of Health Services,* 1989, *19,* 135-155.

Israel, B A., and others. "The Relation of Personal Resources, Participation, Influence, Interpersonal Relationships, and Coping Strategies to Occupational Stress, Job Strains, and Health: A Multivariate Analysis." *Work and Stress,* 1989, *3,* 163-194.

Jackson, S. E. "Participation in Decision Making as a Strategy for

Reducing Job-Related Strain." *Journal of Applied Psychology,* 1983, *68,* 3-19.

Kahn, R. L. *Work and Health,* New York: Wiley, 1981.

Kahn, R., and Antonucci, T. "Convoys Over the Life Course: Attachments, Roles, and Social Support." In P. Baltes and O. Brim (eds.), *Life Span Development and Behavior.* Vol. 3. Orlando, Fla.: Academic Press, 1980.

Kanner, A. D., Coyne, J. C., Schaefer, C., and Lazarus, R. S. "Comparison of Two Models of Stress Measurement: Daily Hassles and Uplifts Versus Major Life Events." *Journal of Behavioral Medicine,* 1981, *4,* 1-39.

Kaplan, H. B. (ed.). *Psychosocial Stress: Trends in Theory and Research.* Orlando, Fla.: Academic Press, 1983.

Karasek, R. A. "Job Demands, Job Decision Latitude, and Mental Strain: Implications for Job Redesign." *Administrative Science Quarterly,* 1979, *24,* 285-308.

Karasek, R. A., and others. "Job Decision Latitude, Job Demands, and Cardiovascular Disease: A Prospective Study of Swedish Men." *American Journal of Public Health,* 1981, *71,* 694-705.

Kasl, S. V., and Cooper, C. L. (eds.). *Stress and Health: Issues in Research Methodology.* New York: Wiley, 1987.

Katz, D., and Kahn, R. *The Social Psychology of Organizations.* (2nd ed.) New York: Wiley, 1978.

Klitzman, S., House, J., and Israel, B. "Work Stress, Nonwork Stress and Health." Forthcoming.

Lawler, E. E. *High-Involvement Management: Participative Strategies for Improving Organizational Performance.* San Francisco: Jossey-Bass, 1986.

Lazarus, R. *Psychological Stress and the Coping Process.* New York: McGraw-Hill, 1966.

Leighton, D. C., and others. "The Character of Danger: Psychiatric Symptoms in Selected Communities." In D. C. Leighton and others (eds.), *The Stirling County Study of Psychiatric Disorder and Sociocultural Environment.* Vol. 3. New York: Basic Books, 1963.

Levi, L. *Preventing Work Stress.* Reading, Mass.: Addison-Wesley, 1981.

Lewis, F. M. "The Concept of Control: A Typology and Health-

Related Variables." *Advances in Health Education and Promotion*, 1987, *2*, 277–309.

Likert, R. *The Human Organization: Its Management and Value.* New York: McGraw-Hill, 1967.

McGrath, J. (ed.). *Social and Psychological Factors in Stress.* New York: Holt, Rinehart & Winston, 1970.

Margolis, B., Kroes, W., and Quinn, R. "Job Stress: An Unlisted Occupational Hazard." *Journal of Occupational Medicine*, 1974, *16*, 659–661.

Menaghan, E. "Individual Coping Efforts: Moderators of the Relationship Between Life Stress and Mental Health Outcomes." In B. H. Kaplan (ed.), *Psychosocial Stress: Trends in Theory and Research.* Orlando, Fla.: Academic Press, 1983.

Mitchell, R. E., and Trickett, E. J. "Social Networks as Mediators of Social Support and Health." *Community Mental Health*, 1980, *16*, 27–44.

Norbeck, J. S., Lindsey, A. M., and Carrieri, V. L. "Further Development of the Norbeck Social Support Questionnaire: Normative Data and Validity Testing." *Nursing Research*, 1983, *32*, 4–9.

Payne, R., and Jones, J. "Measurement and Methodological Issues in Social Support." In S. Kasl and C. Cooper (eds.), *Stress and Health: Issues in Research Methodology.* New York: Wiley, 1987.

Pearlin, L. L. "Role Strains and Personal Stress." In H. B. Kaplan (ed.), *Psychosocial Stress: Trends in Theory and Research.* Orlando, Fla.: Academic Press, 1983.

Pearlin, L. L., and Anesheusel, C. A. "Coping and Social Supports: Their Functions and Applications." In L. Aiken and D. Mechanic (eds.), *Applications of Social Science to Clinical Medicine and Health Policy.* New Brunswick, N.J.: Rutgers University Press, 1986.

Peters, M., and Robinson, V. "The Origins and Status of Action Research." *Journal of Applied Behavioral Science*, 1984, *20*, 113–124.

Rook, K. S. "The Negative Side of Social Interaction: Impact on Psychological Well-Being." *Journal of Personality and Social Psychology*, 1984, *46*, 1097–1108.

Selye, H. *The Stress of Life.* New York: McGraw-Hill, 1956.

Spector, P. "Perceived Control by Employees: A Meta-Analysis of

Studies Concerning Autonomy and Participation at Work." *Human Relations*, 1986, *11*, 1005–1016.

Stokols, D., and others. "Traffic Congestion, Type A Behavior, and Stress." *Journal of Applied Psychology*, 1978, *63*, 467–480.

Susman, G., and Evered, R. "An Assessment of the Scientific Merits of Action Research." *Administrative Science Quarterly*, 1978, *23*, 582–603.

Sutton, R., and Kahn, R. L. "Prediction, Understanding, and Control as Antidotes to Organizational Stress." In J. Lorsch (ed.), *Handbook of Organizational Behavior*. Cambridge, Mass.: Harvard University Press, 1984.

Tannenbaum, A. S. *Control in Organizations*. New York: McGraw-Hill, 1968.

Thoits, P. G. "Dimensions of Life Events That Influence Psychological Distress: An Evaluation and Synthesis of the Literature." In H. B. Kaplan (ed.), *Psychosocial Stress: Trends in Theory and Research*. Orlando, Fla.: Academic Press, 1983.

von Bertalanffy, L. *General Systems Theory*. New York: Braziller, 1968.

Wagner, B., Compas, B., and Howell, D. "Daily and Major Life Events: A Test of an Integrative Model of Psychosocial Stress." *American Journal of Community Psychology*, 1988, *16*, 189–205.

Walker, K. W. "Worker's Participation in Management: Problems, Practice, and Prospects." *International Institute of Labour Studies Bulletin*, 1974, *12* (entire issue).

Zimmerman, M. A. "Empowerment: Forging New Perspectives in Mental Health." In J. Rappaport and E. Seidman (eds.), *The Handbook of Community Psychology*. New York: Plenum, forthcoming.

Chapter 10

Sandra K. Joos
David H. Hickam

How Health Professionals Influence Health Behavior: Patient-Provider Interaction and Health Care Outcomes

Understanding the process of interaction between patients and providers is necessary to help health professionals and patients communicate effectively. Effective communication facilitates decision making and improves patient understanding, satisfaction, and cooperation. Unfortunately, however, disagreement between patients and providers on the nature of health problems, appropriate treatment, and expected outcomes is common (Starfield and others, 1981; Woolley, Kane, Hughes, and Wright, 1978; Zimmerman, 1988), as is lack of provider awareness of patient attitudes, concerns, and perspectives (Holmes and others, 1987; Strull, Lo, and Charles, 1984; Potts, Weinberger, and Brandt, 1984). These discrepancies in perceptions and expectations have a negative effect on patient satisfaction (Woolley, Kane, Hughes, and Wright, 1978), compliance (Sideris and others, 1986), and resolution of problems (Romm, Hulka, and Mayo, 1976; Starfield and others, 1981). Moreover, providers often lack adequate interviewing skills, overestimate the amount of information they provide, underestimate the amount of information patients want (Strull, Lo, and Charles, 1984; Waitzkin, 1985), and have difficulty detecting and resolving compliance problems (Brody, 1980). Patients, in turn, are often reluctant to express

216

their desires or to request information. Thus, poor health care outcomes may result from providers' failure to elicit and provide information in a way that will produce desired changes in patient attitudes, commitment to treatment, and behavior and from patients' inability to relay their expectations for care and information to their providers.

Despite the importance of patient-provider interaction to the delivery of health care, study of this topic is in its infancy. Most research is descriptive and observational in nature, and links to theory are often tenuous and after-the-fact. Moreover, much of the research on interaction and communication between patients and health care providers has focused on physicians. Considerably less attention has been directed to other health care professionals (Zimmerman, 1988; Rorer, Tucker, and Blake, 1988; Swain and Steckel, 1981). The goals of this chapter are to provide a brief historical overview of models of patient-provider relationships, describe current social-psychological perspectives on patient-provider interaction, review the observational and experimental research on patient-provider communication and health care outcomes, and discuss this research in light of these frameworks. Although the "providers" referred to in the literature are usually physicians, the discussion is relevant to other health professionals.

Historical Overview of Models
of Patient-Provider Relationships

Because comprehensive reviews have been published elsewhere (Bloom and Wilson, 1979; DiMatteo and DiNicola, 1982), only a brief historical overview of theories of patient-provider relationships will be provided here. The earliest formulations of interpersonal influence in the medical setting emerged from sociology. Henderson (1935) uses the concept of the *social system* to analyze the doctor-patient relationship. He describes human relationships as patterns that stem from cultural expectations about the social roles of group members, in which the fundamental process of behavior is communication. Parsons (1951) extends this idea further in his study of medicine as a major subsystem of our society. Parsons describes the medical subsystem as one in which the roles, obligations, and privileges of patients and physicians are clearly defined and learned by socialization. The physician's role as a professional is characterized by a high degree of technical skill and knowledge, objectivity, and commitment to the welfare of the patient. In their professional role, physicians legitimize patients' entry into the *sick role,* one that exempts patients from normal obligations and responsibilities. Because the sick role is undesirable and socially disruptive, patients are expected to seek technically competent help, to be motivated to get well, and to cooperate fully with the doctor. A central feature of this view of the doctor-patient relationship is asymmetry. The doctor possesses professional role attributes and greater technical competence, while the patient is passive and dependent on the expert doctor. According to this model, the mutual role expectations of doctors and patients are the primary influence on behavior and are learned as part of socialization into the culture. Thus, doctors give treatment advice to patients on the basis of their expertise, objectivity, and concern, and patients are expected to be motivated to cooperate. Patients who fail to cooperate are considered socially deviant.

Critics of Parson's model argue that it presents a narrow and unrealistic stereotype of what should happen rather than reflecting what actually does happen. Szasz and Hollender (1956) propose that Parson's model of the doctor-patient relationship is only applicable to emergency situations in which the patient is helpless (such as surgery or an accident) or to situations in which decisions about treatment for acute disorders are necessary. They characterize the mode of interaction in these situations as *activity-passivity* and *guidance-cooperation,* respectively. To broaden Parson's concept of the patient-provider relationship, they propose a third model of *mutual participation* that is based on equality between doctor and patient. They argue that this model of the doctor-patient relationship, in which the patient carries out the treatment program and "the physician helps the patient to help himself" (p. 587), is more appropriate for the management of chronic illnesses. Szasz and Hollender predict that problems between doctor and patient will arise when the type of relationship employed is not appropriate to the illness and needs of the patient. For care to be most effective, modes of interaction should correspond to the varying nature of patients' illnesses.

Freidson (1970) also departs from Parsons by viewing the doctor and patient as members of two distinct social systems rather than one homeostatic system. According to Freidson, the doctor-patient relationship is characterized by *conflict* between the professional who "expects patients to accept what he recommends on his terms" and "patients who seek services on their own terms" (1961, p. 171). He argues that a *lay referral system* exerts the greatest influence on patients' opinions about the nature of the problem and what to do about it. This system consists of friends, relatives, and professionals, and the physician is but one of many consultants and sources of diagnosis, treatment, and referral. As a result, patients' expectations may be quite different from those of the physician, and conflict will occur. Interaction in treatment requires the negotiation of conflict between these separate perspectives and understandings (Freidson, 1970, p. 322).

Current Perspectives on Patient-Provider Interaction

Most current theories of patient-provider relationships integrate social and psychological perspectives on interpersonal influence to explain how the characteristics and behavior of others affect a person's attitudes, feelings, and behavior. Social-psychological approaches address various aspects of the patient-provider relationship that influence behavior and outcomes of care. These aspects include the clarity, openness, and effectiveness of patient-provider communication; the quality of the interpersonal relationship; the mutual understanding and recognition of patients' and providers' attitudes, beliefs, expectations, and desires; and awareness of external social factors (organizational setting, patient's socioeconomic status) that influence the patient-provider relationship and behavior (DiMatteo and DiNicola, 1982, pp. 25–26). Psychosocial perspectives that may be especially useful for understanding patient-provider communication are those relating to cognition and information processing, interpersonal interaction, conflict between patients and providers, and social influence. These approaches correspond to the principal factors that appear to affect the quality and effectiveness of communication between patients and providers: cognitive and socioemotional processes in the interaction, congruence between patients' and providers' attitudes and expectations, and strategies utilized to influence behavior (Rodin, 1982; Shuy, 1983).

Cognition and Information Processing. Patients need and desire information regarding diagnosis, etiology, and treatment, and a fundamental purpose of communication in the health care setting is to transmit information. However, the literature shows that a large proportion of patients do not understand and are unable to recall what they are told. Moreover, patients are less satisfied with their care and less likely to adhere to treatment recommendations when understanding and recall are impaired (Ley, 1983, 1986). Theories of cognition point to a number of factors that may interfere with patients' understanding and recall of information in the health care setting. First, oral and written information is often laden with jargon and vocabulary that is too complex for the majority of patients. Second, situational influences such as drug effects, anxiety, illness, and other distractions affect patients' ability to attend to, understand, and recall information. Third, because patients and providers often do not share the same background knowledge and underlying assumptions, their ability to elicit information from and provide it to each other is hampered. Research on cognition and learning shows that providers can enhance the understandability and recall of written and oral information by using shorter words and sentences, presenting the most important information first and stressing its importance, using explicit categories, employing specific rather than general instructions, and summarizing and checking for comprehension of major points (Ley, 1986; Hunt and MacLeod, 1979).

Interpersonal Interaction. Good interpersonal and relationship-building skills are fundamental to the ability of providers to establish rapport, transmit information, elicit patients' expectations, and influence patients' behavior. Research concerning the qualities of effective therapists and therapeutic interaction stems from the work of Carl Rogers (1957). Rogers was an early advocate of a nondirective, client-centered approach to therapy in which patients were helped to verbalize their perceptions and learn more about themselves. By analyzing the behaviors of effective and ineffective therapists (those whose patients' self-concepts did or did not improve), Rogers (1957) identifies specific behaviors that could be communicated to others. Empathy, genuineness, and acceptance of the client are the core conditions Rogers defines as necessary for positive therapeutic change.

Building on Rogers's work, Kagan and colleagues conducted a systematic research program to identify additional interpersonal skills and develop techniques to teach them (Kagan, 1979). Their Interpersonal Process Recall (IPR) method is based on a theoretical perspective that views "behavior as part of a complex interpersonal and intrapersonal process" (p. 469). From this perspective, the attitudes we believe another person has about us are the most influential factors in determining how we will respond to that person and our degree of interpersonal comfort. The key strategies taught in the IPR method are (1) specific response modes that providers can use with patients (for example, exploratory and open-ended responses to elicit a patient's concerns and point of view, listening responses that clarify and paraphrase, and feeling and labeling responses that focus on the patient's affect, attitudes, and behavior), (2) awareness of personal stereotypes and prejudices against certain types of patients, (3) understanding the value of exploring interpersonal issues and patient concerns, and (4) understanding the range of behavior styles that can be used in interpersonal interactions. The IPR method has been widely applied in the training of students and practitioners in the health professions, and it has proven to be a reliable and effective technique for enhancing interpersonal interaction skills.

Conflict Between Patient and Provider Perspectives. Patients' perceptions of illness, prevention, and treatment are primary forces in their behavior, and patients' perceptions may differ substantially from those of their providers. Kleinman (1980) formulated the concept of "explanatory models" (EMs) to analyze problems in clinical communication caused by differences in patients' and providers' perspectives. Explanatory models are the notions about an illness and its treatment that seek to provide explanations for questions of etiology, symptoms, and pathophysiology; degree of severity; type of sick role (acute, chronic); and treatment. Kleinman hypothesizes that the efficacy of clinical communication and health care outcomes will be a function of the extent to which there are discrepancies between patients' and providers' explanatory models. To facilitate disclosure of patients' explanations of their problems, Kleinman suggests that providers ask patients directly about what they think has caused their problem, how severe they think it is, whether its course will be long or short, what concerns them most about it, what difficulties it has posed for them, what kind of treatment they think they should receive, and what results they hope to receive from treatment (p. 106).

Similarly, Leventhal (1985) proposes using a systems approach to identify and assess basic categories of belief that play a key role in guiding patient and provider behavior. According to Leventhal (p. 559), "the encounter is influenced by and influences both the patient's and practitioner's view of the disease and the treatment, their views of one another, and their perception as to how the other views them." Patients' behavior can be predicted by understanding their view of the problem and the coping strategies and appraisal processes they use. Moreover, a patient's system of beliefs changes over time in response to the natural history of the illness, the life course of the patient and family, and historic trends of the culture.

The perspectives advocated by Kleinman and Leventhal constitute a "patient-centered," as opposed to a "provider-centered," approach to care. Patient-centered care emphasizes the patient's perspective and the need to elicit and respond to patients' definitions of their problems, their goals and expectations for outcome, and their requests for information and treatment (Lazare and Eisenthal, 1979; Levenstein and others, 1986). Because patient and provider agendas may differ and patients may make excessive or inappropriate requests, providers must work with patients to prioritize and negotiate requests and develop a mutually acceptable therapeutic plan (Lazare, Eisenthal, and Frank, 1979; Quill, 1983). Strategies for conflict resolution and negotiation include the related processes of persuasion, education, and mutual problem solving.

Negotiation should result in a situation of mutual influence in which the power of both parties is recognized, the patient receives what he or she believes is needed, and the patient accepts what the physician believes to be effective treatment. Even though negotiation is a mutual process, the provider's role requires that he or she take the initiative to determine the nature of the conflict and establish an atmosphere that facilitates negotiation. An atmosphere for negotiation can be fostered by using interpersonal skills, such as communicating an attitude of respect, understanding, acceptance and openness, and establishing expertise by thoroughness and providing information about the problem.

Social Influence. In the course of interaction with patients, providers have the opportunity to exercise a variety of types of social power by which they can influence patients' attitudes, motivations, and behavior. Theories of social power and influence provide a unifying framework for understanding how information delivery, interpersonal skills, and patient-provider conflict affect patients' attitudes, behavior, and health care outcomes. The sources of social power that physicians and other providers may use to influence patients are *expert, legitimate, coercive, reward, informational,* and *referent* power (Raven, 1982). Expert power and legitimate power are based on the patient's acceptance of the provider's credibility, technical knowledge, and formal right to make health-related demands. Coercive power and reward power are based on the provider's ability to mediate punishments and rewards. However, because expert and legitimate power may increase personal distance between provider and patient and because coercive power and reward power rely on external incentives to motivate patients, Rodin and Janis (1982) predict that these sources of influence may be useful only in the short term and will not produce enduring attitude and behavior change.

Informational power is based on the content and persuasiveness of the communication and the cognitive changes that result from the information itself; in this sense, it is largely independent of the personal social influence of the provider. In contrast, referent power is based on a patient's identification with the provider as a person like herself or himself in some respect and feelings of communality, security, and trust. Informational power can be invoked by using techniques to enhance the persuasiveness of the message and to improve information delivery, understanding, and recall similar to those that were described in the earlier section on Cognition and Information Processing. Techniques to establish referent power include emphasizing the patient's well-being as a mutual goal, giving positive feedback, and accepting feedback. Skillful delivery and interpretation of verbal and nonverbal communication are important for implementing referent power and creating its motivating effect (DiMatteo, 1982). The provider also can develop motivating power by encouraging patients to disclose their attributions about the cause(s) of their troubles, beliefs about treatment and recovery, and expectations about the roles of patient and provider and then responding to their views with interest and concern (Rodin, 1982). By responding to patients' self-disclosures with understanding, encouragement, and acceptance, providers enhance patients' self-esteem and lead them to perceive the provider as likeable, benevolent, and caring. A provider who shares, or at least acknowledges and accepts, the patients' beliefs, attitudes, and values is most likely to have referent power for patients (Rodin and Janis, 1982)

Informational power and referent power are probably the most effective sources of social influence for inducing long-term attitude and behavior change because they are hypothesized to promote *internalization* of treatment recommendations and to increase the patient's sense of control and personal influence over outcomes. Internalization is the propensity to carry out a behavior in the absence of the source of influence and involves the patient's acceptance of health information and incorporation of it into his or her own belief system (Kelman, 1958). It is the most enduring response to social influence, and it is essential for any health behavior that requires long-term voluntary action by the patient (Rodin and Janis, 1982).

Rodin and Janis (1982, p. 39) suggest that the factors that promote internalization also function "to increase patients' feelings of choice and control because they perceive themselves to be acting on the basis of internal, self-motivated norms and goals." Informational power and referent power convey respect for patient integrity and can also lead to cognitive changes that result in personal acceptance of the recommendation, with no need for direct surveillance or continuing contact with the provider to ensure compliance. Developing referent power may lead to a two-way communication and influence process and greater involvement of patients in decision making. Likewise, research has shown that informational power affects the extent to which individuals attribute causality to themselves, and greater feelings of personal responsibility increase behavioral commitment and facilitate adherence (Rodin and Janis, 1982; also, see Chapter Five on Attribution Theory). Although informational power is not likely to be effective when patients do not understand the content of the message, when they are too anxious or distracted to attend to the message, or when the message arouses such fear that defensive mechanisms result in rejection of information, appropriate information about available alternatives offers patients some choice and may enhance feelings of self-efficacy. Informational and referent power may interact so that providing information needed for behavior change and adherence to treatment recommendations is likely to be more effective after referent power has been established (Rodin and Janis, 1982). Moreover, the reassurance and interpersonal contact generated by exercising referent power may moderate the impact of fear-inducing information or relieve anxiety and enhance patients' ability to attend to information they receive (Raven, 1982).

Table 10.1 summarizes the primary behaviors to enhance communication that are derived from the four social-psychological perspectives on patient-provider interaction and also illustrates that their features overlap. It suggests that patients respond positively to providers whose affect is concerned and caring and that information giving is enhanced by a positive emotional atmosphere. Furthermore, providers whose affective and interpersonal skills are good will be most able to use cognitive and social influence strategies for changing behavior. Finally, information delivery, interpersonal interaction, and ability to influence behavior are enhanced by awareness of the patient's attitudes, perspectives, and expectations.

Applications: Research on Patient-Provider Interaction and Health Care Outcomes

This section describes observational and experimental research that applies conceptual frameworks for patient-provider interaction.

Table 10.1. Behaviors Suggested by Social-Psychological Perspectives on Patient-Provider Interaction.

1. *Cognition and Information Processing*
   Provide written information
   Use shorter words and sentences
   Present important information first; stress its importance
   Categorize, summarize, check comprehension of information
   Give specific rather than general instructions

2. *Interpersonal Interaction*
   Convey empathy, warmth, concern, genuineness, sincerity, respect, acceptance
   Use exploratory and open-ended questioning skills to elicit and facilitate patient's expression of concerns and point of view
   Use listening skills to clarify, paraphrase, and check understanding
   Be aware of personal reaction to certain patients

3. *Conflict Resolution and Negotiaton*
   Establish atmosphere for negotiation (provide information; communicate respect, understanding, acceptance)
   Elicit patient views about problem, treatment, and outcome
   Elicit patient requests, desires, and expectations
   Prioritize and negotiate requests
   Develop a mutually acceptable plan

4. *Social Influence*
   Develop informational power: use techniques to enhance persuasiveness, cognition, and information processing
   Develop referent power: emphasize patient's well-being as mutual goal; elicit patient's views; respond to patient's disclosures with acknowledgment, interest, concern, acceptance; disclose own views; give positive feedback and accept feedback

While none of the studies was designed explicitly to test a single theory of patient-provider communication, their results are useful for evaluating the applicability of various theoretical perspectives to optimal patient care.

Most research on patient and provider interaction consists of observational studies of the association between patient-provider communication behaviors and a variety of health care outcomes. The few experimental studies have examined the effects of interventions to enhance patient-provider interaction and health care outcomes.

Researchers have used many methods for measuring patient-provider interaction. These can be broadly grouped into methods that attempt to categorize the factual *content* of information communicated by physicians in an encounter and methods that analyze the *process* or function of patient and provider behaviors during an encounter. Most measures of the content of communication have been developed specifically for particular investigations (Bertakis, 1977). Measures of process include Roter's (1977) modification of Bales's Interactional Process Analysis method (Bales, 1950) and Stiles's (1978) Verbal Response Mode system. Interaction coding methods are labor-intensive and expensive to use. Further, most systems merely count the frequency of utterances reflecting specific content or process rather than analyzing the sequence and flow of communication.

The diversity of measurement methods makes comparison and synthesis of results across studies difficult. Because an in-depth discussion of the relative advantages and disadvantages of the various interaction analysis methods is beyond the scope of this chapter, interested readers should refer to other sources. See, for example, Inui, Carter, Kukull, and Haigh (1982); Inui and Carter (1985); and Wasserman and Inui (1983).

Observational Studies. Several recent reviews have summarized research on patient-provider interaction and health care outcomes (Hall, Roter, and Rand, 1981; Roter, Hall, and Katz, 1988; Pendleton, 1983; Inui and Carter, 1985). Measures of communication and outcome, as well as the subjects and settings, vary greatly across studies. Nevertheless, it is clear that both physician and patient communication behaviors are meaningfully related to outcomes such as satisfaction, compliance, and problem resolution.

The most comprehensive review of observational studies is a meta-analysis conducted by Hall, Roter, and Katz (1988) of forty-one independent studies in which the relations between provider (physician) behaviors and health care outcomes were examined. Across studies, they found that the amount of information given by physicians was strongly associated with greater patient recall or understanding and satisfaction and moderately associated with patient compliance. Question asking by physicians was not related to satisfaction and was negatively associated with recall or understanding and compliance. Physician interpersonal competence was strongly correlated with patient satisfaction, whereas technical competence was only moderately correlated with satisfaction. Physician "partnership-building" behavior to enlist patient input was positively associated with recall or understanding, satisfaction, and compliance; however, physician behavior that allowed patients to take a controlling or dominant role was negatively related to compliance.

Patients' behaviors during the consultation also are related to health care outcomes. Research has shown that level of satisfaction is greater when patients explain their history and symptoms in their own words early in the visit ("patient exposition") (Putnam, Stiles, Jacob, and James, 1985), provide more information (Inui and others, 1982), and express agreement with the plan (Freeman, Negrete, Davis, and Korsch, 1971; Eisenthal, Koopman, and Lazare, 1983). Satisfaction is lower when patients express tension or anxiety or use assertive verbal behaviors (Inui, Carter, Kukull, and Haigh, 1982). Level of compliance with treatment recommendations is higher when patients make suggestions and lower when patients make many requests for clarification (Carter, Inui, Kukull, and Haigh, 1982). Finally, when physicians respond to patient requests and when patient and provider agree about the problem and treatment, patient evaluations of care are more positive, cooperation with treatment is better, and health status outcomes are improved (Bass and others, 1986; Eisenthal, Koopman, and Lazare, 1983; Like and Zyzanski, 1987; Romm, Hulka, and Mayo, 1976; Sideris and others, 1986; Starfield and others, 1981; Uhlmann, Inui, Pecoraro, and Carter, 1988; Woolley, Kane, Hughes, and Wright, 1978).

In general, the findings of observational studies are consistent with the theoretical perspectives of information processing, interpersonal interaction, conflict resolution, and social influence. These studies suggest that there is a positive effect on patient care outcomes when the provider establishes rapport, encourages patients to express their concerns and point of view, and provides information. Good interpersonal skills facilitate these tasks and are related to improved patient satisfaction and compliance and outcomes of care.

Experimental Interventions. Experimental interventions to improve the quality of patient-provider communication have used two strategies: educating patients about how to formulate their questions and elicit information from providers, and teaching providers more effective interaction and communication skills. This review is limited to studies of intervention in which the impact upon both patient-provider behavior *and* patient care outcomes were assessed.

Several studies have evaluated the efficacy of interventions to teach patients how to obtain the information they want and to participate more actively in their own care. Roter (1977) developed an intervention to increase patient activation, enhance qualitative and quantitative components of patient-provider interaction, and improve patient satisfaction and compliance with appointment keeping. She hypothesized that if patients were helped to formulate questions for their physicians and encouraged to ask these questions early in the visit, the opportunity for a bilateral pattern of interaction would be created. The experimental intervention was a ten-minute session with a health educator who used a question-asking protocol to help patients identify and write questions for the doctor about their illness and treatment. The educator provided encouragement, support, and approval for asking the questions by saying: "We think that asking questions is an important part of coming to the clinic. This is the only way patients can really find out about their illness" (Roter, 1977, p. 298). Patients in the placebo intervention were given information about the use and availability of emergency and specialty services. Experimental group patients asked significantly more direct questions of their physicians, even though the average length of visits did not differ between the groups. Patients and physicians in the experimental group expressed significantly more anxiety and anger than those in the placebo group. Although experimental group patients were less satisfied with their visits, they had significantly higher locus of control scores and appointment-keeping ratios over a four-month follow-up period. In the experimental group, higher levels of patient anger and anxiety were associated with better appointment compliance, while the opposite associations were observed in the placebo group.

Greenfield and colleagues (Greenfield, Kaplan, and Ware,

1985; Greenfield and others, 1988) also sought to increase patients' information-seeking skills and participation in medical care decisions. Their intervention was a twenty-minute session in which a health educator reviewed with patients their medical records, a treatment algorithm that identified decisions relevant to the care of their condition, and behavior strategies to increase their involvement. The educator helped patients identify options regarding their care, reviewed techniques for overcoming barriers to discussion, and rehearsed specific questions and negotiation issues by using a standard script to reinforce assertive behaviors. To reduce the potential for conflict, the specific behavioral strategies to increase participation were nonadversarial in nature. Patients in the control group received information about their disease. In a study of patients with peptic ulcer disease, length of the encounter did not differ between treatment groups, nor did patients in the experimental group ask more questions after the intervention. However, in the experimental group, physicians made fewer directing and controlling statements, the expression of affect and opinion sharing between patients and physicians increased, and patients' verbal participation and preference for active involvement in decision making increased. More active patient involvement did not increase tension, perhaps because patients in the intervention group used indirect strategies more often than direct questions to alert physicians to their needs for more information. Significantly fewer patients in the experimental group reported role or physical limitations several weeks after the intervention, and greater patient involvement was associated with fewer functional limitations. A study with diabetes patients obtained similar findings. In addition, higher levels of patient involvement were significantly correlated with better postintervention glycemic control, and levels of functional limitation, glycemic control, and perceived health status were significantly improved in the experimental group (Greenfield and others, 1988).

The conclusions of Roter (1977) and Greenfield and colleagues (Greenfield, Kaplan, and Ware, 1985; Greenfield and others, 1988) were similar. Roter suggests that patients in the intervention condition developed a more internal self-view as a result of increased question asking and that this perception of internal control resulted in improved appointment keeping. Likewise, Greenfield and colleagues found that greater patient participation and sharing of information between patient and physician were associated with better outcomes. They suggest that their intervention to increase patient participation might have improved outcomes of care by enhancing patients' feelings of mastery and control and heightening their motivation to improve self-management of their disease. While the researchers did not measure patients' feelings of control, they did find that patients' preferences for active participation increased as a result of their intervention. This hypothesized sequence of events is consistent with the effects predicted by social influence theories.

These studies show that patient education interventions can influence patient-physician interaction and improve patient care outcomes. An alternate strategy is to improve physicians' communication skills. Changing physician behavior may be a more efficient use of resources in the long run and is consistent with the physician's role and responsibility to establish an atmosphere conducive to negotiation. The effect of educational interventions with physicians on their behavior and patient care outcomes was evaluated in the following studies.

Because patients forget much of what the doctors tell them and satisfaction is greater when patients understand and remember the information they are given, Bertakis (1977) conducted an intervention with physicians to increase the amount of information patients retain. At the end of an appointment, physicians in an experimental group asked fifty of their patients to restate the information they had given them. They then gave patients feedback concerning their understanding of what they had been told, reinforced important points, and gave patients an opportunity to ask questions. This usually took no longer than five minutes. Physicians in the control group received no special instructions. Although audiotapes showed that the total amount of information physicians gave did not differ between groups, patients in the experimental group retained significantly more of the information physicians gave them and reported greater satisfaction with the visit than did patients in the control group.

Inui, Yourtee, and Williamson (1976) studied the effect of a physician tutorial on the management and education of patients with hypertension. Physicians in the experimental group received a one- to two-hour tutorial on how to identify and to alter noncompliance. Physicians were advised to spend more time eliciting patients' perceptions and attitudes about hypertension and less time on historical and physical examinations to search for complications. The Health Belief Model (See Chapter Three) was used to discuss the relationship of compliance to patient ideas concerning the seriousness of the illness, susceptibility to complications, and efficacy of treatment. Physicians in the control group were simply told that the medical care of some of their patients was being reviewed. Before the tutorial, experimental and control physicians' behavior and their patients' characteristics were similar. Afterward, tutored physicians' self-reports and chart notes indicated that they spent more time educating patients and discussing their medications than did the nontutored physicians. Patients of tutored physicians were significantly more knowledgeable about hypertension; had more appropriate attitudes about the disease, its complications, and therapy; and were more likely to adhere to their medication regimen and to have adequately controlled blood pressure.

Sideris and others (1986) tested the effect of a behavioral skills program to enhance patient compliance with instructions. Physicians in an experimental group were taught skills for explaining the diagnosis, treatment objectives, and prognosis; providing written and oral instructions; checking comprehension; and conveying positive affect. Physicians in a comparison group received no special instruction. Those who attended the educational program displayed more effective behavior skills and higher concordance with patients about what information had been communicated. Patient compliance was significantly greater among patients of physicians who received the educational program.

On the basis of their observational studies, which showed that interaction patterns involving patient exposition early in the visit and physician explanation at the conclusion were consistently related to patient care outcomes, Putnam, Stiles, Jacob, and James (1988) taught eleven resident physicians how to use listening skills to encourage patients to describe their concerns freely and how to give objective information about illness and treatment. Eight residents in a control group received no training. Audiotapes showed that interviewing behaviors of experimental and control residents did not differ before training. After training, the frequency of physician verbal encouragement and patient exposition increased significantly in the experimental group, without changing the length of interviews, but the training had no effect on patient satisfaction or compliance or on symptom improvement. Methodological problems (for example, small sample sizes, low response variability, insensitivity of the outcome measures) leave unanswered the question of whether training physicians to increase patient exposition and physician explanation affects patient care outcomes, even though the intervention had a sound basis in prior research.

Maiman and others (1988) evaluated a continuing medical education program to teach pediatricians to use simple informational and motivational techniques for improving mothers' compliance. Techniques for increasing adherence included expressing sincere concern and empathy, improving information provision, simplifying the regimen, assessing and modifying health beliefs with components of the Health Belief Model, eliciting and meeting mothers' expectations, and monitoring regimen noncompliance. Compared to physicians in the control group, physicians in the intervention group used more compliance-enhancing behaviors and their patients were more likely to comply with medications and follow-up appointments.

Finally, Ockene and others (1988a, 1988b) examined whether teaching physicians counseling skills affected the smoking behavior of ambulatory clinic patients. Resident physicians were randomly assigned to one of three interventions: (1) simply advising patients to quit smoking, (2) counseling on smoking cessation using patient-centered techniques, and (3) counseling plus prescribing nicotine chewing gum. Counseling training emphasized guided questioning; providing information; eliciting feelings regarding desire, resources, and ability to cease smoking; and giving feedback of relevant information to patients. The intervention was designed to improve physicians' ability to help patients identify skills and resources needed to stop smoking and develop confidence in their ability to do so. With practice, the counseling typically required only four to seven minutes during a patient encounter. The counseling skills of physicians in the training group improved significantly, and at the six-month follow-up a greater proportion of patients who had received counseling (with or without a prescription for nicotine chewing gum) reported they had attempted to stop smoking or had actually stopped.

The physician interventions in these studies varied greatly in their intensity, ranging from simply asking physicians to check patients' understanding of information to comprehensive training programs that addressed all of the major factors in provider-patient communication. Nevertheless, all of the interventions produced changes in physician behavior, and all but one also had a measurable effect on outcomes of care. Only three of the six interventions specifically included interpersonal skills training (Maiman and others, 1988; Putnam, Stiles, Jacob, and James, 1988; and Sideris and others, 1986). However, the content of all of the interventions incorporated information-giving skills, and all promoted conflict resolution by encouraging physicians to elicit the patient's perspective. For example, in the process of checking comprehension by eliciting and responding to patients' understanding of what they had been told, physicians who participated in Bertakis's (1977) intervention no doubt became aware of and had to address differences between their own and their patients' perceptions. More direct approaches used in other interventions to elicit patient perspectives might further enhance physician awareness of patients' perspectives. According to Rodin and Janis (1982), the process of eliciting patient perspectives, responding to them, and resolving differences generates referent power and internalization of recommendations and increases patients' feelings of participation, involvement, and self-efficacy. Internalization of treatment plans and perceptions of greater control result in greater satisfaction, better adherence to recommendations, and improved functional and health status.

The studies of interventions with patients appear to confirm that increased patient involvement in the encounter changes physicians' behavior, augments patients' feelings of control and preferences for active participation, and improves health care outcomes. Interventions with physicians also changed the process and content of patient-physician interaction and in most cases improved health care outcomes. However, because none of these studies actually measured changes in patients' perceptions of control and participation, it is not clear that these feelings are a mechanism by which provider behavior influences health care outcomes. Future studies should measure how patients' perceptions change as a consequence of interventions with physicians. The duration of effect and the relative costs and effectiveness of interventions with patients versus physicians should also be topics of future research.

Conclusion

This chapter has reviewed current theories of patient-provider interaction and communication, with an emphasis on psychosocial perspectives in four areas: cognition and information processing, interpersonal interaction, social influence, and conflict between patient and provider perspectives. These four perspectives overlap and combine to form the conceptual basis for a theoretically sound and empirically effective set of behaviors for use by providers and patients.

While most published research has focused on physicians as health care providers, the concepts and findings discussed here have definite potential for testing and application in health care practice involving other professionals. They can apply to, among others, nurses, dietitians, dentists, and occupational and physical therapists.

As indicated by the historical overview of models of patient-provider relationships, theories of patient-provider interaction and influence reflect the dominant health concerns of a given time period and tend to evolve in concert with the structure and content of health care interactions. The theory, research, and practice implications of models of patient-provider interaction must therefore be continually refined and examined in terms of their suitability and potential for improving health care process and outcomes.

References

Bales, R. F. *Interactional Process Analysis.* Reading, Mass.: Addison-Wesley, 1950.

Bass, M. J., and others. "The Physician's Actions and the Outcomes of Illness in Family Practice." *Journal of Family Practice,* 1986, *23,* 43–47.

Bertakis, K. D. "A Method of Increasing Patient Retention and Satisfaction." *Journal of Family Practice,* 1977, *5,* 217–222.

Bloom, S. W., and Wilson, R. N. "Patient-Practitioner Relationships." In H. E. Freeman, S. Levine, and L. G. Reeder (eds.), *Handbook of Medical Sociology.* (3rd ed.) Englewood Cliffs, N.J.: Prentice-Hall, 1979.

Brody, D. S. "Physician Recognition of Behavioral, Psychological, and Social Aspects of Medical Care." *Archives of Internal Medicine,* 1980, *140,* 1286–1289.

Carter, W. B., Inui, T. S., Kukull, W. A., and Haigh, V. "Outcome-Based Doctor-Patient Interaction Analysis. II. Identifying Effective Provider and Patient Behavior." *Medical Care,* 1982, *20,* 550–566.

Davis, M. S. "Variation in Patients' Compliance with Doctors' Orders: Medical Practice and Doctor-Patient Interaction." *Psychiatry in Medicine,* 1971, *2,* 31–54.

DiMatteo, M. R. "New Perspectives on a Science of the Art of Medicine." In A. Johnson, O. Grusky, and B. H. Raven (eds.), *Contemporary Health Services: A Social Science Perspective.* Boston: Auburn House, 1982.

DiMatteo, M. R., and DiNicola, D. D. *Achieving Patient Compliance: The Psychology of the Medical Practitioner's Role.* New York: Pergamon Press, 1982.

Eisenthal, S., Koopman, C., and Lazare, A. "Process Analysis of Two Dimensions of the Negotiated Approach in Relation to Satisfaction in the Initial Interview." *Journal of Nervous and Mental Disease,* 1983, *171,* 49–54.

Freeman, B., Negrete, V., Davis, M., and Korsch, B. "Gaps in Doctor-Patient Communication: Doctor-Patient Interaction Analysis." *Pediatric Research,* 1971, *5,* 298–311.

Freidson, E. *Patients' Views of Medical Practice.* New York: Russell Sage Foundation, 1961.

Freidson, E. *Profession of Medicine.* New York: Dodd, Mead, 1970.

Greenfield, S., Kaplan, S., and Ware, J. E. "Expanding Patient Involvement in Care." *Annals of Internal Medicine,* 1985, *102,* 520-528.

Greenfield, S., and others. "Patients' Participation in Medical Care: Effects on Blood Sugar Control and Quality of Life in Diabetes." *Journal of General Internal Medicine,* 1988, *3,* 448-457.

Hall, J. A., Roter, D. L., and Katz, N. R. "Meta-Analysis of Correlates of Provider Behavior in Medical Encounters." *Medical Care,* 1988, *26,* 657-675.

Hall, J. A., Roter, D. L., and Rand, C. S. "Communication of Affect Between Patient and Physician." *Journal of Health and Social Behavior,* *22,* 18-30, 1981.

Henderson, L. J. "Physician and Patient as a Social System." *New England Journal of Medicine,* 1935, *212,* 819-823.

Holmes, M., and others. "Women's and Physicians' Utilities for Health Outcomes in Estrogen Replacement Therapy." *Journal of General Internal Medicine,* 1987, *2,* 178-182.

Hunt, E. B., and MacLeod, C. M. "Cognition and Information Processing in Patient and Physician." In G. C. Stone, F. Cohen, and N. E. Adler (eds.), *Health Psychology—A Handbook.* San Francisco: Jossey-Bass, 1979.

Inui, T. S., and Carter, W. B. "Problems and Prospects for Health Services Research on Provider-Patient Communication." *Medical Care,* 1985, *23,* 521-538.

Inui, T. S., Carter, W. B., Kukull, W. A., and Haigh, V. H. "Outcome-Based Doctor-Patient Interaction Analysis. I. Comparison of Techniques." *Medical Care,* 1982, *20,* 535-549.

Inui, T. S., Yourtee, E. L., and Williamson, J. W. "Improved Outcomes in Hypertension After Physician Tutorials: A Controlled Trial." *Annals of Internal Medicine,* 1976, *84,* 646-651.

Kagan, N. "Counseling Psychology, Interpersonal Skills, and Health Care." In G. C. Stone, F. Cohen, and N. E. Adler (eds.), *Health Psychology—A Handbook.* San Francisco: Jossey-Bass, 1979.

Kelman, H. "Compliance, Identification, and Internationalization: Three Processes of Attitude Change." *Journal of Conflict Resolution,* 1958, *2,* 51-60.

Kleinman, A. *Patients and Healers in the Context of Culture: An Exploration of the Borderland Between Anthropology, Medicine, and Psychiatry.* Berkeley and Los Angeles: University of California Press, 1980.

Lazare, A., and Eisenthal, S. "A Negotiated Approach to the Clinical Encounter. I. Attending to the Patient's Perspective." In A. Lazare (ed.), *Outpatient Psychiatry: Diagnosis and Treatment.* Baltimore, Md.: Williams & Wilkins, 1979.

Lazare, A., Eisenthal, S., and Frank, A. "A Negotiated Approach to the Clinic Encounter. II. Conflict and Negotiation." In A. Lazare (ed.), *Outpatient Psychiatry: Diagnosis and Treatment.* Baltimore, Md.: Williams and Wilkins, 1979.

Levenstein, J. H., and others. "The Patient-Centered Clinical Method. 1. A Model for the Doctor-Patient Interaction in Family Medicine." *Family Practice,* 1986, *3,* 24-30.

Leventhal, H. "The Role of Theory in the Study of Adherence to Treatment and Doctor-Patient Interactions." *Medical Care,* 1985, *23,* 556-563.

Ley, P. "Patients' Understanding and Recall in Clinical Communication Failure." In D. Pendleton and J. Hasler (eds.), *Doctor-Patient Communication.* London: Academic Press, 1983.

Ley, P. "Cognitive Variables and Noncompliance." *Journal of Compliance in Health Care,* 1986, *1,* 171-188.

Like, R., and Zyzanski, S. J. "Patient Satisfaction with the Clinical Encounter: Social Psychological Determinants." *Social Science and Medicine,* 1987, *24,* 351-357.

Maiman, L. A., and others. "Improving Pediatricians' Compliance-Enhancing Practices: A Randomized Trial." *American Journal of Diseases of Children,* 1988, *142,* 773-779.

Ockene, J. K., and others. "A Residents' Training Program for the Development of Smoking Intervention Skills." *Archives of Internal Medicine,* 1988a, *148,* 1039-1045.

Ockene, J. K., and others. "The Physician-Delivered Smoking Intervention Project." Paper presented at 116th annual meeting of American Public Health Association, Boston, Nov. 1988b.

Parsons, T. *The Social System.* New York: Free Press, 1951.

Pendleton, D. A. "Doctor-Patient Communication: A Review." In D. A. Pendleton and J. Hasler, (eds.), *Doctor-Patient Communication.* London: Academic Press, 1983.

Potts, M., Weinberger, M., and Brandt, K. "Views of Patients and Providers Regarding the Importance of Various Aspects of an Arthritis Treatment Program." *Journal of Rheumatology,* 1984, *11,* 71-75.

Pratt, L., Seligman, A., and Reader, G. "Physician Views on the Level of Medical Information Among Patients." *American Journal of Public Health,* 1957, *47,* 1277-1283.

Putnam, S. M., Stiles, W. B., Jacob, M. C., and James, S. A. "Patient Exposition and Physician Explanation in Initial Medical Interviews and Outcomes of Clinical Visits." *Medical Care,* 1985, *23,* 74-83.

Putnam, S. M., Stiles, W. B., Jacob, M. C., and James, S. A. "Teaching the Medical Interview: An Intervention Study." *Journal of General Internal Medicine,* 1988, *3,* 38-47.

Quill, T. E. "Partnerships in Patient Care: A Contractual Approach." *Annals of Internal Medicine,* 1983, *98,* 228-234.

Raven, B. H. "Patient-Practitioner Relationships." In A. Johnson, O. Grusky, and B. H. Raven (eds.), *Contemporary Health Services: A Social Science Perspective.* Boston: Auburn House, 1982.

Robinson, E. J., and Whitfield, M. J. "Improving the Efficiency of Patients' Comprehension Monitoring: A Way of Increasing Patients' Participation in General Practice Consultations." *Social Science and Medicine,* 1985, *21,* 915-919.

Rodin, J. "Patient-Practitioner Relationships: A Process of Social Influence." In A. Johnson, O. Grusky, and B. H. Raven (eds.), *Contemporary Health Services: A Social Science Perspective.* Boston: Auburn House, 1982.

Rodin, J., and Janis, I. L. "The Social Influence of Physicians and Other Health Care Practitioners as Agents of Change." In H. S. Friedman and M. R. DiMatteo (eds.), *Interpersonal Issues on Health Care.* Orlando, Fla.: Academic Press, 1982.

Rogers, C. R. "The Necessary and Sufficient Conditions for Therapeutic Personality Change." *Journal of Consulting Psychology*, 1957, *21*, 95-101.

Romm, F. J., Hulka, B. S., and Mayo, F. "Correlates of Outcomes in Patients with Congestive Heart Failure." *Medical Care*, 1976, *14*, 765-776.

Rorer, B., Tucker, C. M., and Blake, H. "Long-Term Nurse-Patient Interactions: Factors in Patient Compliance or Noncompliance to the Dietary Regimen." *Health Psychology*, 1988, *7*, 35-46.

Roter, D. L. "Patient Participation in the Patient-Provider Interaction: The Effects of Patient Question Asking on the Quality of Interaction, Satisfaction, and Compliance." *Health Education Monographs*, 1977, *5*, 281-315.

Roter, D. L., Hall, J. A., and Katz, N. R. "Patient-Physician Communication: A Descriptive Summary of the Literature." *Patient Education and Counseling*, 1988, *12*, 99-119.

Shuy, R. W. "Three Types of Interference to an Effective Exchange of Information in the Medical Interview." In S. Fisher and A. D. Todd (eds.), *The Social Organization of Doctor-Patient Communication*. Washington, D.C.: Center for Applied Linguistics, 1983.

Sideris, D. A., and others. "Attitudinal Educational Objectives at Therapeutic Consultation: Measures of Performance, Educational Approach, and Education." *Medical Education*, 1986, *20*, 307-313.

Starfield, B., and others. "The Influence of Patient-Practitioner Agreement on Outcomes of Care." *American Journal of Public Health*, 1981, *71*, 127-132.

Stiles, W. B. "Verbal Response Modes and Dimensions of Interpersonal Roles: A Method of Discourse Analysis." *Journal of Personality and Social Psychology*, 1978, *36*, 693-703.

Strull, W. M., Lo, B., and Charles, G. "Do Patients Want to Participate in Medical Decision Making?" *Journal of the American Medical Association*, 1984, *252*, 2990-2994.

Swain, M. A., and Steckel, S. B. "Influencing Adherence Among Hypertensives." *Research in Nursing and Health*, 1981, *4*, 213-222.

Szasz, T. S., and Hollender, M. H. "A Contribution to the Philosophy of Medicine. The Basic Models of the Doctor-Patient Relationship." *Archives of Internal Medicine,* 1956, *97,* 585–592.

Uhlmann, R. F., Inui, T. S., Pecoraro, R. E., and Carter, W. B. "Relationship of Patient Request Fulfillment to Compliance, Glycemic Control, and Other Health Care Outcomes in Insulin-Dependent Diabetes." *Journal of General Internal Medicine,* 1988, *3,* 458–463.

Waitzkin, H. "Information Giving in Medical Care." *Journal of Health and Social Behavior,* 1985, *26,* 81–101.

Wasserman, R. C., and Inui, T. S. "Systematic Analysis of Clinician-Patient Interactions: Recent Approaches with Suggestions for Future Research." *Medical Care,* 1983, *21,* 279–293.

Woolley, F. R., Kane, R. L., Hughes, C. C., and Wright, D. D. "The Effects of Doctor-Patient Communication on Satisfaction and Outcome of Care." *Social Science and Medicine,* 1978, *12,* 123–128.

Zimmerman, R. S. "The Dental Appointment and Patient Behavior: Differences in Patient and Practitioner Preferences, Patient Satisfaction, and Adherence." *Medical Care,* 1988, *26,* 403–414.

Chapter 11

Frances Marcus Lewis

Perspectives on Models of Interpersonal Health Behavior

Models of interpersonal health behavior are the focus of the chapters in Part Three. Each of these chapters assumes that people are social beings who derive their sense of power and behavioral competencies from exchanges with significant individuals in their interpersonal environment. This interpersonal environment affects a person's appraisal of potential health threats; provides necessary information and tangible resources or services; predicts a person's health behavior, including his or her level of adherence, self-care practices, satisfaction, and personal control; and ultimately affects a person's health outcomes.

In the chapters of Part Three, people are assumed to analyze cognitively, not respond passively to, their interpersonal environments. This analysis includes anticipating the future and the consequences of one's own behavior and drawing inferences about one's own actions and the actions of others. It further means drawing inferences about the person's own sense of power and influence, personal efficacy, and behavioral competencies. Although Israel and Schurman remind us that the objective properties of the environment may affect both the short- and long-term health outcomes for the individual, it is primarily the subjectively experienced aspects of the interpersonal environment that affect health behavior in the frameworks discussed in Part Three.

242

Social Learning Theory

The conceptual framework in Chapter Eight by Perry, Baranowski, and Parcel, successfully integrates the operant conditioning and cognitive branches of Social Learning Theory (SLT). The authors wisely cast their interpretation of Social Learning Theory beyond the realm of a single concept such as self-efficacy to a broader and more complex theoretical realm. This is not an easy task because these two realms traditionally diverge from each other. Concepts such as reinforcement, from the operant branch of SLT, are integrated with the concepts of self-efficacy and observational learning, from the cognitive branch. These are informed and important choices and provide a conceptual basis for carving out programs for intervention in health education and health behavior. Without such integration, the targets of intervention might be unduly limited. Moreover, the authors draw distinctions between concepts such as expectations and expectancies, environment and situation, and observational learning and operant learning. These distinctions are important for guiding future intervention studies.

Perry, Baranowski, and Parcel summarize two applications of SLT: the A Su Salud project and the Minnesota Home Team study. Each intervention applies the concepts of SLT that are defined in the chapter. Unlike some applications of SLT to individually focused or clinic-based populations, the A Su Salud project uses SLT to guide the components of a multifaceted community-based intervention, an intervention that emphasizes behavioral capability, positive social reinforcement, and performance modeling.

The Minnesota Home Team project is a school-based intervention study that engages both third grade students and their parents in healthy eating behaviors. As with the A Su Salud study, the Minnesota Home Team project derives its rationale from concepts in SLT.

Social Support, Control, and the Stress Process

In Chapter Nine, Israel and Schurman extend concepts from cognitive psychology, organizational sociology, and occupational health into the realm of health behavior. Their conceptual framework analyzes the stress process, control, and social support. Israel and Schurman do the reader a great service by fastidiously integrating these three concepts with both short- and long-term health outcomes. They analyze these concepts in detail, thereby allowing the reader a depth of understanding about the multiple dimensions and definitional distinctions between the three terms. Stress is conceptualized as a process and is defined as an imbalance between demands and resources. Both cognitive and behavioral mediation of stress are critical to the authors' framework. Objective stressful conditions alone do not result in health disruption. Rather, both appraisal and control processes affect the experience of stress. Only when a demand exceeds a person's abilities or resources is the condition experienced as stressful.

Stress is perceptual and has short- as well as long-term physiological, behavioral, and psychological consequences. There are also factors that moderate the stress process. Of critical importance are the particular person's appraisal of the environment and the ways in which that person is able to affect control over his or her immediate conditions, primarily through decision making and participation in influential structures.

Israel and Schurman's conceptual framework is noteworthy in its systematic integration of an exceptionally large theoretical and empirical literature and also in its integration of the literatures of multiple and somewhat disparate disciplines. Each of these disciplines has its own conceptual notation, including definitions; its own research traditions; and its own priority areas for research. For example, Israel and Schurman offer a comprehensive overview of the multiple dimensions of the concept of social support, its distinction from the related concept of social network, methods of measuring social support, and the sources of social support. Where appropriate, the authors detail the multiple interrelationships between the concepts of the framework and also provide a meaningful set of caveats about the assumptions or the direction of the relationships between the concepts in their framework.

Interpersonal Influence

In Chapter Ten, Joos and Hickam underscore the importance of the interpersonal exchanges that occur between clients or patients and health professionals in positively affecting the former's health behavior. This chapter also represents a slight shift of emphasis from general interpersonal models to provider-patient interpersonal models. Here, the authors sketch the underlying assumption in all the models of interpersonal influence: Effective communication between the health professional and the client results in the client's improved decision making and increased understanding, cooperation and adherence, satisfaction, and internalization of responsibility for his or her own health behavior. Basically, the health professional's interchanges with clients help clients help themselves; mutual participation is the goal.

Joos and Hickam organize the interpersonal models of provider-patient influence into four perspectives: cognition and information processing, interpersonal interaction, conflict, and social influence. Each of these perspectives corresponds, the authors' analysis reveals, to the major factors affecting the quality and effectiveness of communication between patients and providers. Conflict, power, influence, and role negotiation are basic to all four perspectives. Ultimately, Joos and Hickam suggest, informational power and referent power are the most effective sources of social influence. These types of power result in long-term changes in health behavior, including changes in attitudes. The authors further hypothesize that informational power and referent power result in a person's heightened sense of control and personal influence over outcomes.

The applications in Chapter Ten focus on research on patient-provider frameworks that measure health outcomes. This research is dominated by observational studies of patient-provider communication and health care outcomes; only a few experimental studies exist.

Core Concepts from the Chapters

Core concepts emerge from the first three chapters in Part Three. All highlight the importance of a person's sense of confidence and behavioral and personal control over his or her environment. In Chapter Eight, Perry, Baranowski, and Parcel do this through the concepts of behavioral capability and self-efficacy; in Chapter Nine, Israel and Schurman do this through the concepts of decision making and participatory control; and in Chapter Eleven, Joos and Hickam do this through the concepts of influence and power processes.

In many ways, the preceding chapters in Part Three redefine both the sources and the legitimacy of power for health. The interpersonal environment, whether within a school, community, work site, or clinic setting, is being challenged to endorse, sustain, and otherwise enhance the individual's ability to carry out self-care and health-promoting activities. The essence of the chapters lies in the interpersonal environment's development of the individual's own capacity for health enhancement. At the level of the organization and the patient-provider relationship, empowering processes are emphasized. As a result, the health professional is best viewed not as an individually focused "interventionist" or "fixer" as much as the change agent of the client or patient's environment. By mobilizing critical elements of the interpersonal environment, including social support and sources of positive reinforcement, the health professional alters or assists the participants to modify their interpersonal environment in ways that foster positive health behavior. In the process, personal levels of power and control, including self-efficacy, are enhanced.

Dynamic, reciprocal determinism is relevant to all three chapters. Multiple theoretical perspectives are introduced in each chapter in order to depict the causes, the explanatory processes or mechanisms, and the consequences of health behavior. Chapters Eight, Nine, and Ten successfully challenge the reductionist perspective of simple, single-variable explanations. In the theories, parsimony is balanced against the more rigorous criterion of explanation. Efficiency of prediction is important, but not at the expense of understanding the underlying processes and multidirectional relationships between the concepts of interest. Parsimony is limited by the necessary constraints of capturing the essence of a complex situation.

Future Research in Interpersonal Models of Health Behavior

Future research in any of the frameworks included in Part Three will rely increasingly on multivariate data analytic strategies. Such strategies assist in the analysis of multiple variables while statistically controlling for others. Multiple regression methods are only one small component of such analytic strategies (McCuan and Green, forthcoming). Additional analytic strategies, especially path analysis and structural equation modeling, will be particularly important in future work (Boyd, Frey, and Aaronson, 1988; Donaldson, McCorkle, Georgiadou, and Benoliel, 1986; Timko and Janoff-Bulman, 1985; Lewis, Woods, Hough, and Bensley, 1989; Joreskog, 1973; Lewis-Beck, 1974). Such analytic methods require the investigator to specify carefully the relationships between the intervention components and health behavior and health outcomes. The methods allow the researcher to test the adequacy of the underlying measurement model and a set of interrelated predictive equations about the relationships between the concepts. The best explanatory model is identified by fitting alternative and competing models of explanation with a set of data. Such processes distinguish between the development and testing of a theoretical framework, the fitting of a framework to a set of data, and the respecification of the framework on the basis of a set of data (Pedhazur, 1982; Namboodiri, Carter, and Blalock, 1975). Only by positing a set of interrelationships such as those proposed between social support, control, and the stress process can investigators begin to test competing or alternative models of explanation for short- and long-range health outcomes. Thus, model development, testing, and respecification processes are fundamental to developing and refining theories in health behavior and health education.

Future research with structural equations will also assist investigators in examining the specific links between each of the program or intervention components and the explanatory variables or processes (Leinhardt, 1980). It is insufficient merely to state that an arm of a clinical trial intervention achieved a statistically significant effect. We need to know why or through what processes such effects were achieved; we need to know more about the links between the program components and their effects (Perloff, Perloff and Sussna, 1976). In the A Su Salud project, what aspects of the media modeling resulted in the obtained results? What do we need to know about the social reinforcements and their relationship to efficacy levels before using such reinforcements in a community? In studying interpersonal influence processes, to what extent does the transfer of power to the client result in increased levels of internalized responsibility for his or her own health or treatment plan? Does this hypothesized internalization or some alternative explanation provide the best explanation of health behavior and positive health outcomes? We need more studies whose emphasis is on explanation, not mere statistical significance.

It is clear that multicomponent frameworks such as those discussed in Part Three raise a host of issues and questions that are not realistically handled in only large-scale studies or in single confirmatory studies using experimental designs. We need to guard against both an overreliance on experimental designs or large-scale studies and an overly simplified or reduced form of reporting study results.

An overreliance on experimental design represents an oversimplified view of cause and effect and the dynamic, not static, nature of intervention programs in health education and health behavior. In confirmatory studies, programs are assumed to be sealed tightly with little or no variation (Stanford Evaluation Consortium, 1976). The program, in all of its rich complexities, is essentially treated as a constant independent variable, and the health-related outcomes are treated as the dependent variables. The problem is that such studies cast the research question in oversimplified terms. Typically, a health education intervention is not a tightly sealed intervention. It is often fluid and ranges within boundaries; often, too, it is altered in the field or received by the participants in differing levels or doses (Green and Lewis, 1986). Both this program variability and the differing levels of exposure or implementation deserve measurement in future studies (Leinhardt, 1980).

If studies are to improve future programs, details are needed about what part(s) of the intervention among the set of components contributed to changed health behavior in which population. The typical confirmatory study inappropriately casts aside such additional information that would help us better serve programs and better inform policy (Green and Lewis, 1981). Such studies are often more interested in whether the program achieved a significant level of change in the participants than in a detailed examination of the processes that caused the change.

The multivariate nature of the frameworks requires more core studies with substudies built into them (Cronbach and others, 1980, p. 219). Such core studies might occur at one site or across multiple sites (Windsor and Orleans, 1986). Multiple core studies would cast tests of the frameworks as a program of evolving studies rather than as a single, large-scale confirmatory study. Such studies could also help accumulate diverse data across diverse sites, as well as gather grounded data by means of a combination of qualitative and quantitative models (Cook and Reichardt, 1979; Mullen, McCuan, and Iverson, 1986). This seems particularly important in diverse settings such as communities and work sites. It also seems particularly important in essentially understudied populations, including the vulnerable. As Cronbach and others (1980, p. 221) remind us, "The wealth of wisdom that can alleviate a social problem is no lone explorer's cargo; it can be drawn only from a treasure room that many expeditions have stocked." The further development and utility of interpersonal models of health behavior are dependent on multiple explorers using multiple frameworks.

References

Boyd, C. J., Frey, M. A., and Aaronson, L. S. "Structural Equation Models and Nursing Research: Part I." *Nursing Research,* 1988, *37,* 249-252.

Cook, T. D., and Reichardt, C. S. *Qualitative and Quantitative Methods in Evaluation Research.* Newbury Park, Calif.: Sage, 1979.

Cronbach, L. J., and others. *Toward Reform of Program Evaluation.* San Francisco: Jossey-Bass, 1980.

Donaldson, G., McCorkle, R., Georgiadou, F., and Benoliel, J. Q. "Distress, Dependency, and Threat in Newly Diagnosed Cancer and Heart Disease Patients." *Multivariate Behavioral Research,* 1986, *21,* 267-298.

Green, L. W., and Lewis, F. M. "Issues in Relating Evaluation to

Theory and Practices in Health Education." *Mobius*, 1981, *1*, 46–58.

Green, L. W., and Lewis, F. M. *Measurement and Evaluation in Health Education and Health Promotion.* Mountain View, Calif.: Mayfield, 1986.

Joreskog, K. G. "A General Method for Estimating a Linear Structural Equation System." In A. S. Goldberger and O. D. Duncan (eds.), *Structural Equation Models in the Social Sciences.* New York: Seminar Press, 1973.

Leinhardt, G. "Modeling and Measuring Education Treatment in Evaluation." *Review of Educational Research*, 1980, *50*, 393–420.

Lewis, F. M., Woods, N. F., Hough, E. S., and Bensley, L. S. "The Family's Coping and Functioning in Chronic Illness: The Partner's Perspective." *Social Science and Medicine*, 1989, *29*, 1261–1269.

Lewis-Beck, M. S. "Determining the Importance of an Independent Variable: A Path Analytic Solution." *Social Science Research*, 1974, *3*, 95–107.

McCuan, R. A., and Green, L. W. "Multivariate Analysis in Evaluation of Health Education and Health Promotion Programs." *Advances in Health Education and Promotion*, forthcoming.

Mullen, P. D., McCuan, R. A., and Iverson, D. C. "Evaluation of Health Education and Promotion Programs: A Review of Qualitative Approaches." *Advances in Health Education and Promotion*, 1986, *1*, 467–498.

Namboodiri, N. K., Carter, L. F., and Blalock, H. M. "Recursive Models and One-Way Causation." *Applied Multivariate Analysis and Experimental Designs.* New York: McGraw-Hill, 1975.

Pedhazur, E. J. *Multiple Regression in Behavioral Research.* (2nd ed.) New York: Holt, Rinehart & Winston, 1982.

Perloff, R., Perloff, E., and Sussna, E. "Program Evaluation." *Annual Review of Psychology*, 1976, *27*, 569–594.

Stanford Evaluation Consortium. "Review Essay: Evaluating the Handbook of Evaluation Research." In G. V. Glass (ed.), *Evaluation Studies.* Vol. 1. Newbury Park, Calif.: Sage, 1976.

Timko, C., and Janoff-Bulman, R. "Attributions, Vulnerability,

Psychological Adjustment: The Case of Breast Cancer." *Health Psychology*, 1985, *4*, 521-544.

Windsor, R. A., and Orleans, C. T. "Guidelines and Methodological Standards for Smoking Cessation Intervention Research Among Pregnant Women: Improving the Science and Art." *Health Education Quarterly*, 1986, *13*, 131-162.

▲ ▲ ▲

PART FOUR

GROUP INTERVENTION MODELS OF HEALTH BEHAVIOR CHANGE

An understanding of the functioning of groups, organizations, large social institutions, and communities is vital to health enhancement. Designing programs to reach *populations,* not merely individuals, is at the heart of a public health orientation. The collective well-being of communities can be fostered by creating structures and policies that facilitate health-promoting actions by individuals or, more directly, by reducing or eliminating health hazards in the social and physical environment. Both approaches require an understanding of how social systems operate, how change occurs within and among systems, and how systemwide, community, and organizational changes influence people's health behavior and health.

Health promotion today faces rapid technological change and important policy debates. Health concerns such as AIDS prevention and education, smoking control, and technologically sophisticated medical treatments raise issues that cannot be addressed adequately through individual or small group interventions alone. Rather, health professionals need to view and understand health behavior and organizational changes in the context of social institutions. The theories and frameworks in this part of *Health Behavior and Health Education* can help professionals understand the health behavior of large groups, communities, and organizations and can guide organization-wide and community-wide health education interventions. These social systems are both viable and essential units of practice when widespread and long-term maintenance of behavior change are important goals.

The chapters in this section represent state-of-the-art descriptions of five models for health behavior change in social systems or large populations. Some of the chapters address theoretical perspectives on changing the health behavior of populations, whereas other chapters are concerned primarily with conceptual frameworks for intervention methods that are *based on* theoretical foundations from the social sciences.

In Chapter Twelve, Meredith Minkler provides a comprehensive overview of the principles and methods of community organization as applied to health education. She discusses the main theoretical and conceptual bases of community organization, the process of community organization, and three distinct models of community organization. Minkler then describes two case studies of community organization. The Tenderloin Senior Organizing Project (TSOP) for low-income elderly in San Francisco demonstrates community organization in a relatively strict sense of the term, and the Minnesota Heart Health Program (MHHP) illustrates how health practitioners can adapt community organizing methods to heighten community participation and increase the effectiveness of a community health promotion campaign.

In Chapter Thirteen, Mario Orlandi and colleagues present diffusion of innovations theory, which addresses how new ideas, products, and social practices spread within a society or from one society (or social system) to another. They then focus on how the diffusion of innovations framework was integrated with a linkage model and applied to enhance the successful dissemination of cholesterol control interventions in a multicultural community setting.

Next, Robert Goodman and Allan Steckler, in Chapter Fourteen, analyze two theories of organizational change: Stage Theory and Organizational Development Theory. Both of these theories suggest specific intervention strategies that are directed at levels of the organization at which health education can be influential. Further, strategies based on each of the two theories can be used simultaneously to produce optimal effects. Goodman and Steckler then illustrate how these theories can be used as a basis for health promotion and health care intervention, both in a school setting and in a health care setting.

William Novelli introduces applications of social marketing to health promotion and disease prevention in Chapter Fifteen. Social marketing is best described as a *process* that draws its methods from theories of marketing, consumer behavior, information processing, and decison making. Novelli uses two examples of successful health and social interventions to demonstrate the success of social marketing in the Metro Manila Measles Immunization Campaign and the National High Blood Pressure Education Program. He concludes by introducing some provocative thoughts about evaluating whether an organization has conditions that will be hospitable to social marketing strategies.

In Chapter Sixteen, Lawrence Wallack introduces the strategies of media advocacy, which complement social marketing concepts as a means of using the mass communication system to promote health. Media advocacy uses media access and issue-framing strategies, which are often used in political campaigns, to increase the prospects for developing supportive public policies and social-environmental change. Media advocacy also provides alternative mechanisms for public education that build a case for countering misleading information promulgated by for-profit interests. Wallack describes the application of media advocacy to a community antismoking program in Utica, New York.

Part Four concludes with a summary, comparison, and critique of group, organizational, and community interventions in health education. Chapter Seventeen discusses common theoretical bases, parallel elements in concepts and strategies, and converging applications of group intervention models of health behavior change.

An understanding of theory, research, and practice to promote change in systems, communities, and organizations will be critical to wide improvement of health in the future. This part of *Health Behavior and Health Education* provides a diverse set of frameworks and applications for the consideration of both researchers and practitioners.

Chapter 12

Meredith Minkler

Improving Health
Through Community Organization

The principles and methods for effecting change that are loosely referred to as community organization are central to the practice of health education and related fields. For the purpose of this chapter, community organization will be defined as the process by which community groups are helped to identify common problems or goals, mobilize resources, and in other ways develop and implement strategies for reaching the goals they have set.

Implicit in this definition is the concept of empowerment, viewed as an enabling process through which individuals or communities take control over their lives and their environment (Rappaport, 1984). Indeed Murray Ross (1955), widely regarded as the father of community organizing practice, argued that community organization cannot be said to have taken place unless community competence or problem-solving ability has been increased in the process.

Strict definitions of community organization also suggest that the needs or problems around which community groups are organized must be identified by the community itself, not by an outside organization or change agent. Thus, while a health professional may borrow some principles and methods from community organization to help mount an AIDS organizing effort in the community, he or she cannot be said to be doing community organiza-

257

tion in the pure sense unless the community itself has identified AIDS as the problem area it wishes to address.

In this chapter, these and other concepts of community organization will be examined for their relevance to health education and related disciplines. Following a brief historical overview of the field and process of community organization, the concept of community will be examined, and three models of community organization will be presented. Key theoretical and conceptual bases of community organization will be explored, with examples used to illustrate their applications in practice. Finally, two case studies will be described, one demonstrating community organization in a relatively strict sense of the term and a second illustrating the ways in which different strategies and methods of community organization can be adopted usefully in externally initiated health or social service program efforts.

Community Organization in Historical Perspective

The term *community organization* was coined by American social workers in the late 1800s in reference to a specific field of activity in which they were engaged. This was the period of history marked by the mushrooming of charity organizations and settlement houses for new immigrants and the poor, and "community organizing" was the phrase used to describe social workers' efforts to coordinate services for these various groups (Mowat, 1961; Garvin and Cox, 1987).

Because most histories of community organization have been written by social workers and professionals in related disciplines, they understandably portray community organization as having been born of the settlement house movement. Yet as Garvin and Cox (1987) have pointed out, several important milestones in the history of community organization took place well before and outside of social work and related fields. These antecedent and concurrent developments include such occurrences as the post–Reconstruction period organization of blacks by blacks in this country, to try to salvage newly won rights that were rapidly slipping away. The Populist movement in the American South, which began as an agrarian revolution and became a multisectoral coalition and a major political force, was also an important contributor, as was the labor movement of the 1930s and 1940s, which taught the value of forming coalitions around issues, the importance of full-time professional organizers, and the use of conflict as a means of bringing about change.

Within the field of social work, early definitions of community organization as a process of bringing about a more effective adjustment between social welfare resources and social welfare needs had been replaced by the 1940s with new visions of social work as a means of helping people change, not merely adjust to, the status quo. The concept of a professional organizer as a change agent working "with" rather than "on" communities also gained popularity at this time, and the appearance of Ross's (1955) classic textbook on community organization practice in the early 1950s helped shape and popularize this new approach (Garvin and Cox, 1987).

While Ross's approach to community organization stressed methods of consensus and cooperation, a new brand of community organization was also gaining popularity in the 1950s and 1960s and stressed confrontation and other conflict strategies as equally valid—and often more useful—approaches to social change. Saul Alinsky, the individual most identified with this newer brand of community organization, gained early notoriety for his role in organizing white ethnic workers in an area of Chicago known as the "back of the yards" (Reitzes and Reitzes, 1980). Although Alinsky argued that there was no such thing as an "Alinsky method" of organizing, his landmark books, *Rules for Radicals* (1972) and *Reveille for Radicals* (1969), reveal a clear set of operating principles and methods of practice that define his philosophy and approach. Alinsky stressed the need for "disorganizing" communities before they can be organized (stirring discontent, creating a dissatisfaction with the status quo); identifying and "freezing" targets that are winnable, specific, and local; and using nonviolent conflict to build community-wide identification and participation (Alinsky, 1972). Alinsky also made valuable contributions to our understanding of the concept of community and its relevance as a base from which effective social change can take place (Reitzes and Reitzes, 1980).

By the late 1950s and early 1960s, a new dimension of community organization practice was realized in the form of the civil rights movement and other national movements that applied the strategies and tactics of community organization to the achievement of broader social change objectives. The brilliant organizing approaches of Martin Luther King, Jr., and other civil rights leaders helped effect a major social transformation in legislation, politics, and other arenas and further laid the groundwork for subsequent national organizing efforts such as the women's movement, the gay rights movement, and the anti–Vietnam War movement.

Alongside these major social movements were efforts within government and the helping professions to apply some of the lessons of effective community organization practice in other arenas. The late 1960s and early 1970s, for example, witnessed a call for "community participation" in everything from antipoverty programs to health care decision making, ideally toward the end of helping democratize institutions, agencies, and programs suffering from public apathy and noninvolvement. While for the most part these efforts at "maximum feasible participation" failed in their attempts and indeed often created instead what Moynihan (1969) calls "maximum feasible misunderstanding," there were a few notable successes. In rural Mt. Bijou, Mississippi, for example, a truly community-based and community-controlled health center was established in the late 1960s. This included the first cooperative of landless peasants, an effective public transportation system, training and education for future health workers, and other features in keeping with a vision of community health in the broadest sense (Geiger, 1969). While subsequent cutbacks eventually caused the stripping away of some of the key features of the center, it nevertheless became an "ideal model" and helped inspire many of the positive features of the neighborhood health center movement that followed.

On an international scale, growing appreciation of the importance of community organization and participation in health and related fields led to a major new emphasis, in the late 1970s and 1980s, on community participation as an integral part of health and health care (United Nations International Children's Emergency Fund/World Health Organization, 1981; World Health Organization, 1983). The International Conference on Primary Health Care held in Alma Ata, USSR, in 1978, was heralded as a turning point in the international health field, in part for giving new meaning and emphasis to the role of community organization and participation in health. Cosponsored by WHO and UNICEF, the conference resulted in the adoption by 134 countries of a bold new document known as the Alma Ata Declaration. The declaration states in part, that "people have the right and the duty to participate individually and collectively in the planning and implementing of their health care" (World Health Organization, 1978, p. 20). Further, it argues that real community participation implies a sharing of power and responsibility, not simply getting people to do what health and social service professionals feel they ought to be doing. Subsequent documents by WHO and other international bodies have reflected this new appreciation of the primacy of community organization and community participation in achieving health and social goals on a broad scale (World Health Organization, 1983); more importantly, they have been reflected in practice.

The term *community organization* has emerged from a narrowly conceived field within the social work profession into a broad process that stresses working with people as they define their own goals, mobilize resources, and develop action plans for addressing problems they collectively have identified. While frequently occurring on the local level, effective organizing also was a hallmark of such national social change efforts as the civil rights movement. Finally, concepts originally identified with community organizing (for example, the importance of increasing a community's participation in and control over the institutions and programs designed to serve it) were also borrowed by government, health care agencies, and international bodies such as WHO with varying degrees of success. Following an examination of the concept of community and a typology of community organization practice, some key concepts will be discussed in more detail.

The Concept of Community

Integral to a discussion of community organization practice is an examination of the underlying concept of community. While typically viewed in geographic terms, communities may also be nonlocality identified and based instead on shared interests or characteristics, such as ethnicity, sexual orientation, or occupation (Fellin, 1987). Communities indeed have been defined as social units that are at least one of the following: (1) functional spatial units meeting basic needs for sustenance, (2) units of patterned social interaction, and (3) symbolic units of collective identity (Hunter, 1975).

Fellin (1987) identifies two sets of theories relevant to the concept of community. The first of these, the ecological system perspective, is particularly useful in the study of geographic communities, focusing as it does on population characteristics such as size, density, and heterogeneity, the physical environment, the social organization or structure of the community, and the technological forces impacting upon it. As Choldin (1985) notes, human ecology as a theoretical framework for studying communities draws attention to such key phenomena as the community's changing age structure, the degree of integration or segregation of different subsets of the population, and the existing means of transportation and communications.

In contrast, the social systems perspective focuses primarily on the formal organizations that operate within a given community, exploring the interactions of community subsystems (economic, political, and so on) both horizontally within the community and vertically as they relate to other, extra-community systems (Fellin, 1987).

Warren's (1963) widely held approach to community clearly fits within the latter perspective, envisioning communities as entities that change their structure and function to accommodate various social, political, and economic developments. These changes occur along either a horizontal (local) or a vertical axis, with the latter involving relationships between the immediate community and its external organizations, institutions, or political entities (Warren, 1963).

The view of communities as operating not merely on a horizontal but also on a vertical axis is also in keeping with Alinsky's notion of the importance of viewing local communities as reflecting "the social problems and processes of an urban society" (Reitzes and Reitzes, 1980, p. 40). While earlier models of community tended to view the latter as complete, self-contained, and autonomous (Effrat, 1974), the social systems perspective, and Alinsky as an early proponent of that theoretical frame, view community as intimately interconnected with the larger units of the social structure.

Clearly, the perspective on community that one adopts (for example, community as autonomous versus interdependent) will influence what are viewed as the appropriate domains and functions of community organization. Community development specialists (such as agricultural extension workers) thus have focused over the years on helping people identify with and bring about changes within their own geographic community, implicitly defining the latter as a unit unto itself (Khinduka, 1975). By contrast, proponents of a broader approach, typified by Alinsky and other social action organizers, have encouraged organizing around issues such as public housing and unemployment in recognition of the tremendous impact those larger socioeconomic issues have on local communities (Alinsky, 1941).

The typology of community organization described below examines in more detail the alternative assumptions that shape and determine how community organization is conceptualized and practiced.

Models of Community Organization

While community organization frequently is treated as a singular model of practice, several typologies of community organization have been developed on the premise that this phenomenon is in fact comprised of various alternative change models. The best known of these typologies is Rothman's (Rothman and Tropman, 1987) categorization of community organization as consisting of three distinct models of practice: locality development, social planning, and social action. These are summarized in Table 12.1. Locality development is a heavily process-oriented model, stressing consensus and cooperation and building group identity and a sense of community. By contrast, social planning is heavily task oriented and stresses rational-empirical problem solving—usually by an outside expert—as a means of ameliorating or solving selected problems. In Rothman and Tropman's words (1987, p. 94), the concern in social plan-

Table 12.1. Three Models of Community Organization Practice According to Selected Practice Variables.

	Model A (Locality Development)	Model B (Social Planning)	Model C (Social Action)
1. Goal categories of community action	Self-help; community capacity and integration (process goals)	Problem solving with regard to substantive community problems (task goals)	Shifting of power relationships and resources; basic institutional change (task or process goals)
2. Assumptions concerning community structure and problem conditions	Community eclipsed, anomie; lack of relationships and democratic problem-solving capacities; static traditional community	Substantive social problems; mental and physical health, housing, recreation	Disadvantaged populations, social injustice, deprivation, inequity
3. Basic change strategy	Broad cross section of people involved in determining and solving their own problems	Fact gathering about problems and decisions on the most rational course of action	Crystallization of issues and organization of people to take action against enemy targets
4. Characteristic change tactics	Consensus: communication among community groups and interests; group discussion	Consensus or conflict	Conflict or contest: confrontation, direct action, negotiation
5. Salient practitioner roles	Enabler-catalyst, coordinator; teacher of problem-solving skills and ethical values	Fact gatherer and analyst, program implementer, facilitator	Activist advocate: agitator, broker, negotiator, partisan

6. Medium of change	Manipulation of small task-oriented groups	Manipulation of formal organizations and data	Manipulation of mass organizations and political processes
7. Orientation toward power structure(s)	Members of power stucture as collaborators in a common venture	Power structure as employers and sponsors	Power structure as external target of action: oppressors to be coerced or overturned
8. Boundary definition of the community client system or constituency	Total geographic community	Total community or community segment (including "functional" community)	Community segment
9. Assumptions regarding interests of community subparts	Common interests or reconcilable differences	Interests reconcilable or in conflict	Conflicting interests which are not easily reconcilable: scarce resources
10. Conception of the client population or constituency	Citizens	Consumers	Victims
11. Conception of client role	Participants in an interactional problem-solving process	Consumers or recipients	Employers, constituents, members

Source: Rothman and Tropman, 1987, pp. 3-26.

ning "is with establishing, arranging and delivering goods to people who need them. Building community capacity or fostering radical or fundamental social change does not play a central part."

The third model, social action, is both task and process oriented. It is concerned with increasing the problem-solving ability of the community and with achieving concrete changes to redress imbalances of power and privilege between an oppressed or disadvantaged group and the larger society.

Rothman argues that while none of these models is mutually exclusive, community organization efforts nevertheless appear to exhibit a central tendency that places them most appropriately within one of the three categories. Thus, an effort to increase a sense of community and mutual aid among cancer patients would appear most closely aligned with the locality community development model, even if on occasion it displayed aspects of social action organizing. Similarly, an effort by people with AIDS to fight for increased insurance coverage would fall under the heading of social action, even though an increased sense of community might well constitute an important by-product of their efforts.

While Rothman's typology of community organization practice remains widely accepted, it has at least two important limitations. First, use of the term *locality development* may be unnecessarily restrictive, limiting consideration of the process-oriented model of community organization to geographically identified communities. The earlier term *community development* may well be a useful replacement for *locality development* since it has many of the same characteristics and emphases described by Rothman yet is not limited to geographic communities.

A second and more serious limitation of this typology is its characterization of social planning as a model of community organization. If the spirit of community organization is to increase the problem-solving capacities of the community or group, then a method that relies heavily on expert technical assistance to achieve specific objectives probably will not meet this important criterion.

Key Concepts in Community Organization Practice

While no single unified model of community organization exists, several key concepts are central to this approach to effecting change on the community level. Six of these concepts—empowerment, community competence, the principles of participation and "starting where the people are," issue selection, and creating critical consciousness—are discussed below.

Empowerment. The term *empowerment* represents a central tenet of community organization practice. Defined by Rappaport (1984, p. 1) as "a process by which individuals, communities and organizations gain mastery over their lives," it builds upon the Latin root *passe*, from which we derive both the word *power* and the word *freedom*. If power is the ability to predict, control, and participate in one's environment (Kent, 1970), then empowerment is the process by which individuals and communities are enabled to take such power and act effectively in transforming their lives and their environments.

Within community organization practice, the concept of empowerment operates on two levels simultaneously. First, the individual involved in a community organizing effort may experience increased social support, which is defined by Cohen and Syme (1985) as the resources, both tangible and intangible, derived from his or her web of social ties. Such social support may contribute to a more generalized sense of control or "coherence" (Antonovsky, 1979), and this increased sense of control may in turn have positive health benefits. Studies have shown, for example, that community involvement may be a significant psychosocial factor in improving perceived personal confidence, individual coping capacity, and life satisfaction (Leighton and Stone, 1974). The physical health benefits of such activity also have been demonstrated; research suggests that social participation can affect the body's defense system and decrease susceptibility to illness (Cohen and Syme, 1985; Thomas, Goodwin, and Goodwin, 1985; see also Chapter Nine for a detailed analysis of the concepts of social support and participation).

Individual-level empowerment through involvement in community organizing is in marked contrast to "learned helplessness," a psychological phenomenon that occurs when individuals who are made to feel inadequate and unable to master certain tasks become actually unable to perform these and other tasks that are objectively well within their grasp (Garber and Seligman, 1980). By providing opportunities for individuals to experience an increased sense of control and self-confidence, community organization can help counter some of the environmentally induced loss of control that frequently causes or exacerbates health and social problems on the individual level.

On a broader level, community organization can contribute to community-level empowerment, operationalized in part as increased community competence. As communities become empowered and are better able to engage in collective problem solving, key health and social indicators may reflect this with rates of alcoholism, divorce, suicide, and other social problems beginning to decline. Moreover, the empowered community that works effectively for change can bring about changes in some of the very problems that contributed to its ill health in the first place (Minkler, 1985; Israel, 1985; Thomas, Israel, and Steuart, 1985).

Community Competence. The notion of community competence is closely related to the concept of empowerment as a central goal and outcome of community organization practice. Coined in the 1970s in reference to the community's ability to engage in effective problem solving (Iscore, 1980), the term *community competence* has much earlier roots. In one of the first and best-known definitions of community organization, for example, Ross (1955) described the process as one in which the ability of the community to function effectively as a unit of problem solving was increased.

Cottrell (1983, p. 403) provides a more detailed definition of the competent community as "one in which the various component parts of the community are able to collaborate effectively on identifying the problems and needs of the community; can achieve a working consensus on goals and priorities; can agree on ways and means to implement the agreed upon goals; [and] can collaborate effectively in the required actions."

While Cottrell (1983) and others (Barbarin, Good, Pharr, and Siskind, 1981; Fellin, 1987) have applied this concept primarily to geographic communities, its relevance to nongeographic communities is also apparent. Indeed, whether the community is a neighborhood in the South Bronx, a union local in Ohio, or the family care givers of victims of Alzheimer's disease working together for change, increasing the community's capacity for collective problem identification and problem solving is of paramount importance if the community is effectively to reach both its current objectives and whatever goals it may set for the future.

Many principles and concepts basic to health education and community psychology have relevance for increasing community competence. Israel (1985) notes that key principles and approaches within the areas of social network theory and social support may be applied usefully in the development of competent communities. Social network techniques by which one can "map" the web of social ties in which individuals are embedded may help identify natural helpers or leaders within a community and help such natural leaders identify their own networks, understand community patterns, identify high-risk groups within the community, and involve network members in undertaking their own community assessment and actions necessary to strengthen networks within the community. A number of network assessment tools are available for mapping personal and community networks (McCallister and Fischer, 1978; Heitzmann and Kaplan, 1988) and may be useful to health education professionals.

Leadership development is a key aspect of developing competent communities. In particular, the development of leaders able to fulfill the roles of animator (stimulating people to think critically and to identify problems and new solutions) and facilitator (providing a process through which the group can discuss its own content in the most productive possible way) is key to building group competence and effectiveness (Hope and Timmel, 1984).

Using these and other approaches, the health or social service practitioner as community organizer can play a key role in helping communities increase their problem-solving ability and hence realize one of the most important outcomes of community organization practice.

The Principles of Participation and "Starting Where the People Are." Two principles central to community organization practice are the principle of participation and the principle of relevance or "starting where the people are." While both precepts have been "rediscovered" in recent decades (for example, in conjunction with the War on Poverty in the United States and the primary health care movement internationally), both have far earlier roots in social learning theory and in the field of adult education.

Individuals must experience a felt need to change or to learn before learning and change can take place. Kurt Lewin (1958) postulated in the mid-1940s that individuals must experience an "unfreezing" of old attitudes and beliefs before they can consider and try out new ones. Lewin's concept of "unfreezing" the old as a prerequisite to the new had an important parallel in Hochbaum's (1960) emphasis on the need to create "a psychological state of readiness to learn" before a particular change can occur. For Allport (1945), unfreezing takes the form of catharsis, which he describes as a necessary first step in the breaking down of prejudice (1945). In the field of social action organizing, unfreezing finds a further adaptation in Alinsky's (1972) articulation of the need to disorganize communities (stirring frustration, creating dissatisfaction with the status quo) before they can be organized or, more properly, reorganized. In short, Hochbaum, Allport, Alinsky, and others share with Lewin the view that change is not a single event but a complex process in which old attitudes and practices must be opened to reexamination (unfrozen) before change can take place (Lewin, 1958).

Health education leader Dorothy Nyswander built on this notion when she articulated the principle of *relevance* or "starting where the people are" as perhaps the most fundamental tenet of health education practice. In health education, as in other helping professions, the change agent who begins with the individual's or the community's felt needs and concerns rather than with a personal or agency agenda will be far more likely to experience success in the change process than if he or she were to impose an agenda from outside (Nyswander, 1966).

As important as this tenet is in theory, however, its implementation can be difficult. In the field of health education, for example, Grossman (1971) notes that the health educator's role in helping people set their own goals often in reality means helping them set their goals *within the context of preexisting goals*. To the extent that the agenda of a health or social service agency or employer fails to correspond to the needs and desires of the community, the practitioner may face difficult decisions concerning conflicting loyalties.

Within community organization practice, the paramount importance of having the community identify the needs and issues to be addressed is widely acknowledged. Yet even in "pure" community organizing, strict adherence to this principle is difficult. If community organizing is to be effective, the issues selected for attention must be winnable and specific. When a community selects as an issue a problem it cannot hope to solve, the organizer has a responsibility to pose questions and in other ways help the group refocus its objectives so that a more specific and winnable issue is identified. Only when issues are selected by the community itself can a real sense of "ownership" emerge, and this sense of ownership of the organization is critical to empowerment and to the ultimate development of competent communities.

Closely related to the principle of relevance, the principle of participation also has its roots in social psychology theories of learning and adult education. The fact that learners should be active rather than passive participants in the learning process, participants who "learn by doing," thus is grounded in some of the earliest stimulus-response theory (Hilgard and Bower, 1975) and is reinforced by principles from cognitive theory that stress the importance of feedback and learning with understanding rather than by formula.

Lewin's classic experiments during World War II (for example, in studying the factors involved in getting housewives to support the war effort by purchasing and using less-popular cuts of meat) also provided important empirical validation for the principle of participation. In the above-mentioned studies, women who were actively involved in group learning and decision making were much more likely to change their attitudes and practices with respect to trying a new behavior than were those for whom the educational situation was undimensional and authoritarian in nature (Lewin, 1958).

In the field of adult education, the principle of participation receives special attention in the work of Dewey (1946) and Lindeman (1926). Indeed, the very notion of adult education as a process of enlarging people's understandings, activating them, and helping them make and implement decisions for themselves is congruent with the community organization principle of facilitating true involvement and participation by community members at all stages of the organizing process.

The two studies presented later in this chapter illustrate alternative approaches to applying the principle of participation in a practice setting. In both, the overall success of the programs in meeting their stated objectives lies in part in their adherence to this important community organization principle.

Issue Selection. One of the most important steps in community organization practice involves the effective differentiation between *problems,* or things that are troubling, and *issues,* or problems that the community feels strongly about (Miller, 1985). A good issue must meet several other important criteria: it must be winnable, simple, and specific. If a campaign is winnable, working on it does not cause disappointment or reinforce fatalistic attitudes and beliefs. A good issue must be simple and specific so that any member of the group can explain it clearly in a sentence or two. It must unite members of the group and must involve them in a meaningful way in achieving issue resolution. It should affect many people and build up the community or organization (giving leadership experience, increased visibility, and so on), and it should be part of a larger plan or strategy (Miller, 1985).

A variety of methods familiar to health and social service professionals can be used to help a community group acquire the data needed for issue selection. Nominal group process (Delbecq, Van de Ven, and Gustafson, 1975), door-to-door surveys, and the use of Freire's (1973) problem-posing dialogical methods may thus all be effective for this purpose. Of the many methods that may be utilized to assess community needs while in the process increasing participation, few have had the dramatic results of the problem-posing method developed by Brazilian educator Paulo Freire. In light of its influence on community organization practice both in the United States and internationally, Freire's approach will be examined in more detail below.

Creating "Critical Consciousness." One of the most important recent contributions to community organization practice has come from Paulo Freire (1973), whose concept of *contientizacion,* or creating critical consciousness, has added an important dimension to more traditional organizing approaches. Freire developed a methodology for teaching illiterate peasants to read while at the same time teaching them to "read" the political and social situation in which they found themselves. This method stressed a relationship of equality and mutual respect between group members or "learners-teachers" and the facilitators or "teacher learners" who engaged them in problem-posing dialogue designed to help them elucidate the root causes of problems they had identified. Working together in small groups, the men and women discussed common problems, and then were challenged to look for the root causes or "problems behind the problems" they initially had identified. Finally, they were helped to explore the interconnection between various aspects of their reality, and to devise action plans, based on critical reflection, to help transform that reality (Freire, 1973).

The Freire method is widely used in health and related fields in Third World countries and has also been adopted for use in a number of health education projects in the United States (Minkler and Cox, 1980; Wallerstein and Bernstein, 1988; Auerbach and Wallerstein, 1987).

In rural Honduras, for example, it was used in the 1970s by Catholic priests involved in the training of local women as village health workers, or *promotores de salud.* As the women discussed common problems (for example, worms in children) and such "problems behind the problems" as poverty and lack of education, they devised action plans, including the building, by the women themselves, of a village school (Minkler and Cox, 1980). The Freire method also was used to secure land reforms and more recently to help Salvadoran refugees in Honduras attain the skills and self-confidence needed as they prepare to return to a new life in their war-torn country (Minkler, 1983).

In the United States, an unusual application of the Friere method is taking place in Albuquerque, New Mexico, in conjunction with a substance abuse program for high-risk teenagers. The low-income Native American, Hispanic, and Anglo youth in Albuquerque, experience drinking and driving, suicide, and other problems at rates far higher than the national average (Wallerstein and

Bernstein, 1988). The Alcohol and Substance Abuse Prevention Program (ASAP) was established in 1982 as a community- and school-based prevention project, cosponsored by the University of New Mexico School of Medicine. Its goal is to empower teenagers in this high-risk community through a program that has them visit local hospital emergency rooms and jails and then discuss in a safe environment the meaning of this experience and the many other issues that emerge from it. The students are encouraged to engage in critical thinking with hospital patients and each other and to explore the root causes of problems in their communities, as well as their own role in seeking and implementing possible solutions. In the latter regard, for example, students involved with ASAP have made presentations at two tribal councils, one of which went on to plan a drug and alcohol campaign for the Pueblo as a result (Wallerstein and Bernstein, 1988).

The significance of the Freire method for community organization practice lies not only in providing an effective methodological refinement (problem-posing dialogue) but, more importantly, in its requirement that community organization efforts be grounded in a deeper understanding of the root causes of problems and issues being addressed.

The two case studies described below illustrate the application of concepts and principles of community organization in practice settings.

Tenderloin Senior Organizing Project

For the low-income elderly in America's single-room occupancy (SRO) hotels, poor health, social isolation, and powerlessness are often intimately connected. This case study describes an attempt by health educators and graduate students in health education and related disciplines to address these interrelated problems by fostering social support and social action organizing among elderly residents of San Francisco's Tenderloin hotels.

The Tenderloin Senior Organizing Project (TSOP) is a useful example of the ways in which health professionals functioning as community organizers can help a community identify and address its own issues and concerns and in the process increase its ability to function effectively as a unit of solution (Minkler, 1985).

Originally known as the Tenderloin Senior Outreach Project, TSOP was established in 1979 with the dual goals of (1) improving physical and mental health by reducing social isolation and providing relevant health education and (2) facilitating through dialogue and participation a process through which residents were encouraged to work together to identify common problems and to seek solutions to these shared problems and concerns.

Student volunteers began in a single Tenderloin hotel, encouraging resident interaction and eventually forming an informal group that met weekly and included a core of twelve residents and two outside facilitators. As trust and rapport increased, group members began to share personal concerns regarding such issues as fear of crime, loneliness, rent increases, and their own sense of powerlessness.

Student facilitators used a combination of organizing and educational approaches to help foster group solidarity and social action organizing. A modified Freirian problem-posing process thus was used to help residents engage in dialogue about shared problems and their causes and to generate potential action plans. In addition, Alinsky's (1972) admonitions to create dissatisfaction with the status quo, channel frustration into concrete action, and help people identify specific, winnable issues were among the community organization precepts followed. Finally, drawing on social support theory that stresses the importance of social interaction opportunities, the facilitators tried to create a group atmosphere conducive to meeting the purely social needs of residents as well as the more political and task-oriented concerns of some group members (Minkler, 1985).

As the first hotel group evolved into an established entity, seven additional groups were organized in other Tenderloin hotels. As in the first hotel, the project director and student facilitators employed a variety of educational and organizational strategies and sought a delicate balance between meeting the political/task-oriented and the strictly social needs of residents.

Although each hotel group developed and retained its own unique character over time, several common trends among the groups were evident. In most hotel groups, for example, decreased reliance on outside facilitators developed over time, with broader resident participation in discussion and decision making.

A second trend observed in the groups, and one critical to TSOP's evolution, was the residents' realization of the need for looking beyond hotel boundaries and working with residents of other hotels and community groups on shared problems. TSOP residents in several hotels identified crime and safety as their key area of concern and formed an interhotel coalition to begin work on the problem. The coalition in turn started the Safehouse Project, recruiting forty-eight neighborhood businesses and agencies to serve as places of refuge, demarcated by colorful posters, where residents could go for help in times of emergency. Coalition members also convinced the mayor of San Francisco to increase the number of beat patrol officers in the neighborhood and through this and other measures, helped effect a dramatic reduction in crime in their community.

Encouraged by the success of the Safehouse Project, TSOP members later addressed the problem of hunger and poor food access, establishing minimarkets in three hotels and a cooperative breakfast program in a fourth and renovating a shabby basement room in a fifth hotel to provide an attractive area for congregate dining (Minkler, 1985).

TSOP also has engaged in significant leadership training, stressing both one-on-one and small group activities through which residents work on improving interpersonal skills, learning to facilitate meetings, and discovering ways of working through bureaucracies to bring about change.

As Tenderloin residents have become increasingly willing and able to take control of this project, TSOP staff and volunteers have played a less visible role, serving primarily as resource people and "sounding boards" for residents' ideas and strategy discussions. The organization changed its name in 1988 from the Tenderloin Senior "Outreach" Project to the Tenderloin Senior "Organizing" Project to reflect this change in orientation. The key mechanism of action within the project has changed over time from health educator–facilitated support groups to resident-run tenant associations (Goldoftas, 1988). Currently, TSOP-related tenant organizations operate in five Tenderloin hotels, with a total of 800 residents. Some 250 residents are regularly involved in tenant organizing activities with 30 to 50 of them playing key leadership roles in the project.

TSOP is not without problems, including resident burnout on some issues they had earlier decided to tackle, occasional power conflicts within the groups, and leadership turnover as a consequence of illness, transiency, and other problems. Evaluation of the project has been difficult because many residents harbor an understandable distrust of outside researchers and because project staff members are committed to avoiding data-gathering activities, which might confuse residents as to the true mission of the organization. However, community indicators such as a reduced crime rate and qualitative changes in the health and life satisfaction of participating residents suggest that TSOP has been effective in meeting its goals and in leaving behind a more competent community.

Minnesota Heart Health Program

The case study presented above was used to illustrate an attempt at "true" community organizing in which group members themselves identified the problems they wished to address and the outside organizers played a facilitative role in helping the community group as it devised methods and strategies for achieving its objectives. The next case study illustrates the ways in which health and social service practitioners can adapt certain community organizing methods to heighten community participation and increase the effectiveness of a major community health program. While not technically "doing" community organizing, the health educators in this case study have improved the project's chances for success by taking seriously several key precepts of community organizing practice.

A major development in the field of health promotion and disease prevention in the last decade has been the design and implementation of several large-scale research and demonstration programs to address major health problems by intervening on a broad community level (Mittlemark and others, 1986). One of these, the Minnesota Heart Health Program, is discussed here as an example of an ambitious health promotion project that has relied heavily on community organization principles and approaches with encouraging results.

The ten-year-old Minnesota Heart Health Program (MHHP) is a large community study involving approximately 250,000 residents of three communities and an equal number of controls in comparison locales. Its ambitious objectives include (1) developing and implementing coordinated community-wide health education strategies, (2) improving community health behavior and reducing related risk factors, and (3) reducing the incidence of premature disability and death from cardiovascular disease (Carlaw, Mittlemark, Bracht, and Luepker, 1984). The focus of individual and community intervention has been in three areas: smoking cessation, detection and control of hypertension, and changes in patterns of diet and exercise (Blackburn, 1983; Mittlemark and others, 1986).

Integral to the program since its inception has been a commitment to developing "community partnerships" for health through which community members work with the research team in decision making and program implementation. As Carlaw, Mittlemark, Bracht, and Luepker (1984, p. 245) have stated, "The hypothesis was that educational interventions planned with, through, and for communities would lead to changes in individual and family behaviors conducive to heart health."

While community organization has in fact been only one of three educational approaches used in this project, the others being media and direct face-to-face education, community organizing principles have been apparent in virtually all aspects of program development. Community analysis and "mapping," gathering of data from community leaders, and the early formation of a community advisory board in each community thus were among the early steps taken to ensure that community input and involvement was assigned a high premium.

MHHP researchers have argued that the program represents a blend of social planning and locality development (Carlaw, Mittlemark, Bracht, and Luepker, 1984). They further have noted that the MHHP has had to walk a fine line between being a *scientific* project (requiring a degree of investigator control to ensure measurable results) and being a *community-based* program, emphasizing local ownership and responsibility. On balance, however, the

MHHP appears to have been successful in addressing both sets of commitments and needs and in combining the strengths of its two community organizing approaches.

The MHHP was implemented by means of a sequential design in which the three communities were added at one-year intervals, with each community having the intensive educational intervention for a period of five years. In each community, the program has moved through two major phases, the first facilitating the development of increased community awareness of the heart health concept and the second stressing the development of opportunities to practice behaviors conducive to improved cardiovascular health (Carlaw, Mittlemark, Bracht, and Luepker, 1984).

Community participation and involvement has been critically integrated into each step of the process by means of a series of small group structures (board membership, functional task forces, and committees) used as vehicles through which residents have played major roles in generating action areas to be addressed, specific activities to be undertaken, and appropriate groups to be targeted. Moreover, participation on task forces and committees has not only enabled community residents to share their knowledge of community needs and resources in the design of concrete strategies but also promoted the continued diffusion of awareness of and interest in heart disease prevention in the community (Mittlemark and others, 1986; Finnegan, Murray, Kurth, and McCarthy, 1989).

As the program has moved from the development of task forces and committees into the nurturance of a wider support system and the strengthening of community norms and values supportive of heart health behaviors, another important change has occurred as well. The researchers have stepped back from their early position as "initiating partners," and community members increasingly have served this catalytic role. Of particular importance in this regard is the fact that the three groups formed at the beginning of the project as "advisory boards" to the University of Minnesota School of Public Health have all become autonomous, private nonprofit [501 (c)(3)] organizations (Bracht, 1988). The latter not only played key decision-making (as opposed to advisory) roles, but also have begun to plan ahead to provide for continuity once federal funding for the MHHP is terminated. The MHHP's director of community organization reports that all three organizations have already developed mission statements for the period 1990–1995, when they will be without government support (Bracht, 1988).

Through the development of an effective network of community groups and support systems that show great promise for outliving the formally funded program, the MHHP has increased community competence by enhancing the problem-solving capacity of the group. Moreover, as the research team progressively has served as "consultants and program resources" with the community boards assuming "planning and even funding roles" (Blackburn, 1983), the program has moved increasingly from a social planning model toward a community development approach.

In this and other ways, the program has contributed to individual and community empowerment. As Carlaw, Mittlemark, Bracht, and Luepker (1984, p. 248) note, "Sustained volunteer interest and assertiveness of community leadership for heart health" coupled with an increased community role as the "initiating partner" in the program are among the indications of empowerment that can be readily observed.

Because the MHHP was initiated from outside the community and because the research team entered with a clear idea of the problem to be addressed (cardiovascular health), the MHHP does not demonstrate the principle of starting where the people are in its pure form. Within the context of a previously defined problem area, however, clear efforts were made to ensure resident involvement in the setting of specific objectives, the choosing of particular issues around which to mobilize, and so on. While not a "pure" community organizing project, the MHHP appears to have drawn effectively on many key principles of community organization practice, tailoring and applying them in this community-based action research program.

The overall evaluation goals of the MHHP are "to measure the changes in disease, risk factor distributions, and behavior and to relate these changes to components of the educational program" (Blackburn, 1983, p. 415). From a community organization perspective, several early indicators of success can be identified. As Bracht (1988) notes, leadership retention rates have been high, with over 50 percent of the current executive committee members of each community's nonprofit organization having been founding members of the MHHP in their communities in the early 1980s. Forty-two percent of the heart health programs within the communities are now being run by local community sponsors, with another one-third making the transition toward this goal.

Thus, in terms of volunteer retention rates, community ownership, and continuity over time, the Minnesota Heart Health Program has achieved a high level of success that it is hoped will also be reflected in the achievement of community-wide risk factor reduction rates and related outcomes (Bracht, 1988).

Conclusion

While a number of promising new approaches and change processes have been adopted by health professionals in recent years, community organization remains an important method of health education practice. Moreover, the pivotal role of this change approach reflects not only its time-tested efficacy as a methodological tool but also its high degree of philosophical fit or congruence with the most fundamental principles of effective community work. Both change theory and community organization practice, for example, stress the principle of relevance, or starting where the people are, the principle of participation, and the importance of empowering individuals and communities as a vital part of the change process.

The way in which community organizing is envisioned and practiced, of course, depends in part on how "community" is conceptualized. Health education professionals who adopt an ecological systems perspective on community are most likely to regard community organization in geographic terms and to apply methods and approaches accordingly. In contrast, a social systems perspective may enable practitioners to see community organizing in terms of either geographic or interest-group identification and stress working across communities as well as within them. Similarly, whether the practitioner views a community as autonomous or interdependent and as essentially harmonious and homogeneous or heterogeneous and competitive will influence the model of community organization practice that he or she is most likely to adopt. While Rothman's three models of community organization practice—locality development, social planning, and social action—reflect these and other underlying assumptions and are frequently used to classify alternative approaches to practice, considerable overlap occurs in their actual application.

Regardless of the particular approach employed, the health education professional who is functioning specifically as a community organizer is in a unique position to help members of a community identify common goals, develop strategies, mobilize resources, and in other ways collectively address their shared concerns. Frequently, however, health and social service professionals are not employed by the community itself but by an agency with specific agendas and often with categorical funding. The practitioner in this setting may find that he or she cannot undertake community organizing in the strictest sense of the word because the agency rather than the community has identified the specific health problem(s) to be addressed. Yet as the Minnesota Heart Health Program experience demonstrates, professionals in such situations can effectively apply many of the core principles and approaches of community organization practice. They thus can elicit high-level community participation or involvement in every aspect of program planning, implementation, and evaluation; moreover, they can strive to build leadership skills and increase community competence as an integral part of the overall health education project. In addition, while the overall health problem area (for example, AIDS or hypertension) may initially have been identified by an outside agency, the health education professional using community organization skills and approaches can help communities identify within this broader framework those specific issues they feel are of greatest relevance. He or she can help both professional colleagues and members of the community understand the importance of working in a partnership toward the eventual goals of community ownership of projects and increased empowerment and community competence.

In sum, community organization is one of the oldest tools within the helping professions, one that remains central to the practice of health education in a wide variety of settings.

References

Alinsky, S. D. "Community Analysis and Organization." *American Journal of Sociology*, 1941, *46*, 797–808.

Alinsky, S. D. *Reveille for Radicals.* Chicago: University of Chicago Press, 1969.

Alinsky, S. D. *Rules for Radicals.* New York: Random House, 1972.

Allport, G. W. "Catharsis and the Reduction of Prejudice." In K. Lewin and P. Grabbe (eds.), "Problems of Re-Education." *Journal of Social Issues,* 1945, *1,* 3-10.

Antonovsky, A. *Health, Stress, and Coping.* San Francisco, Calif.: Jossey-Bass, 1979.

Auerbach, E. R., and Wallerstein, N. *ESL for Action Problem Posing at Work,* Teacher's Guide. Reading, Mass.: Addison-Wesley, 1987.

Barbarin, O., Good, P. R., Pharr, O. M., and Siskind, J. A. (eds.). *Institutional Racism and Community Competence.* U.S. Department of Health and Human Services Publication no. ADM, 1981, pp. 81-907.

Blackburn, H. "Research and Demonstration Projects in Community Cardiovascular Disease Prevention." *Journal of Public Health Policy,* 1983, *4,* 398-421.

Bracht, N. (Director of Community Organization, Minnesota Heart Health Program). Personal communication, June 25, 1988.

Carlaw, R. W., Mittlemark, M., Bracht, N., and Luepker, R. "Organization for a Community Cardiovascular Health Program: Experiences from the Minnesota Heart Health Program." *Health Education Quarterly,* 1984, *11,* 243-252.

Choldin, H. M. *Cities and Suburbs.* New York: McGraw-Hill, 1985.

Cohen, S., and Syme, S. L. (eds.). *Social Support and Health.* Orlando, Fla.: Academic Press, 1985.

Cottrell, L. S., Jr. "The Competent Community." In R. Warren and L. Lyon (eds.), *New Perspectives on the American Community.* Homewood, Ill.: Dorsey Press, 1983.

Delbecq, A., Van De Ven, A. H., and Gustafson, D. H. *Group Techniques for Program Planning: A Guide to Nominal Group and Delphi Processes.* Glenview, Ill.: Scott, Foresman, 1975.

Dewey, J. *The Public and Its Problems: An Essay in Political Inquiry.* Chicago: Gateway Books, 1946.

Effrat, M. "Approaches to Community: Conflicts and Complementarities." In M. Effrat (ed.), *The Community: Approaches and Applications.* New York: Free Press, 1974.

Fellin, P. *The Competent Community*. Itasca, Ill.: Peacock, 1987.

Finnegan, J. R., Murray, D. M., Kurth, C., and McCarthy, P. "Measuring and Tracking Education Program Implementation: The Minnesota Heart Health Program Experience," *Health Education Quarterly*, 1989, *16*, 77-90.

Freire, P. *Education for Critical Consciousness*. New York: Seabury Press, 1973.

Garber, J., and Seligman, M. (eds.). *Human Helplessness: Theory and Applications*. Orlando, Fla.: Academic Press, 1980.

Garvin, C. D., and Cox, F. M. "A History of Community Organizing Since the Civil War with Special Reference to Oppressed Communities." *Strategies of Community Organizing*. (4th ed.) Itasca, Ill.: Peacock, 1987.

Geiger, H. J. "Community Control—Or Community Conflict?" *Bulletin of the National Tuberculosis and Respiratory Disease Association*, 1969, *55*, 4-11.

Goldoftas, B. "Organizing in a Gray Ghetto: The Tenderloin Senior Organizing Project." *Dollars and Sense*, Jan./Feb. 1988, pp. 18-19.

Grossman, J. "Health for What? Change, Conflict, and the Search for Purpose." *Pacific Health Education Reports*, 1971, *2*, 51-66.

Hatch, J. W., and Eng, E. "Community Participation and Control: Or Control of Community Participation?" In V. W. Sidel and R. Sidel (eds.), *Reforming Medicine: Lessons of the Last Quarter Century*. New York: Pantheon, 1984.

Heitzmann, C. A., and Kaplan, R. M. "Assessment of Methods for Measuring Social Support." *Health Psychology*, 1988, *7*, 75-109.

Hilgard, E. R., and Bower, G. H. *Theories of Learning*. (4th ed.) Englewood Cliffs, N.J.: Prentice-Hall, 1975.

Hochbaum, G. "Modern Theories of Communication." *Children*, 1960, *7*, 13-18.

Hope, A., and Timmel, S. *Training for Transformation: A Handbook for Community Workers*. Gweru, Zimbabwe: Mambo Press, 1984.

Hunter, A. "The Loss of Community: An Empirical Test Through Replication." *American Sociology Review*, 1975, *40*, 537-552.

Iscore, I. "Community Psychology and the Competent Community." *American Psychologist*, 1980, *29*, 607–613.

Israel, B. "Social Networks and Social Support: Implications for Natural Helper and Community Level Interventions." *Health Education Quarterly*, 1985, *12*, 66–80.

Kent, J. "A Descriptive Approach to a Community Clinic." Unpublished report, Denver, Colo., 1970.

Khinduka, S. K. "Community Development: Potentials and Limitations." In R. M. Kramer and H. Specht (eds.), *Readings in Community Organization Practice*. (2nd ed.) Englewood Cliffs, N.J.: Prentice-Hall, 1975.

Leighton, D. C., and Stone, I. T. "Community Development as a Therapeutic Force: A Case Study with Measurement." In P. M. Roman and H. M. Trice (eds.), *Sociological Perspectives on Community Mental Health*. Philadelphia: F. A. Davis, 1974.

Lewin, K. "Group Decision and Social Change." In E. Maccoby and others (eds.), *Readings in Social Psychology*. (3rd ed.) New York: Holt, Rinehart & Winston, 1958.

Lindeman, E. *The Meaning of Adult Education*. New York: New Republic, 1926.

McCallister, L., and Fischer, C. S. "A Procedure for Surveying Personal Networks." *Sociological Methods and Research*, 1978, *7*, 131–148.

Miller, M. "Turning Problems into Actionable Issues." Unpublished report, Organize Training Center, San Francisco, 1985.

Minkler, M. "Theory into Action: Health Education in a Honduras Refugee Camp." Paper presented at the 111th annual meeting of the American Public Health Association, Dallas, Nov. 1983.

Minkler, M. "Building Supportive Ties and Sense of Community Among the Inner-City Elderly: The Tenderloin Senior Outreach Project." *Health Education Quarterly*, 1985, *12*, 303–314.

Minkler, M., and Cox, K. "Creating Critical Consciousness in Health: Applications of Freire's Philosophy and Methods to the Health Care Setting." *International Journal of Health Services*, 1980, *10*, 311–322.

Mittlemark, M., and others. "Community-Wide Prevention of Cardiovascular Disease: Education Strategies of the Minnesota Heart Health Program." *Preventive Medicine,* 1986, *15,* 1-17.

Mowat, C. L. *The Charity Organization Society, 1869-1913.* London: Methuen, 1961.

Moynihan, D. P. *Maximum Feasible Misunderstanding: Community Action in the War on Poverty.* New York: Free Press, 1969.

Nyswander, D. "The Open Society: Its Implications for Health Educators." *Health Education Monographs,* 1966, *1,* 3-13.

Rappaport, J. "Studies in Empowerment: Introduction to the Issue." *Prevention in Human Services,* 1984, *3,* 1-7.

Reitzes, D. C., and Reitzes, D. C. "Saul Alinsky's Contribution to Community Development." *Journal of the Community Development Society,* 1980, *11,* 39-52.

Ross, M. *Community Organization: Theory and Principles.* New York: Harper & Row, 1955.

Rothman, J., and Tropman, J. E. "Models of Community Organization and Macro Practice: Their Mixing and Phasing." In F. M. Cox, J. L. Erlich, J. Rothman, and J. E. Tropman (eds.), *Strategies of Community Organization.* (4th ed.) Itasca, Ill.: Peacock, 1987.

Thomas, P. D., Goodwin, J. M., and Goodwin, J. S. "Effect of Social Support on Stress-Related Changes in Cholesterol Level, Uric Acid Level, and Immune Function in an Elderly Sample." *American Journal of Psychiatry,* 1985, *142,* 735-737.

Thomas, R. P., Israel, B., and Steuart, G. W. "Cooperative Problem Solving: The Neighborhood Self-Help Project." In H. P. Cleary, J. M. Kichen, and P. G. Ensor (eds.), *Advancing Health Through Education.* Mountain View, Calif.: Mayfield, 1985.

United Nations International Children's Emergency Fund/World Health Organization Joint Committee on Health Policy. "Community Involvement." *National Decision Making for Primary Health Care.* Geneva, Switzerland: World Health Organization, 1981.

Wallerstein, N., and Bernstein, E. "Empowerment Education: Freire's Ideas Adapted to Health Education." *Health Education Quarterly,* 1988, *15,* 379-394.

Warren, R. *The Community in America.* Chicago: Rand McNally, 1963.

World Health Organization/United Nations International Children's Emergency Fund. International Conference on Primary Health Care. Alma Ata, Union of Soviet Socialist Republics, 1978.

World Health Organization. *New Policies for Health Education in Primary Health Care.* Background document no. A36 for the 36th World Health Assembly. Geneva, Switzerland: World Health Organization, 1983.

Chapter 13

Mario A. Orlandi
Cassie Landers
Raymond Weston
Nancy Haley

▲ ▲ ▲

Diffusion of
Health Promotion Innovations

During the past three decades, the way in which we think about health and disease has changed dramatically.* This change is a result of the realization that individuals can significantly influence their health and longevity and that they can prevent the onset of chronic disease by changing their life-styles. The translation of this recent epidemiological understanding into the widespread reduction of avoidable morbidity and mortality through behavior change has rapidly become a common theme for the public health community (Green, 1979).

However, many individuals and in fact large segments of society continue to engage in behaviors that are known to lead to premature disability and death (Yankauer, 1988). The gap between what health professionals believe people should do and what the general population actually does has become one of the principal challenges of public health today (Baquet and Ringen, 1987).

In response to this challenge, public health researchers have begun to study systematically the barriers to bridging this gap in an attempt to identify more effective and more cost-efficient intervention strategies. One important perspective that has only recently been explored within the context of health promotion research for

*This work was supported in part by a grant from the National Heart, Lung and Blood Institute (HL-40688).

chronic disease prevention and management is the area of diffusion theory (Winett, 1986; Rogers, 1983). The process of translating new health-related research findings or effective interventions into widespread behavior change for the good of society is a classic example of the general process defined as the diffusion of innovations.

This chapter discusses various aspects of diffusion theory that have direct applicability to the problem of bridging the health promotion gap. In doing so, the chapter focuses on three key areas: First, it reviews the concept of a generic diffusion system and notes some limitations of the classic diffusion model. Second, the chapter describes an alternative research framework that enhances standard approaches to both innovation development and diffusion planning by incorporating methods for increasing target group participation. Third, the chapter provides an example of this research framework in the form of a community-based health promotion study that utilizes this approach during all phases of program planning and implementation. The chapter concludes with an analysis of questions that are left unanswered and directions for future research.

Contemporary Perspectives on Classical Diffusion Theory

Diffusion is defined as the process by which an innovation is communicated through certain channels over time among members of a social system (Rogers, 1983). An *innovation* is an idea, practice, service, or other object that is perceived as new by an individual or other unit of adoption. Classical diffusion theory developed as an attempt to explain this communication process in a rigorous and scientific way that would have predictive validity from one innovation situation to another (Rogers, 1983, p. 333). The original model was also an attempt to determine the most consistently effective way to apply solutions that are developed in test settings to problems in real-world settings.

The study of diffusion of innovations has its roots in rural sociology, and early applications included investigations of how new agricultural technologies spread (or failed to spread) among farmers. Subsequent work applied diffusion theory to a wide variety of practices and technologies, including family planning and the use of medical screening tests and new pharmaceutical products. Diffusion research spans many countries, cultures, and issues (Rogers, 1983). In three separate books over nearly three decades, Everett Rogers has synthesized thousands of diffusion studies and advanced the understanding of diffusion theory and its utility in many settings (Rogers, 1962, 1983; Rogers and Shoemaker, 1971).

A basic assumption underlying the early work in this area was that diffusion patterns and adoption rates of particular innovations are determined primarily by the scientific attributes of the innovation and the unique characteristics of the adopter. Following this line of reasoning therefore led to the assumption that a thorough analysis of innovations that had been adopted and of the organizations or individuals that had adopted them would result in formulas for successful diffusion that could be applied to other innovations in other settings.

Features of Successful Diffusion Efforts. Though such variables have been redefined and modified over time, several of them have been consistently identified as attributes of successful diffusion efforts (Kolbe and Iverson, 1981). These include the following:

> *Compatibility.* When innovations are consistent with the economic, sociocultural, and philosophical value system of the adopter, adoption is more likely to take place.
>
> *Flexibility.* Innovations that can be unbundled and used as separate components will be applicable in a wider variety of user settings.
>
> *Reversibility.* If for any reason, the adopting individual or organization wants to revert to its previous practices, it is desirable that an innovation be capable of termination. Innovations that are not are less likely to be adopted.
>
> *Relative advantage.* If an innovation appears to be beneficial when compared to current and previous methods, adoption is more likely.
>
> *Complexity.* Complex innovations are more difficult to communicate and to understand and are therefore less likely to be adopted.
>
> *Cost-efficiency.* For an innovation to be considered desirable,

its perceived benefits, both tangible and intangible, must
outweigh its perceived costs.

Risk. The degree of uncertainty introduced by an innovation
helps determine its potential for adoption. Innovations
that involve higher risk are less likely to be adopted.

This classical approach also established specific roles for different interest groups that interact as part of the overall diffusion
system. Innovations were seen as originating from a *resource system*
that has the knowledge and expertise required to create the new
concept. The innovation was viewed as a uniform, intact entity that
moves from the resource system to the adopting individual and/or
organization, which were described collectively as the *user system.*

Though the classical diffusion model has contributed greatly
to our understanding of this important research area, it has been
challenged in the recent past in a number of ways (Rogers, 1983;
Basch, Eveland, and Portnoy, 1986). First, the characterization of
the innovation as an intact package directs attention toward the user
system and the adoption decision and away from the concept of
innovation refinement as a means of improving the "fit" betweeen
innovation and user. Second, this orientation does not provide an
adequate means of evaluating the potential contribution of efforts
on the part of the resource system or the user system to influence the
diffusion process. In this sense, as a rule, the process is viewed as
static rather than dynamic. Third, the classical model fails to recognize the fact that the adoption decision is only one step in a multistep process that ranges from the first phases of innovation
development to a point beyond adoption at which the innovation
either succeeds or fails in achieving a lasting and meaningful impact. This point is critical, for example, when the innovation under
consideration is a health promotion intervention. As the next section of this chapter indicates, a significant impact from a public
health perspective requires maintenance of intervention effects that
extend far beyond the adoption decision.

Potential System Failure Points. With respect to the multistep process, modern conceptualizations of the diffusion process typically
and more realistically view each step as a potential failure point—a

critical barrier that must be overcome for the overall system to achieve a lasting and meaningful impact. These potential system failure points include the following:

Innovation failure. The system can fail if the innovation does not bring about its intended effect. For example, this might occur if an innovation, though highly touted, had been poorly designed, inadequately evaluated, or dishonestly represented.

Communication failure. An innovation can be genuinely efficacious and have the potential to achieve its intended effect yet fail to do so because it was communicated ineffectively. Failure at this stage normally means that the user subsystem was either unaware of the innovation or was improperly informed as to its availability or applicability.

Adoption failure. Though efficacious and properly communicated, an innovation may not be adopted because of a host of factors ranging from differing value and belief systems to a lack of necessary resources.

Implementation failure. Despite being successfully adopted, an innovation may not be implemented properly or even implemented at all. This frequently occurs when specific program components (such as instructor training) that are considered instrumental to the program's efficacy are omitted or drastically abbreviated. This is more likely to occur when programs are adopted at the organizational level (for example, the corporation or school level) and then implemented by the organization among its members.

Maintenance failure. Even though an efficacious program may be successfully communicated, adopted, and initially implemented, it can lose its momentum and dissipate rapidly over time. From a health promotion perspective, program maintenance over time is critical.

The Innovation-Development Process. As this overview indicates, diffusion theory begins conceptually with an innovation that has the potential for communication and adoption. The relationship between diffusion theory and health promotion innovation development can best be understood as a specific application of the *innovation-development process*. This process includes all the decisions and the activities and their impacts that occur from the early stage of an idea through its development and its production, diffusion, adoption, and consequences (Rogers, 1983, p. 135). A six-stage innovation-development process includes these main steps: (1) recognition of a problem or need; (2) basic and applied research; (3) development to put a new idea into a form that is expected to meet the needs of an audience of potential adopters; (4) commercialization that involves production, marketing, and distribution of the innovation; (5) diffusion and adoption; and (6) consequences (Rogers, 1983).

Federally sponsored health promotion innovation research has been described according to a five-phase model that parallels the general innovation-development process and includes basic research, applied research and development, clinical investigation, clinical trials, and demonstration and education research (U.S. Department of Health and Human Services, 1987). However, despite the value that has been placed upon this paradigm, there is little evidence that innovations that result from this process are necessarily more successfully diffused than those that do not (Kolbe and Iverson, 1981; Patton, 1978). A number of factors contribute to this inconsistency, including the limited involvement of user systems in developing innovations and the gaps in translating knowledge acquired in controlled research studies into real-world settings. A further limitation is that research usually focuses on short-term intervention effects and fails to consider longer-term issues such as program maintenance that are critical to improvements in public health.

Innovation Development and Diffusion:
A Conceptual Integration

Health promotion innovation development is a process that begins with basic research and hypothesis testing and leads ultimately to demonstrations in real-world settings. The heart of diffusion theory begins, essentially, where innovation development leaves off in an attempt to characterize the success of an innovation as it moves out of research and development settings and into real-world settings. If this system functioned flawlessly, there would be many more health promotion innovations in operation in settings where they could potentially have a significant impact (Yankauer, 1988).

As noted earlier, a significant number of barriers have the potential, if left unaddressed, to undermine the objectives of either the innovation-development or the innovation-diffusion process. The fact that many of these barriers frequently are left unaddressed and that the gap frequently remains is evidenced by the number of health promotion innovations that remain "on the shelf" after considerable development effort (Iverson and Kolbe, 1983). Though diffusion and application are the goals of these efforts, they typically are not the outcomes.

In some respects, the problem can be viewed as a gap that is frequently left unfilled between the point where innovation-development ends and diffusion begins. Some of the factors that contribute to innovation efficacy and diffusion success are very similar, and there are strategies that can be used to address these factors simultaneously. The purpose of doing so is to attempt to bridge the gap that often remains when innovation-development barriers and diffusion barriers are considered separately, as though they were aspects of unrelated problems.

One strategy that attempts to bridge this gap is the linkage approach to innovation-development and diffusion planning. The key to this approach lies in its reliance on increased target group participation in all aspects of the process.

A methodology for bridging the health promotion diffusion gap that enhances both the innovation-development process *and* the diffusion planning process is the *linkage approach*. This perspective was first described by Havelock (1971) and later expanded by Kolbe and Iverson (1981) and Orlandi (1986a, 1987). It involves the integration of three separate but interactive systems into a single general systems model (see Figure 13.1).

In addition to the resource and user systems, in which innovations originate and are ultimately adopted (or not adopted), a linkage system that represents the cooperative exchanges and inter-

Figure 13.1. Overview of the Linkage Approach to Innovation Diffusion.

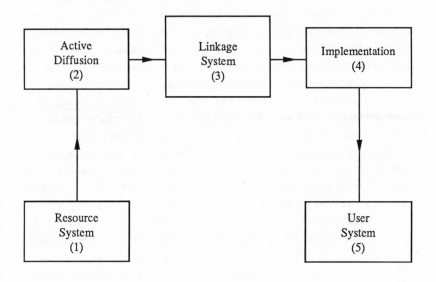

1. The resource system consists of researchers, developers, trainers, consultants, services, products, and materials.

2. The diffusion process is the range of activities carried out specifically to result in the spread of an innovation to specific target groups.

3. The linkage system consists of representatives of the resource system, representatives of the user system, change agents, and strategic planning activities.

4. The implementation process may be carried out either by members of the user system who have received training or by members of the resource system. The important point is that the implementation process and the innovation itself have been developed through collaboration, thus increasing the likelihood that efficacious approaches will be used in a culturally sensitive manner whenever possible.

5. The user system consists of the individuals, organizations, agencies, groups, and networks.

actions required to collaboratively develop user-relevant innovation and diffusion strategies is defined. The individuals who interact within the linkage subsystem include representatives of the user and resource subsystems plus *change agents,* who facilitate the collaboration. The role of change agent does not have to be filled by an independent third party; members of the user or resource subsystems can also operate in this facilitative capacity.

The most critical aspect of this approach is the perspective that defines the information exchange that takes place within the linkage subsystem. This perspective incorporates elements of community organization (see Chapter Twelve) and theories of organizational change (see Chapter Fourteen); however, it is most closely aligned with social marketing (Bloom and Novelli, 1981), an area that is described in depth in Chapter Fifteen of this book. Several characteristics of the social marketing perspective are critical to the area of innovation diffusion in general and to the linkage approach to innovation-development and diffusion planning in particular.

According to this perspective, the role of the resource system is to collaborate with the user system in the innovation planning process by helping the user system determine its needs, expectations, and limitations. Optimally effective innovation messages and strategies must take into consideration a variety of socioculturally relevant communication factors. Therefore, data must be collected to help define these communication characteristics in ways that are likely to enhance the efficacy of the intervention message.

The techniques of social marketing research, which include a variety of methods for gathering relevant quantitative and qualitative data, are designed specifically to optimize the effectiveness of the innovation-development and diffusion planning processes by addressing issues such as user group preferences, perceived needs, and limitations. The two key concepts directing these formative research activities are *segmentation* of a general population into relevant subgroups and *tailoring* an innovation to the particular characteristics of the targeted segments (Orlandi, 1986b).

The preceding discussion describes a promising line of reasoning for approaching the development of health promotion innovations and suggests methods for designing innovation-development research studies. Three ideas are central. First, the multiple objectives of modern diffusion theory are kept in mind as are the various steps at which such a process can fail. Second, the five-phase innovation-development research model discussed earlier (U.S. Department of Health and Human Services, 1987) is employed, with careful attention to the objectives of each phase. Third, the known limitations and gaps of these approaches are addressed and, one hopes, minimized through the use of a linkage approach and social marketing research methods to enhance the quality and quantity of target group (user system) participation in the program development and research process. The next section provides one example of how this theoretical framework is being carried out.

The Mount Vernon CARES Project

The American Health Foundation is involved in the design and implementation of innovative community-based cholesterol screening, education, and referral strategies. The overall goal of this effort is to design, implement, and evaluate strategies to enhance the effectiveness of a community-based cholesterol screening system and to elicit participation of members of the Black American population who have traditionally been unresponsive to such efforts. The intervention system includes components to (1) enhance cholesterol awareness, (2) increase participation in cholesterol screening activities, and (3) motivate those identified as at risk to comply with referral for further treatment.

Elevated Blood Cholesterol and Health Promotion Innovation. Elevated blood cholesterol is a major risk factor for coronary heart disease and a significant public health problem, affecting as many as 50 percent of all adults in the United States ("Report of the National Cholesterol Education Program Expert Panel," 1988). Control of elevated cholesterol to reduce the risk of heart disease involves detection of high-risk groups, diagnosis, and effective treatment. The primary treatment approach for high blood cholesterol levels is dietary change. The recent promulgation of guidelines for detecting and lowering high cholesterol has spurred important community and patient health education efforts to improve awareness, detection, and adherence to dietary guidelines to reduce elevated cholesterol levels (Ernst and Cleeman, 1988).

Both the public's and health professionals' awareness and concern about the problem of elevated cholesterol are rapidly gaining momentum (Schucker and others, 1987a, 1987b). Information about cholesterol management is now flooding all forms of media. However, gaps in knowledge, attitudes, and practices of health care providers and at-risk individuals present major challenges for health care and health education (Glanz, 1988). The set of health promotion innovations that is most effective and can be refined and diffused is in an early stage. The challenge is to develop this set of innovations and to achieve its successful adoption, diffusion, and maintenance in defined communities. The Mount Vernon CARES (Cholesterol Awareness, Risk Education, and Screening) Project is an effort to accomplish these goals effectively.

Overview of Project Components. The intervention community is Mount Vernon, a biracial community in Westchester County that is thirteen miles north of New York City. The project is a collaborative effort initiated by the American Health Foundation (AHF) and involving the health, cultural, civic, industrial, and religious organizations serving the Mount Vernon community. The broad program goal is to implement a cholesterol education, screening, and referral program for Mount Vernon residents aged eighteen and older over a three-year period. As indicated in Figure 13.2, several components of the Mount Vernon CARES Project are being designed, implemented, and evaluated:

> *Community assessment and analysis.* A sample of resident and community leaders are being interviewed at baseline and at years two and three of the project to determine changes in community knowledge, attitudes, and practices regarding cholesterol as a result of the intervention.
> *Community education and recruitment.* Educational materials designed specifically to meet the needs of the target population are being developed. In addition, innovative recruitment strategies to elicit community participation are being devised.

Figure 13.2. Mount Vernon CARES: Overview of Intervention
Development and Implementation.

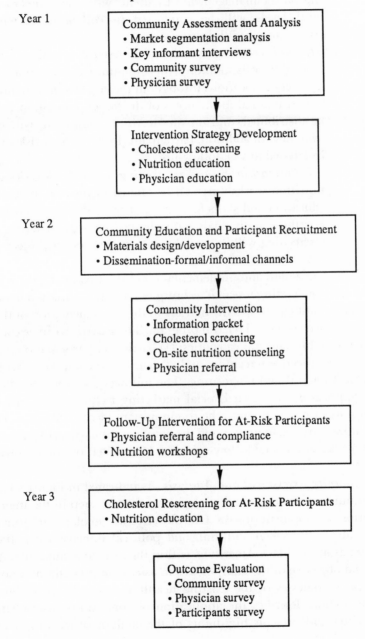

Year 1

Community Assessment and Analysis
• Market segmentation analysis
• Key informant interviews
• Community survey
• Physician survey

Intervention Strategy Development
• Cholesterol screening
• Nutrition education
• Physician education

Year 2

Community Education and Participant Recruitment
• Materials design/development
• Dissemination-formal/informal channels

Community Intervention
• Information packet
• Cholesterol screening
• On-site nutrition counseling
• Physician referral

Follow-Up Intervention for At-Risk Participants
• Physician referral and compliance
• Nutrition workshops

Year 3

Cholesterol Rescreening for At-Risk Participants
• Nutrition education

Outcome Evaluation
• Community survey
• Physician survey
• Participants survey

Physician education. A physician education program focusing on the management of patients with elevated cholesterol levels will be conducted in collaboration with community health institutions.

Cholesterol screening. A series of cholesterol screenings will be held in collaboration with community organizations at a variety of locations throughout the city. An information packet tailored to the needs of the target population will be distributed, and on-site nutrition counseling will be available. In addition, participants found to be at risk will be advised to seek follow-up.

Nutrition workshops and rescreening activities. A series of nutrition workshops will be offered to provide in-depth education and skills for modification of dietary behavior. For those individuals with elevated cholesterol levels, a rescreening will be available in year three of the project.

In the design and implementation of these components, various social marketing research techniques are being employed in an attempt to anticipate specific barriers to the implementation of the proposed screening and referral program. These barriers can be classified into three general categories: (1) barriers to participation, (2) barriers to effective screening, and (3) barriers to compliance with physical referral and rescreening. The following section describes the application of selected social marketing techniques in an attempt to gain insights into the community residents and pertinent organizations and to understand the nature of the barriers to participation, screening, and follow-up in the Mount Vernon community.

Community Assessment and Analysis. As indicated in Figure 13.2, community assessment and analysis was the first step in the intervention development process. One objective was to obtain information about the social, cultural, and political dimensions of the target group of Black Americans within the general community. A second objective of the analysis was to assess the strengths and potential weaknesses of the existing health service delivery system. This section describes the application of community assessment activities and presents highlights of the analysis of existing data sources, semistructured interviews with key informants, and telephone surveys of community residents and physicians.

Sociodemographic indicators were obtained through the *analysis of census and other archival data sources.* From this information, we learned that Black Americans comprise 48.7 percent of the 67,000 residents in Mount Vernon and that this proportion appears to be increasing. The median age is thirty-five years, and much of the working population is made up of skilled and semiskilled blue-collar workers.

Analysis of selected characteristics along racial lines revealed important differences in the population. White residents of Mount Vernon tend to have higher incomes, less unemployment, and more formal education. Both blacks and whites have relatively stable periods of residence in the community.

Analysis of the twenty-one census tracts comprising Mount Vernon helped to identify three distinct groups. Group 1 is predominantly black (72.8 percent), is less often high school educated (50.9 percent), and has a significant proportion (23.9 percent) of female-headed households. Group 2 is a racially mixed population, with somewhat higher levels of high school education (66.8 percent) and fewer female-headed households (15.7 percent) than Group 1. Group 3 is of higher income, predominantly white, has a higher educational level, and tends to use health and recreation facilities outside of Mount Vernon proper. The segmentation that was revealed by this census tract analysis was an important basis for tailoring specific intervention components to specific population subgroups.

A second type of data collection activity involved a series of *semistructured interviews with community representatives* of health, civic, industrial, and religious organizations. The interviews, conducted by trained AHF personnel, focused on three major themes: organizational objectives; obstacles encountered in accomplishing these objectives; and social, economic, and cultural strengths and weaknesses of the community. A secondary objective of these interviews was to gain insight into the feasibility of the proposed cholesterol intervention and the potential obstacles that might be encountered. In addition to serving as a means for data collection, the interviews identified potential collaborators and provided an initial entry point into the power structure in the community.

The third set of data collection activities during the intervention planning phase involved *telephone surveys* of a random sample of *community residents* as well as *physicians* practicing in Mount Vernon. The strategies for each of these surveys will be discussed briefly.

In order to obtain baseline data on the pertinent knowledge, attitudes, beliefs, and practices of Mount Vernon residents, we conducted a telephone survey with a random sample of 550 residents from Groups 1 and 2 (the two community segments with most of the black population). The survey will be repeated during years two and three of the project to help determine the ability of the intervention to penetrate the target community and to monitor its impact. A panel of 100 black residents will be followed throughout the three years of the project to determine the impact of the intervention on these individuals over time.

The survey included thirty-five closed-ended questions and took about ten minutes to complete. Questions addressed personal background information and knowledge of cholesterol and its relationship to cardiovascular disease. The survey also asked about dietary practices known to affect cholesterol levels as well as exercise patterns, smoking, and other life-style factors. This survey provided both baseline data for the evaluation *and* important insights for development of educational messages.

In addition to the community survey, a physician telephone survey addressed the beliefs, attitudes, and practices of physicians regarding the management and treatment of individuals with elevated cholesterol levels. The survey also provided an initial entry point into the health care system and an opportunity to introduce the program to the medical community. Physicians surveyed included internists, cardiologists, and family practitioners affiliated with either of the two health care facilities serving Mount Vernon.

Before the telephone survey, we sent an introductory letter to physicians about the community cholesterol program as well as the survey. Despite these efforts, the initial survey response rate was less than 20 percent. While physician resistance to community-based screening programs is common, physicians' cooperation is critical to the design of effective referral strategies. Therefore, we identified the need to pursue alternative strategies to elicit the support and commitment of physicians serving the community. These strategies included providing information at grand rounds, distributing information flyers, and eliciting the support of a key physician from each institution to act as a project facilitator. In addition, we conducted interviews with physicians in the health care setting. Through these efforts the physician response rate was increased to 60 percent. Additional attempts to further increase this participation are in progress.

Intervention Strategy Development. This section describes the sequence of activities involved in developing strategies for the cholesterol screening, nutrition education, and physician education components of the intervention.

Because we recognized the need to involve the community in the initial planning phases, the Community Advisory Board was established. The board consists of eight community leaders and, among other things, provides continual insights into the sociological, cultural, and political dimensions of the community. The first responsibility of the committee was to create a project theme, name, and logo. Following this activity, the board has played a pivotal role in identifying community organizations capable of successfully carrying out the screening events.

We recognized the need to develop a range of complementary strategies in order to reach the black population, which has been unresponsive to traditional recruitment strategies (Wynder, Harris, and Haley, 1989; Wynder, Field, and Haley, 1986). Through an elaborate negotiation process with representatives from prospective interested institutions, fourteen participating community institutions were identified. The *cholesterol screening sites* included health institutions, work sites, community service organizations, churches, and low-income housing projects.

The selection of these sites was guided by the census tract analysis performed during the community assessment phase of the project. The segment of the population least likely to participate in community-based health promotion events resides in the area defined by Group 1. In an effort to attract the participation of this segment, we selected five screening sites including the Neighborhood Health Center, a YMCA, a large Baptist church, and two low-income housing projects. Nine screening sites are located within the geographical boundaries comprising Group 2. These include the Mount Vernon Hospital, two community service organizations, city hall, two work sites, and three churches.

The *nutrition education component* has been developed partly on the basis of data collected during the community assessment phase, which underscored the need for community-based nutrition resources. The two-part nutrition component includes on-site nutrition counseling at screening locations and a series of follow-up workshops on nutrition for those individuals identified with elevated cholesterol levels. The AHF will complete initial design of the follow-up workshops, which will be implemented by nutritionists from five community service organizations within Mount Vernon. This approach ultimately will strengthen the community's nutrition education resources and will also foster commitment to the program from within the community.

The *physician education* component consists of a two-part lecture program that is being integrated into the continuing medical education program of the community's two health care institutions. The lectures address barriers identified by the physician survey and provide a clear, concise, and action-oriented approach to patient management. They are delivered by a cardiologist with expertise in the management of patients with elevated cholesterol. The lecture content and timing parallels the community program: The first lecture focused on diagnosis and management of elevated cholesterol and was delivered several months prior to the screening program. A second lecture addressing dietary management immediately follows implementation of the screening program.

Physicians have noted the need for follow-up information to help monitor patient compliance. Thus, in addition to the lecture series, physicians will receive "booster materials" during the intervention phase of the program. A physician survey during year three of the project will determine the impact of the program on physicians' attitudes and practices related to cholesterol management.

Community Education and Participant Recruitment. The sequence of tasks involved in the design and development of intervention materials and communication through formal and informal dissemination channels is depicted in Figure 13.3.

The first step was to review available cholesterol education materials. A review of existing printed materials revealed a serious lack of information tailored specifically to the needs of Black American populations (U.S. Department of Health and Human Services, 1989). It further showed that available materials failed to recognize implementation barriers unique to this minority group.

With these barriers in mind, we developed a set of complementary educational materials tailored to the needs of Mount Vernon's black population. This process began with the identification of a series of eductional "themes" or messages that comprised the basic educational objectives of the intervention. Once identified, these messages would be continually reinforced and disseminated through a variety of formal and informal message channels. The development of the message design strategy attended to factors such as content, design, persuasion, and memorability. On the basis of commonly asked cholesterol-related questions, a message campaign using a question-and-answer format was created. Focus groups were conducted to test the effectiveness of these messages both with members of the target population and with technical experts in nutrition and health promotion. Through these focus groups, the content, format, and structure of the messages were refined.

In addition to printed materials, we designed a video to increase awareness of cholesterol as a risk factor for members of the black population. The video was filmed within Mount Vernon; its content focuses on the reaction of a young child to the death of her father from cardiovascular disease. Both the complete video and one-minute abbreviated versions will contribute to the recruitment and education of the particularly hard to reach segments of the black community.

In order to overcome the barriers to participation common to members of the target population, identification and selection of effective *information dissemination strategies* was important. A variety of complementary dissemination strategies utilizing both

Figure 13.3. Mount Vernon CARES: Community Education and
Participant Recruitment.

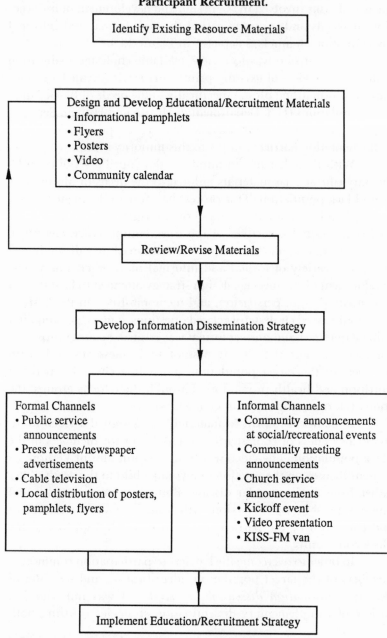

formal and informal communication channels was developed according to the subpopulations that had been identified through census tract analysis. Factors related to message selection were matched with a particular dissemination channel in order to reach a specific subgroup of the target audience. Through this approach, intervention messages have the best potential to penetrate all segments of the community.

The *formal dissemination channels* comprising the education and recruitment component for the program include public service announcements, press releases, newspaper advertisements, direct mail inserts, community bulletin announcements, cable television announcements, bus shelter posters, and locally distributed posters, pamphlets, and flyers.

In addition to these distribution channels, a variety of informal strategies are being implemented. Promotion of a health innovation through word-of-mouth contacts provides opportunities for feedback that is not possible through the printed word. Given the inability of media campaigns alone to motivate desired behavior changes, a series of informal promotional events has been designed to complement the formal distribution channels. The *informal channels* include announcements at community, social, and recreational events; church service announcements and discussions; video presentations and group discussion; presentations at community meetings; and a phone-a-thon.

The screening implementation phase will begin with a kickoff press event, featuring the mayor of Mount Vernon as the first Mount Vernon resident to receive a cholesterol screening test. One additional recruitment and communication technique utilizes the participation of a very popular radio station in the community. The station's promotional van will be located at a major screening site and will make live radio announcements throughout the screening event.

The education and recruitment activities described in this section will be implemented during the six weeks prior to initiation of the screening activities. Intensified recruitment will take place within the last few days immediately prior to the screening and will continue throughout the screening period. The program is expected to elicit the participation of at least 10,000 adult Mount Vernon residents.

Cholesterol Screening and Follow-Up. When participants enter the screening site, they will be given a *participant information packet.* The packet includes the pamphlet with the project's key educational messages, including "Cholesterol: Know the Facts," "Watch What You Eat," and "Get the Total Picture." Participants will also receive a cookbook that was designed to address the dietary practices of the target audience and includes multiethnic low-fat, low-cholesterol recipes; information on understanding nutrition labels; tips for meal preparation; and tips for choosing low-cholesterol meals in restaurants. In addition to specially developed materials, the packet includes the AHF's "Health Passport," an AHF cholesterol information pamphlet, a dietary information brochure from the Westchester County Department of Health, a survey form, and a consent form.

At each of the screening sites, volunteers will work with supervision from AHF cholesterol screening personnel to guide participants through the screening process. Participants will complete a consent form and then proceed to the blood sampling section. Next, their blood will be drawn by trained and certified technicians using a finger-stick method. Blood samples will be analyzed on-site with Kodak Ektachem DT60 analyzers, and participants will receive the results of their cholesterol screening within approximately thirty minutes. During this waiting period, participants will be asked to complete a survey questionnaire.

The information requested on the *self-administered survey* includes background data on ethnicity, age, socioeconomic level, marital status, and educational level. Additional questions address prior knowledge of the respondent's cholesterol level, previous illnesses, dietary practices, and life-style factors, including physical activity and smoking. The information obtained through this survey will provide insight regarding factors associated with the distribution of cholesterol levels within and between population subgroups.

The same survey will be readministered to all participants with elevated cholesterol levels who participate in a *cholesterol re-*

screen at a twelve-month follow-up. This follow-up screening activity will allow for comparison of individuals over time to determine the effectiveness of the physician referral and nutrition education components in helping to lower cholesterol levels of the at-risk population. A unique identification code will allow tracking of participants and matching of survey forms with blood samples.

An additional strategy to obtain accurate and complete contact information for participants involves attachment of a "health lotto" form to each survey. The participants will be asked to provide their phone numbers and addresses so that winners can be notified; this will enhance long-term participant tracking for the project evaluation.

In addition to the self-administered survey, fifteen-minute *face-to-face interviews* will be conducted with a random sample of 1,000 Black Americans. The goal of these interviews is to develop a behavioral prediction model by identifying individual characteristics that are often associated with the capacity for self-change. The interview content and format, based on Prochaska and DiClemente's (1983) model of stages and processes of change, will utilize a transtheoretical model involving ten processes of change within a five-stage change model.

Both before their blood samples are drawn and while they are waiting for the results, participants will have the opportunity to view a series of cholesterol education videos. When the screening results are ready, participants with cholesterol levels placing them at moderate to high risk will be invited to proceed to the nutrition information area, where they may receive *on-site nutrition counseling* and the *high cholesterol pamphlet* designed specifically for this program. The pamphlet uses a simple question-and-answer format and provides information on the interpretation of cholesterol scores as well as recommendations for behavior change.

All patients with moderate to high cholesterol levels will be *referred for additional physician follow-up*. Referral messages delivered at the screening will emphasize that screening cholesterol scores alone should not be used for diagnostic purposes. High-risk individuals will receive physician referral information for both the Neighborhood Health Center and the Mount Vernon Hospital. In addition, information on the time and place of the nutrition follow-up workshops will be available, along with a nutrition telephone hot-line number to obtain detailed information.

Mount Vernon CARES as an Application of Theory: Prognosis for Success. Because the Mount Vernon CARES Project is in the early stage of program implementation, screening participation and impact data are not yet available. However, progress toward developing an innovation that will be effectively adopted and diffused among blacks in Mount Vernon is already evident. The process of collaboration with community members is marked by the establishment of the Community Advisory Board, identification and cooperation of feasible screening sites, involvement of community members in assessment surveys, and the increased participation of physicians in the project survey.

Most importantly, the linkage approach has been put into action through collaboration of the resource system (the AHF) with the user system to enhance innovation planning. Social marketing research methods have been invaluable in refining the AHF's understanding of the target population. The careful and continuing use of the processes that have begun will assure a cholesterol screening and management program that is compatible, flexible, advantageous, cost-efficient, and low risk. The innovation is viewed as a dynamic and evolving "package" rather than a fixed product to be accepted or rejected.

The ultimate success of Mount Vernon CARES will also require vigilance in attending to potential system failure points: innovation failure, communication failure, adoption failure, implementation failure, and maintenance failure. Success of the program is further dependent upon the ability of the AHF and collaborating institutions to negotiate and cooperate carefully. Within the limits imposed by the research design, the AHF recognizes and accommodates the needs of community organizations. The willingness and interest of the community to participate in the program stems in part from the perception of community ownership generated by this process. Representatives from the various sites are motivated by the opportunity to be perceived as providers of a particular set of services, thereby enhancing their own sense of involvement and personal and organizational efficacy.

The art of community negotiation is a process that must proceed cautiously, building upon and continuously reinforcing a foundation of trust and credibility. Only then can an effective health promotion program be designed and successfully diffused.

Conclusion

One of the factors that will significantly influence worldwide health promotion efforts in the 1990s and beyond is the diffusion of viable innovations from those who have them to those who need them. Without widespread diffusion of health promotion innovations, advances in our understanding of chronic disease prevention and management will realize only a fraction of their potential in preventing avoidable disease and premature death.

The brief theoretical overview presented here suggests that increasing target group participation is one strategy for improving the efficiency of innovation development and the effectiveness of diffusion efforts. The example from the Mount Vernon CARES Project supports the feasibility of this approach.

There are, however, many questions that remain unanswered and need to be addressed if critical public health goals for the future are to be met. For example, if a collaborative linkage approach is to be employed, who should initiate it? How should the problem of user groups who do not want to participate in a collaborative exchange process be anticipated and dealt with? How can quality control and implementation integrity best be maintained after diffusion has taken place? What factors contribute most to a community's sense of ownership, and how can these factors be enhanced? How can a community's (or an organization's or an individual's) readiness to change be assessed, and how can such information be utilized by health promotion planners to enhance the diffusion process? How can health promotion providers conduct meaningful and useful community analyses with limited resources?

The framework and strategies described in this chapter suggest an approach for beginning to address some of these issues.

References

Baquet, C., and Ringen, K. "Health Policy: Gaps in Access, Delivery, and Utilization of the Pap Smear in the United States." *Milbank Quarterly*, 1987, *65*, 322–347.

Basch, C. D., Eveland, J. D., and Portnoy, B. "Diffusion Systems for Education and Learning About Health." *Family and Community Health*, 1986, *9*, 1-26.

Bloom, P. N., and Novelli, W. D. "Problems and Challenges in Social Marketing." *Journal of Marketing*, 1981, *45*, 79-88.

Ernst, N. D., and Cleeman, J. "Reducing High Blood Cholesterol Levels: Recommendations from the National Cholesterol Education Program." *Journal of Nutrition Education*, 1988, *20*, 23-29.

Glanz, K. "Patient and Public Education for Cholesterol Reduction: A Review of Strategies and Issues." *Patient Education and Counseling*, 1988, *12*, 235-257.

Green, L. W. "National Policy in the Promotion of Health." *International Journal of Health Education*, 1979, *12*, 161-168.

Havelock, R. *Planning for Innovation Through Dissemination and Utilization of Knowledge*. Ann Arbor, Mich.: Institute for Social Research, 1971.

Iverson, D., and Kolbe, L. "Evolution of the Disease Prevention and Health Promotion Strategy: Establishing a Role for the Schools." *Journal of School Health*, 1983, *5*, 294-302.

Kolbe, L. J., and Iverson, D. C. "Implementing Comprehensive School Health Education: Educational Innovations and Social Change." *Health Education Quarterly*, 1981, *8*, 57-80.

Orlandi, M. A. "The Diffusion and Adoption of Worksite Health Promotion Innovations: An Analysis of the Barriers." *Preventive Medicine*, 1986a, *15*, 522-536.

Orlandi, M. A. "Community-Based Substance Abuse Prevention: A Multicultural Perspective." *Journal of School Health*, 1986b, *56*, 394-401.

Orlandi, M. A. "Promoting Health and Preventing Disease in Health Care Settings: An Analysis of Barriers." *Preventive Medicine*, 1987, *16*, 119-130.

Patton, M. *Utilization-Focused Evaluation*. Newbury Park, Calif.: Sage, 1978.

Prochaska, J. O., and DiClemente, C. C. "Stages and Processes of Self-Change of Smoking: Toward an Integrative Model of Change." *Journal of Consulting and Clinical Psychology*, 1983, *51*, 983-990.

"Report of the National Cholesterol Education Program Expert

Panel on Detection, Evaluation and Treatment of High Blood Cholesterol in Adults." *Archives of Internal Medicine*, 1988, *148*, 36–69.

Rogers, E. M. *Diffusion of Innovations*. New York: Free Press, 1962.

Rogers, E. M. *Diffusion of Innovations*. (3rd ed.) New York: Free Press, 1983.

Rogers, E. M., and Shoemaker, F. F. *Communication of Innovations: A Cross-Cultural Approach*. New York: Free Press, 1971.

Schucker, B., and others. "Change in Public Perspective on Cholesterol and Heart Disease: Results from Two National Surveys." *Journal of the American Medical Association*, 1987a, *258*, 3527–3531.

Schucker, B., and others. "Change in Physician Perspective on Cholesterol and Heart Disease: Results from Two National Surveys." *Journal of the American Medical Association*, 1987b, *258*, 3521–3526.

U.S. Department of Health and Human Services. *Guidelines for Demonstration and Education Research Grants*. U.S. Department of Health and Human Services Publication no. 61116, 1987, pp. 181–296.

U.S. Department of Health and Human Services. *Directory of Cardiovascular Resources for Minority Populations*. U.S. Department of Health and Human Services Publication no. 89-2975, 1989.

Winett, R. A. "Diffusion from a Behavioral Systems Perspective." In R. A. Winett, *Information and Behavior: Systems of Influence*. Hillsdale, N.J.: Erlbaum, 1986.

Wynder, E. L., Field, F., and Haley, N. J. "Population Screening for Cholesterol Determination." *Journal of the American Medical Association*, 1986, *256*, 2839–2842.

Wynder, E. L., Harris, R. E., and Haley, N. J. "Population Screening for Plasma Cholesterol: Community-Based Results from Connecticut." *American Heart Journal*, 1989, *117*, 649–656.

Yankauer, A. "Disease Prevention: Still a Long Way to Go." *American Journal of Public Health*, 1988, *78*, 1277–1278.

Chapter 14

Robert M. Goodman
Allan B. Steckler

Mobilizing Organizations for Health Enhancement: Theories of Organizational Change

Organizational theory is like an oriental box puzzle. When the key is found and the box is unlocked, another box is revealed within and requires a different key. In the smaller box is another, and another still, each requiring a separate key. Organizational theory, like the box puzzle, can be penetrated on many levels.

Organizations are layered. Their strata range from the surrounding environment at the broadest level, to the overall organizational structure, to the management within, to work groups, to each individual member. Change may be influenced at each of these strata (Tichy and Beckhard, 1982; Harrison, 1987; Kaluzny and Hernandez, 1988), and health education strategies that are directed at several levels simultaneously may be most durable in producing the desired results (McLeroy, Bibeau, Steckler, and Glanz, 1988; Simons-Morton, Parcel, and O'Hara, 1988). The health professional who understands the ecology of organizations and who can apply appropriate strategies has powerful tools for affecting change.

Because organizations may be influenced at the many levels comprising their ecology, no single theory is sufficient for explain-

*This work was supported in part by the National Cancer Institute (R01 CA 45997–02).

ing how and why organizations change. In this chapter we analyze two theories of organizational change: Stage Theory and Organizational Development Theory. These theories were selected for three reasons. First, both suggest specific intervention strategies. Thus, the health educator can translate these theories into prescriptions for action. Second, the strategies that extend from these theories are directed at levels of the organization at which health education may be most influential. Third, the strategies can be used simultaneously, thus creating a synergy in the effects that are produced.

Two cases are presented in this chapter to illustrate how the theories may be used together and at the different organizational strata. Before the cases are presented, the origins and elements of the two theories are described.

Stage Theory of Organizational Change

Stage Theory of organizational change explains how organizations innovate new goals, programs, technologies, and ideas (Kaluzny and Hernandez, 1988). Stage Theory is so named because organizations, as they innovate, are thought to pass through a series of steps or stages. Each stage requires a unique set of strategies if the innovation is to grow and to mature. Strategies that are effective at one stage may be misapplied at the next, thereby disabling the innovation. Therefore, the skillful application of Stage Theory requires an accurate assessment of an innovation's current stage of development and the selection of strategies that are appropriate for that stage.

History of Stage Theory

Stage Theory emerges from two research traditions. The first extends from the work of Lewin, who developed one of the earliest stage models (Lewin, 1951). Lewin's model, which emphasizes factors resisting change efforts, has three stages: (1) unfreezing past behaviors and attitudes; (2) moving by exposure to new information, attitudes, and theories; and (3) refreezing through processes of reinforcement, confirmation, and support for the change. As is shown in the next section, Lewin's work was also instrumental in defining theories of organizational development.

The second influence on the development of Stage Theory is Diffusion of Innovation Theory. (See Chapter Thirteen for further analysis of Diffusion Theory.) In the 1950s, Diffusion Theory focused on how individuals such as farmers, teachers, and physicians adopted innovations (Rogers, 1983). In the 1960s, innovation theorists realized that individuals often adopt innovations as members of organizations and that such individuals seldom adopt an innovation until it is first accepted by the organization. Rogers (1983) terms this "contingent innovation-decisions" because the adoption and implementation of an innovation by individuals is contingent on organizational adoption. For example, a teacher often cannot use a new curriculum until it is officially adopted by the school district.

As research on diffusion in organizations grew, two types of studies resulted. In the first type, the characteristics of innovative organizations were examined by gathering cross-sectional data from a large sample of organizations. In the second type, which began in the mid 1970s, case studies were used to provide "insights into the nature of the innovation process and the behavior of organizations as they change" (Rogers, 1983, p. 348). These latter studies of diffusion processes in organizations led to the development of Stage Theory.

Zaltman, Duncan, and Holbek (1973) proposed one of the earliest stage models as applied to organizations. It consists of two main stages. During the first stage, initiation, the organization becomes aware of a proposed innovation, forms attitudes toward it, and makes a decision about implementation. The second major stage, implementation, occurs when the organization actually carries out and sustains the change. Since the development of this model, several other models have been formulated for innovations in policy (Berman, 1978), technical programs (Yin, 1979; Scheirer, 1983), health services (Scheirer, 1981; Kaluzny, Warner, Warren, and Zelman, 1982), and community health education (Schiller, Steckler, Dawson, and Patton, 1987).

Modern Stage Theory

A comprehensive, well-defined, and contemporary model of Stage Theory was developed by Beyer and Trice (1978) and consists of seven stages.

1. *Sensing of unsatisfied demands on the system.* Some part of the system receives information indicating a problem or potential problem with organizational functioning.
2. *Search for possible responses.* Elements in the system consciously or unconsciously try to find alternative ways of dealing with the issues sensed in the first stage.
3. *Evaluation of alternatives.* Desired outcomes, probable outcomes of the various alternatives, and costs are compared.
4. *Decision to adopt a course of action.* An alternative is chosen from among those evaluated. Operative goals and means are specified; that is, a strategy is adopted.
5. *Initiation of action within the system.* A policy or other directive for implementing the change is formulated. The initial diffusion of information about the change takes place within the system. Resources necessary for implementation are acquired.
6. *Implementation of the change.* Resources are allocated for implementation. The innovation is carried out. Attitudinal reactions among organizational members occur, and changes in roles occur.
7. *Institutionalization of the change.* The innovation becomes entrenched in the organization. It is part of routine organizational operations. The new goals and values surrounding the innovation become internalized within the organization.

The Beyer and Trice (1978) model provides a finely grained division of stages. For instance, implementation is divided into two stages: initiation and implementation. Initiation implies a preparatory stage, which can be useful in honing strategies to an innovation's current level of development. The model also includes a maintenance, or institutionalization, stage. This stage, often omitted in other models, indicates that the entrenchment of valued programs is an important goal.

All models of Stage Theory have certain characteristics in common. First, the stages occur "in sequence or as successive iterations or reiterations" (Kantor, 1983, p. 217). Movement from one stage to the next does not imply an inexorable march but allows for the possibility that innovations can move either forward or backward or be abandoned at any point in the process (Beyer and Trice, 1978; Rogers, 1983). Also, each stage has a unique set of actors, variables, and circumstances that propel one stage to the next (Berman, 1978; Scheirer, 1981; Mohr, 1982).

How Stage Theory Operates

How innovations "move" from one stage to the next is still an open question. As Rogers (1983) points out, only a dozen or so investigations of the innovation process in organizations had been completed by the mid 1980s. Most of these studies measure the dynamics within stages, but only a few suggest what mechanisms might lead from one stage to the next (Scheirer, 1981; Huberman and Miles, 1984; Goodman and Steckler, 1987–88). For example, Zaltman, Duncan, and Holbek (1973) found that innovations are more readily initiated when complex organizations have decentralized and have informal mechanisms for decision making. But these same structural characteristics make it difficult for an organization to implement an innovation because implementation often requires strict adherence to rules and procedures. For the innovation to develop, different strategies are selected for the initiation and implementation stages.

In their study of innovations in schools, Huberman and Miles (1984) demonstrate that different actors play leading roles at different innovation stages: Senior-level administrators are important at the problem definition and early adoption stages; midlevel administrators, such as curriculum coordinators and principals, are important actors at the adoption and early implementation stages; teachers are instrumental at the implementation stage; and senior-level administrators once again play a key role in the institutionalization stage. The Huberman and Miles (1984) study suggests that decisions to adopt and to institutionalize are essentially political in nature, and therefore administrators take a leading role. Implementation appears to be a more technical enterprise and involves professional skills such as teaching ability more than administrative and political skills. Thus, health education practitioners might direct strategies at different actors, depending on the innovation stage.

Future Challenges for Stage Theory

Stage Theory holds promise for guiding the practitioner's efforts to nurture health promotion programs, but more precise specification of the number of stages within the model is necessary. Currently, the number of stages varies, depending on which model is employed. As mentioned, the authors prefer Beyer and Trice's (1978) seven-stage model, yet the first case to be presented later in this chapter uses four stages. Better definition of the stages will lead to greater precision of strategies for each stage.

Second, the completeness of stage models has been questioned. To date no models extend beyond institutionalization. Yet evidence indicates that beyond institutionalization is renewal, a stage during which well-established programs evolve to meet changing demands (Goodman and Steckler, 1989a). Additional research is required to extend the stage model through renewal.

Third, those factors known to enable a program's development at each stage should be expanded. The foregoing discussion identifies certain structural characteristics (for example, formalization and centralization of decision making) and different actors within organizations as important at different stages of an innovation's development. As additional factors are identified as important at each developmental stage, both researchers and practitioners will find a greater array of strategies for enhancing program development.

Organizational Development Theory

Organizational Development (OD) is defined as the application of behavioral sciences to improve organizational effectiveness (Tichy and Beckhard, 1982). OD has the dual goals of improving organizational performance and improving the "quality of work life" (Sashkin and Burke, 1987). These goals are generally accomplished through interventions directed at organizational processes and structures and at worker behaviors (Brown and Covey, 1987). The interventions are often stimulated by an OD consultant who is engaged by management and who implements a set of strategies to help the organization diagnose, evaluate, and address its perceived concerns.

History of Organizational Development Theory

The theory of Organizational Development is rooted in the "human relations" perspective that emerged in the 1930s. Prior to that time, organizational effectiveness was equated with structural efficiencies, such as establishing precise lines of authority (Fayol, 1949; Weber, 1964). In the 1920s and 1930s, research known as the Hawthorne studies (Roethlisberger and Dickson, 1939) demonstrated that increasing the attention paid to workers also increases productivity. Therefore, the Hawthorne studies resulted in an expanded view of organizational effectiveness as influenced largely by worker motivation.

Developments in social science in the late 1940s and 1950s provided the theoretical and philosophical basis for management that is worker concerned (Margulis and Adams, 1982). Paramount is Lewin's scientific and humanizing influence on the field of organizational behavior. In emphasizing practical applications, Lewin's "action research" converted organizations into vibrant laboratories for scientific discovery and self-discovery (Argyris, Putnam, and Smith, 1985; Cooperrider and Srivastva, 1987). His model is the basis for action research and the precursor of most contemporary change theories. His view that individual behavior is influenced by the characteristics of the individual coupled with the surrounding environment stimulated others whose writings have defined Organizational Development (Greenberger, Strasser, Lewicki, and Bateman, 1988).

The works of Argyris, MacGregor, and Likert are foremost examples of Lewin's influence (Margulis and Adams, 1982). Argyris (1957) rejected classical bureaucracy, arguing that individual needs must be fulfilled in the contexts of work and organization. MacGregor (1960) also rejected bureaucratic organization, which he termed Theory X, a set of axioms which holds that managers must exert control if workers are to comply with organizational goals. MacGregor proposed an alternative, Theory Y, which holds that work is natural to human activity and that workers will readily fulfill the management's requirements given a supportive environment. Likert (1961) added that managers serve as "linking pins" among semiautonomous work groups into which the individual worker is integrated.

A Typology of Modern Organizational Development Theory

By the 1960s, the term *Organizational Development* emerged in the literature and was characterized by interventions aimed at either the organization's design and technologies or its human processes (Sashkin and Burke, 1987). Today, greater emphasis is directed at environmental influences and how the norms and values of entire organizations are transformed (Beer and Walton, 1987; Brown and Covey, 1987; Bartunek and Louis, 1988). In the past several years, increased attention has been devoted also to the development of OD theory (Bullock and Batten, 1985; Porras and Hoffer, 1986; Porras and Robertson, 1987). Porras and Robertson (1987) describe a typology, depicted in Figure 14.1, into which OD theories may be categorized. Porras and Robertson divide OD theory into two main branches, change process theories and implementation theories. These are summarized below.

Change Process Theories. Change process theories specify the underlying dynamics of change. That is, they define the causal relationships among variables that the practitioner may influence, mediator variables or intermediate stages of the change process, and moderator variables or other influences on intended outcomes. Porras and Robertson (1987) note that few such theories exist and those that do have not been integrated into a coherent explanation of the change process.

Implementation Theories. In contrast to change process theories, implementation theories are relatively well defined. They concern the activities that practitioners employ to ensure that change is successful. Implementation theory is actually an umbrella term for three levels of theories: strategy, procedure, and technique. Strategy

Figure 14.1. Typology of Organizational Change Theory.

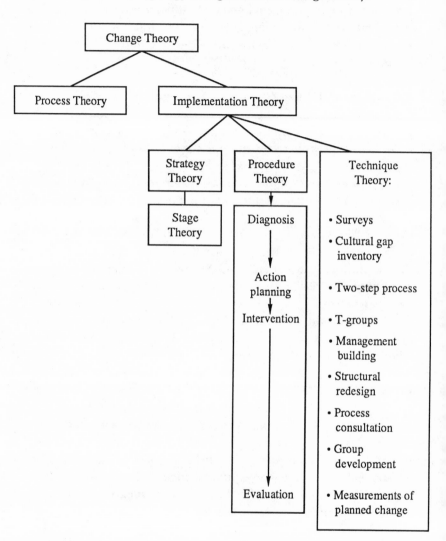

Source: Adapted from Porras and Robertson, 1987.

theories provide broad perspectives for implementing change but generally do not specify guidelines for intervening. Strategy theories describe rather than prescribe: They describe how organizational and other factors may contribute to change but offer few prescriptions for affecting change. Stage Theory is an example of a strategy theory.

Procedure theories identify a sequence of actions for producing change that are missing from strategy theories. Thus, procedure theories are more prescriptive than strategy theories. Action research, which is discussed below, is an example of a procedure theory.

Technique theories are specific to the individual steps within procedure theories. Technique theories consist of a set of activities that practitioners may employ at each step derived from a procedure theory. These activities enable the change process to move from one step to the next.

An Expanded View of Implementation-Procedure Theory. Porras and Robertson (1987) analyze the steps common to several prominent implementation-procedure theories. They conclude that the four steps of diagnosis, action planning, intervention, and evaluation are the core in effecting change. These steps, which are described below, are analogous to the model for action research first developed by Lewin (Argyris, Putnam, and Smith, 1985).

Step 1, diagnosis, can be equated with Lewin's unfreezing. Diagnosis aids an organization in identifying problems or gaps that may impede its functioning. The diagnosis is often conducted by an outside consultant who helps the organization identify its most salient problems. The most traditional diagnostic technique is a formal survey of members of the organization (Sommer, 1987). A more recent technique examines cultural gaps between management and work groups in order to reduce such gaps (Kilmann, 1986). Variables commonly studied include environmental factors; the organization's mission, goals, policies, procedures, structures, technologies, and physical setting; social and interpersonal factors; desired outcomes (Porras and Robertson, 1987); and readiness to take action (Weisbord, 1988).

Step 2, in implementation-procedure theory, *action plan-*

ning or the development of strategies or interventions for addressing the diagnosed problems, often follows diagnosis. Porras and Robertson (1987) describe a two-stage process for selecting interventions. In the first stage, several possible interventions are identified on the basis of the gaps or problem areas that have been diagnosed. In the second stage, the number of interventions is narrowed on the basis of three criteria: the organization's readiness to adopt a proposed strategy (for example, sufficiency of resources, time commitment, and administrative support); the availability of "leverage points," that is, where and how to intervene within the organization; and the skill of the OD practitioner in applying the chosen interventions. The two-stage process contains the essential ingredients of action planning: The practitioner and members of the organization assess the feasibility of different strategies for change. By so doing, the practitioner helps to raise the organization's commitment to the chosen course of action.

Step 3 involves *OD interventions,* and it is on this step in implementation-procedure theory that Lewin is credited with the development of T-groups, originally used to encourage managers to become more aware of their interpersonal style and impact. Other OD interventions include management building (Lippitt, 1961), structural redesign (Galbraith, 1977; Plovnick, 1982), process consultation (Schein, 1969), and group development (Bradford, 1978). In process consultation, the consultant helps members of the organization identify problems, questions, and barriers to a desired change and then works with the organization to address these potential impediments (Schein, 1969; French and Bell, 1973; Lippitt, Langseth, and Mossop, 1985). The consultant usually does not offer specific solutions but rather facilitates problem solving among members. Face-to-face contact and group interaction are integral to this approach. Process consultation is employed in the first case application described below.

Team building, which is employed in the second case, is a form of group development. Team building often utilizes process consultation to improve communication and coordination among members of a work group.

Step 4, the final step in implementation-procedure theory, is *evaluation,* which assesses the planned change effort. Several evaluation techniques measure planned change in organizations (Randolph, 1982). An essential feature of evaluation is that the organization takes stock of its progress in moving to a new state and determines whether additional alterations are needed. Evaluation often allows the changes in an organization to settle, or refreeze.

Future Challenges for Organizational Development Theory

Organizational Development can benefit from refinements in both theory and practice. First, change process theories require greater development; they are not yet well defined.

Second, while more developed than change process theories, implementation theories of change require further refinement. To illustrate, Weisbord (1988) questions Lewin's premise that organizations that are stuck can become unfrozen. This challenges one of the basic assumptions upon which implementation theory rests: Under which conditions are implementation theories of change applied to best advantage? Today most organizations dwell in uncertain environments, and implementation theories of change also must account for the effects of such conditions on the change process (Beer and Walton, 1987; Brown and Covey, 1987; Cooperrider and Srivastva, 1987).

Third, several scholars question whether OD interventions are truly effective (Plovnick, 1982; Cooperrider and Srivastva, 1987). To date, most OD research is based on case studies, and few studies have tested OD strategies in randomized controlled trials. Additional research that uses experimental designs is necessary to demonstrate the effectiveness of OD interventions.

Finally, most OD interventions are not specific to the stage of development of the organizations at which they are directed (Bartunek and Louis, 1988). Although the two cases presented in this chapter are quite distinctive, the first being experimental and the second being a case study, they both demonstrate how OD strategies may be tailored to fit an organization's stage of readiness.

Integrating Tobacco-Use Prevention into School Systems

The negative health consequences associated with tobacco use are well recognized (U.S. Department of Health and Human Services,

1986). Since tobacco use often begins early in life, several school curricula for preventing tobacco consumption have been developed and evaluated (Flay, 1985). Despite their availability, such effective curricula reach only a small proportion of young people in the United States.

In 1987, a study was initiated to explore how to improve the dissemination of tobacco-use prevention curricula. Twenty-two randomly selected public school districts throughout one southeastern state agreed to participate in the study. These districts were then randomly assigned to either a treatment or control group. The treatment group received intensive intervention strategies, while the control districts were provided with just enough attention to retain them in the study.

Four-Stage Model

Stage Theory informed the interventions for disseminating the new tobacco prevention curricula into the schools. In the study, a four-stage model was used, and different strategies were deployed at each of the four stages: awareness, adoption, implementation, and institutionalization. Organizational Development Theory was the basis for the strategies used during the adoption and institutionalization stages.

Awareness Stage. Since senior-level administrators are most influential in decisions to adopt new programs (Huberman and Miles, 1984), the tobacco-use project directed its initial strategies at increasing administrator awareness and concern for tobacco prevention programs. For example, the research team invited administrators and teachers to attend a "Seaside Conference" (Passwater, Trisch, and Slater, 1981). The conference involved a week of well-defined health-related activities that required an intense level of involvement on the part of school personnel. Such activities usually raise attendees' levels of awareness and concern for school health programs (Schaller, 1981; Drolet, 1982). To bolster participation in the tobacco-use study, staff members from the tobacco project also conducted individual awareness meetings with the senior administration of each target school district. Project staff members provided the administrators with a written overview of the project and used this overview to raise the district's level of commitment to the project.

The awareness intervention was evaluated by questionnaires that were administered to conference participants as pretest and posttest measures. Measures included items on demographic characteristics, current role and position in the school district, perceived importance of health as a content area, perceived importance of various components of the comprehensive school health program, attitudes toward tobacco prevention education, and ratings of specific sessions of the conference.

Adoption Stage. Once the decision makers agreed to participate, the research team offered each school district several health curriculum options. So that schools could make an informed selection, process consultation was provided at the adoption stage. The research team conducted a four-hour workshop with each school district in the experimental group. The workshop helped school representatives identify what additional information and decision-making steps were necessary to adopt (or not adopt) one of the available curricula. Since senior- and middle-level administrators often make adoption decisions, participants at each workshop included an assistant superintendent for instruction, a health coordinator, and principals, as well as teachers. Consultation continued through weekly phone calls until an adoption decision was reached.

Evaluation of the adoption intervention included questionnaires that measured participant satisfaction with the process consultation workshop, and five other variables for predicting adoption on the basis of Rogers's (1983) work: the relative advantage of the proposed new curriculum over the old, the new curriculum's technical complexity, its fit with the school district's current practices, the observability of the curriculum's outcomes, and the ability to implement the curriculum on a trial basis. Case studies of individual districts were also conducted to explore processes that influenced adoption decisions.

Implementation Stage. During implementation, technical aspects of a program are addressed and interventions are directed at those who actually run the program. Effective strategies at the implementation stage include teacher training in the chosen curriculum and guidance and support of teachers after training (Huberman and Miles, 1984; Connell, Turner, and Mason, 1985). The tobacco project hired nationally recognized trainers in school health to conduct curriculum workshops for teachers and health education coordinators. After training, project staff members continued to visit each implementing school system to review the progress made toward implementation. School health coordinators and teachers were also encouraged to use a telephone hot line staffed by the project to address questions concerning any aspect of curriculum implementation.

The implementation workshops were evaluated by a questionnaire of participant satisfaction. The overall implementation intervention was evaluated with two questionnaires. The first was adapted from the work of Hall and Loucks (1977) and measured the degree to which teachers used the new curriculum. The second questionnaire was adapted from the work of Dowling (1982) and measured the degree to which school administrators were satisfied with the implementation of the new curriculum. Case studies of selected districts were also conducted to increase understanding of implementation.

Institutionalization Stage. In moving beyond implementation to institutionalization, administrators once again became leading actors. Administrators may champion a program by cultivating active coalitions for the program's continuance (Goodman and Steckler, 1989b). To increase institutionalization in the tobacco curriculum study, process consultation was redeployed. Project staff members aided administrators in identifying barriers to institutionalization and strategies for overcoming such impediments. The research team also added a skill development component to the consultation for building the needed coalitions. Skill development consisted of techniques for recognizing potential supporters of the program, developing incentives to offer to supporters, and inducing supporters to form coalitions for the program's continuation (Goodman and Steckler, 1989b).

The level of institutionalization was assessed by a scale that measured how integrated the new curriculum became with other school district operations (Goodman and Steckler, 1988). As with earlier stages, case studies of selected districts were conducted for the institutionalization stage.

Application of Organizational Change Theories to the Case

Use of a Prospective Experimental Design. The tobacco curriculum dissemination study applied Stage Theory and Organizational Development in several innovative ways. In previous research, strategies informed by these theories have been examined primarily through retrospective case studies. By using an experimental design, the tobacco project had randomized intervention and control school districts. Thus, the effectiveness of the strategies could be compared across two similar groups in which only one received an intervention. The interventions were therefore evaluated prospectively. Thus, bias that often influences retrospective explanations for a program's outcomes was reduced.

Combined Stage and Organizational Development Theories. Perhaps the project's most important contribution is in the way that Stage and OD Theories were combined. In the tobacco curriculum study, Stage and OD Theories were intertwined, and the related strategies were directed at multiple levels. The theories were most directly combined by using process consultation as the intervention at both the adoption and institutionalization stages.

The application of process consultation illustrates how OD techniques can be applied to specific stages. At the adoption stage, the tobacco study had to overcome three major impediments: The project was sponsored by outsiders who were trying to influence schools to adopt a new health curriculum; school personnel had limited knowledge about the curricula being offered and the requirements for instruction; and tobacco prevention was not a priority in schools (and sometimes was considered risky in a "tobacco state" such as North Carolina). Cummings and Mohrman (1987) argue that OD techniques are most relevant at adoption, when an innovation is vaguely defined and its implementation and skill requirements are unclear. Therefore, the process consultation was used to help introduce schools to the curriculum and to clarify the training and commitment required.

At the institutionalization stage, the curriculum had already been implemented. Process consultation was therefore no longer directed at familiarization as in the adoption stage. Process consultation focused instead on the political skills of those individuals who championed the program. Skill development centered on building coalitions of program advocates so that the program could become entrenched within the school system.

Intervention at Multiple Organizational Levels. In addition to contouring OD techniques to fit specific stages, the tobacco study intervened at different organizational levels. For instance, at the awareness stage, the Seaside Conference was directed at both administrators and teachers. The process consultation for adoption also included administrators and teachers, while implementation was mainly teacher oriented. At institutionalization, the focus was once again on administrators. The intervention also influenced the environment surrounding schools because the research team, which supported the innovation, were outsiders. Hence, the interventions were sensitive to the organizational strata that could influence the innovation's movement to its next stage of development.

Project Weaknesses. Despite the tobacco project's strengths in conceptualization and design, it also illustrates areas in which the application of theory can be improved. For instance, in the process consultation for adoption, the research team had a preplanned agenda. Project staff members began with the goal of getting schools to adopt a tobacco-use prevention curriculum. The traditional approach to OD is less directed in that the consultant is more generally interested in identifying gaps between actual and desired practice (Porras and Robertson, 1987). Once the gaps are identified, the consultant and organization work together to select the areas that are important to address. Such an open-ended approach to problem identification is more consistent with the action research model that is depicted in Figure 14.1. It is also consistent with the tenets of community organization; see Chapter Twelve.

In actuality, the tobacco study did not adhere to the action research model. Action research extends from procedure theory (Figure 14.1) and therefore outlines the steps along which change occurs. Stage Theory, as applied in the tobacco study, functioned as a strategy theory. That is, it provided broad parameters for influencing change at each stage while not in itself identifying specific steps. Process consultation at the adoption and implementation stages is an application of technique theory. The study was missing the middle layer, procedure theory, which is sandwiched between strategy and techniques. Had the action research model been more closely followed, the research team would have included a more detailed diagnosis of each school system, followed by action planning, an intervention such as process consultation, and finally, an evaluation of the change effort. To its detriment, the tobacco-use curriculum study did not adhere to such a procedure theory.

Because the action research model was omitted, schools did not participate in a thorough diagnosis. Therefore, much of the unfreezing that begins to take place when diagnosis is used remained unaddressed. Had action planning been employed as a consequence of such a diagnosis, perhaps a strategy other than process consultation might have been selected for influencing schools to implement the tobacco prevention program. The point is that in not using a procedure theory as the action research model, the research team may have missed important opportunities to involve the schools in deciding how to approach the innovation of tobacco-use prevention programs. Had the schools been more involved from the beginning in diagnosis, the resulting strategies might have been more durable in producing the desired changes.

A Team Approach to Patient Care in a Teaching Hospital

Cohen (1982) describes the team development efforts of a group of residents at an urban teaching hospital. The residents were concerned that the quality of patient care suffered because it was disjointed and did not include patient input. On the basis of prior experience with OD techniques in a community clinic, the residents decided that patient care could be improved if teams consisting of the patient, the patient's family, attending and house physicians, nurses, and aides were formed. The residents identified a floor of the hospital on which to initiate their experiment with team building and obtained the hospital administration's permission to be assigned together to that floor. The residents' goal was to create team care within four months, the duration of their assignment on the target floor.

To form the teams, the residents employed OD consultants who were not part of the hospital staff. The consultants applied an action research strategy and recommended that interviews be conducted with the relevant groups on the experimental floor. The interviews identified the perceived barriers to optimum patient care. On the basis of the interview data, a floorwide meeting was held to discuss the barriers. They included factors such as arrogance and poor communication by physicians, demoralized and intemperate attitudes of nurses, and inconsistent support from attendants. The meeting initially resulted in silence and tension. But with the support of the consultants, the lead residents and nursing supervisors agreed to continue biweekly meetings of the entire floor and to organize three task forces to address some of the barriers to improved care.

Over the next several months, only one task force met, and only one additional floor meeting occurred. Rivalries for recognition surfaced among the residents. The chief of medicine was lukewarm to the experiment. The interns who were present at the initial floor meeting were rotated to other service areas, and the new interns had a mixed reaction to team care. Time pressures did not permit extended group development efforts between staff members and consultants. All of these factors contributed to the delay of team formation.

Out of frustration with the delays, the residents and staff members most committed to the experiment moved the patients into a new configuration that was meant to facilitate team care. The move resulted in anger because the admitting office was not consulted, confusion because the patients and their families were not consulted, and embarrassment because the hospital administration was not informed. Thus, the very actions meant to cause team building resulted in further tension.

Although the staff's action caused conflict, benefits also resulted from the crisis. Meetings continued among the nursing supervisors, residents, and interns. Physicians and nurses accompanied each other on rounds, which led to greater communication. In general, the staff became more sensitive to the feelings of others, so morale improved. However, these benefits were short lived. The next group of interns and residents who were rotated onto the floor did not support the team concept. When nurses tried to interact as team members, they received curt answers, and nurses were no longer allowed on physician rounds. Nursing morale dropped, and the team concept was over.

Application of Organizational Change Theories to the Case

What went wrong with the team-building effort? Cohen (1982) argues that the culture of the hospital works against traditional OD efforts such as team development: Hospitals thrive on a status hierarchy in which physicians are at the pinnacle; and OD techniques, such as process consultation, require time that hospital staff members do not have. Also, rapid staff turnover limits the continuity necessary for OD strategies to take hold. Cohen argues that a collaborative diagnosis between consultants and clients may simply not be feasible given the cultural constraints of hospitals. Therefore, he suggests that OD consultants may need to be more assertive in identifying and lobbying for desired changes.

While Cohen is accurate in identifying the unique constraints in the hospital setting, a more assertive approach by OD consultants may not be the answer. Practitioners often do not have the luxury of outside consultants as advocates for desired change. Where consultants are available, their position outside the organization can actually work against change occurring, and a more proactive position may increase resistance (Argyris, 1987). In the following discussion, a different perspective is offered, one that is informed by Stage Theory.

Allowing Time for Nurturing. Radical departures from traditional practice require time. Such a perspective is imbedded in Stage Theory, which accounts for the cultivation of appreciation, acceptance, adoption, implementation, and sustenance necessary to nurture innovations. The major limitation of the hospital team-building case was the four-month time period that was imposed for team development. Four months is simply too short a time to actualize such a far-reaching change.

Developing Awareness. The second limitation was that residents were an inappropriate group to be the main champions of the team concept. Stage Theory suggests at least two reasons why this is so. First, the residents were relatively short-term members of the hospital staff and therefore lacked the continuity required to nurture the change through the necessary stages. Second, the residents were not in a strategic position to orchestrate the desired changes. Administrators have the authority and can dedicate resources to facilitate change. In this case, the chief of medicine was not fully supportive of team building. While the residents may be applauded for their ideals, their strategy was not likely to endure.

Fostering Adoption. A possible third factor in limiting success at team building involves the way in which the residents set up their experiment. They selected the floor on which to implement the team concept. Both Stage Theory and diffusion of innovation theory from which it derives maintain that some units will adopt sooner than others. Therefore, rather than selecting a particular floor, the residents, in concert with the chief of medicine, might have publicized the experiment and selected a floor that had a staff and patients who were eager to participate. Such volunteerism might have reduced resistance. Once the team approach was tested under favorable conditions, other floors might have joined the experiment. Success is more likely if new programs are not imposed on an organizational unit.

Smoothing Implementation. A fourth and glaring deficiency in the hospital case concerns the implementation of team care by the shifting of beds. According to Stage Theory, implementation requires the use of a new repertoire of skills and practices, support and monitoring by midlevel managers, and feedback to the staff that reinforces the new activities. Action planning was needed and not done in this case. Such planning allows staff members to identify and phase in strategies that are likely to increase the implementation of a new program. Change is then palatable, not overwhelming. Moreover, if adoption of the team building in the hospital had been more voluntaristic, implementation might have been more by plan than by fiat. Alienation could have been minimized.

Enhancing Institutionalization. A fifth and final critique concerns the institutionalization of the team concept. In the hospital case, the experiment died when the physician staff rotated. Even the most desired programs can falter when new actors come on the scene. They are not part of the history of the program and often do not hold a stake in seeing it continue. For institutionalization to occur, a program's legacy must be transmitted from one generation of the staff to the next. In this case, institutionalization failure was almost preordained. If middle- to upper-level administrators had been advocates during the awareness and adoption stages, support could have been provided ultimately to sustain the program.

Conclusion

This chapter has offered some of the prerequisites for successfully guiding organizational change. Two theories of organizational change were analyzed: Stage Theory and Organizational Development Theory. Both theories were applied to two distinct cases. The first case, a randomized experimental study, illustrates how OD techniques may be used to intervene at different stages of an innovation's development. The second, a case study, illustrates how attention to stages can improve OD interventions such as team building. Taken together, the two cases support the value of applying theories of organizational change in concert.

In both cases, change was influenced by individuals outside the innovating organization. In the curriculum dissemination project, university researchers influenced change; and in the hospital team-building effort, OD consultants guided the change process. Health educators are often in a position to influence change from the outside. They may try to affect the adoption of work site health promotion programs as consultants to the organization. In such cases, the theories and strategies presented in this chapter are directly applicable. In other instances, health educators play the role of internal organizational change agents. While working in hospitals, they may try to develop innovative programs. The strategies for organizational change discussed in this chapter may be applied effectively by those influencing change from the inside.

Whether directing change strategies originating within or outside an organization, health practitioners are presented with unique challenges. Health care organizations, such as hospitals, may be dominated by professionals who are skeptical about health promotion programs (Orlandi, 1987). Other organizations, such as schools, may not view health promotion as a priority issue. Organizational change theories offer a foundation for skills to mediate such challenges.

References

Argyris, C. *Personality and Organization.* New York: McGraw-Hill, 1957.

Argyris, C. "Reasoning, Action Strategies, and Defensive Routines." In R. W. Woodman and W. A. Pasmore (eds.), *Research in Organizational Change and Development.* Vol. 1. Greenwich, Conn.: JAI Press, 1987.

Argyris, C., Putnam, R., and Smith, D. M. *Action Science: Concepts, Methods, and Skills for Research and Intervention.* San Francisco: Jossey-Bass, 1985.

Bartunek, J. M., and Louis, M. R. "The Interplay of Organization Development and Organizational Transformation." In R. W. Woodman and W. A. Pasmore (eds.), *Research in Organizational Change and Development.* Vol. 2. Greenwich, Conn.: JAI Press, 1988.

Beer, M., and Walton, A. E. "Organization Change and Development." *Annual Review of Psychology,* 1987, *38,* 339–367.

Berman, P. "Study of Macro-Implementation and Micro-Implementation." *Public Policy,* 1978, *26,* 157–184.

Beyer, J. M., and Trice, H. M. *Implementing Change: Alcoholism Policies in Work Organizations.* New York: Free Press, 1978.

Bradford, L. P. (ed.). *Group Development.* (2nd ed.) La Jolla, Calif.: University Associates, 1978.

Brown, L. D., and Covey, J. G. "Development Organizations and

Organization Development: Toward an Expanded Paradigm for Organization Development." In R. W. Woodman and W. A. Pasmore (eds.), *Research in Organizational Change and Development.* Vol. 1. Greenwich, Conn.: JAI Press, 1987.

Bullock, R., and Batten, D. "It's Just a Phase We're Going Through: A Review and Synthesis of OD Phase Analysis." *Group and Organization Studies,* 1985, *10,* 383–412.

Cohen, A. R. "Organizational Development as Radical Surgery: An Experiment in Delivering Better Patient Care." In N. Margulis and J. Adams (eds.), *Organizational Development in Health Care Organizations.* Reading, Mass.: Addison-Wesley, 1982.

Connell, D. B., Turner, R. R., and Mason, E. F. *School Health Education Evaluation.* Vol. 1: *Final Report.* Cambridge, Mass.: ABT Associates, 1985.

Cooperrider, D. L., and Srivastva, S. "Appreciative Inquiry in Organizational Life." In R. W. Woodman and W. A. Pasmore (eds.), *Research in Organizational Change and Development.* Vol. 1. Greenwich, Conn.: JAI Press, 1987.

Cummings, T. G., and Mohrman, S. A. "Self-Designing Organizations: Towards Implementing Quality-of-Work-Life Innovations." In R. W. Woodman and W. A. Pasmore (eds.), *Research in Organization Change and Development.* Vol. 1. Greenwich, Conn.: JAI Press, 1987.

Dowling, A. F. *A Measure for Determining the Success of Medical Computer-Based Information Systems.* Cleveland, Ohio: Weatherhead School of Management, Case Western Reserve University, 1982.

Drolet, J. "Evaluation of the Impact of the Seaside Health Education Conferences and the Nutrition Education Training Programs in the Oregon School Systems." Unpublished doctoral dissertation, Department of Education, University of Oregon, 1982.

Fayol, H. *General and Industrial Management.* London: Pitman, 1949. (Originally published 1916.)

Flay, B. R. "Psychosocial Approaches to Smoking Prevention: A Review of Findings." *Health Psychology,* 1985, *4,* 449–488.

French, W. L., and Bell, C. H., Jr. *Organization Development: Be-*

havioral Science Interventions for Organization Improvement. Englewood Cliffs, N.J.: Prentice-Hall, 1973.

Galbraith, J. *Organization Design.* Reading, Mass.: Addison-Wesley, 1977.

Goodman, R. M., and Steckler, A. "The Life and Death of a Health Promotion Program: An Institutionalization Perspective." *International Quarterly of Community Health Education,* 1987–88, *8,* 5–21.

Goodman, R. M., and Steckler, A. *Assessing the Institutionalization of Health Promotion Programs: Or, You Can't Tell the Program Without a Scorecard.* Chapel Hill: Department of Health Behavior and Education, University of North Carolina, 1988.

Goodman, R. M., and Steckler, A. "A Framework for Assessing Program Institutionalization." *Knowledge in Society: The International Journal of Knowledge Transfer,* 1989a, *2,* 52–66.

Goodman, R. M., and Steckler, A. "A Model for the Institutionalization of Health Promotion Programs." *Family and Community Health,* 1989b, *11,* 63–78.

Greenberger, D., Strasser, S., Lewicki, R. J., and Bateman, T. S. "Perception, Motivation, and Negotiation." In S. M. Shortell and A. D. Kaluzny (eds.), *Health Care Management: A Text in Organization Theory and Behavior.* (2nd ed.) New York: Wiley, 1988.

Hall, G. E., and Loucks, S. F. "A Developmental Model for Determining Whether the Treatment Is Actually Implemented." *American Educational Research Journal,* 1977, *14,* 263–276.

Harrison, M. I. *Diagnosing Organizations: Methods, Models, and Processes.* Newbury Park, Calif.: Sage, 1987.

Huberman, A. M., and Miles, M. B. *Innovation Up Close: How School Improvement Works.* New York: Plenum, 1984.

Kaluzny, A. D., and Hernandez, S. R. "Organization Change and Innovation." In S. M. Shortell and A. D. Kaluzny (eds.), *Health Care Management: A Text in Organization Theory and Behavior.* (2nd ed.) New York: Wiley, 1988.

Kaluzny, A. D., Warner, D. M., Warren, D. G., and Zelman, W. N. *Management of Health Services.* Englewood Cliffs, N.J.: Prentice-Hall, 1982.

Kantor, R. *The Change Masters.* New York: Simon & Schuster, 1983.

Kilmann, R. H. "Five Steps for Closing Culture-Gaps." In R. H. Kilmann, M. J. Saxton, R. Serpa, and Associates (eds.), *Gaining Control of the Corporate Culture.* San Francisco: Jossey-Bass, 1986.

Lewin, K. *Field Theory in Social Science.* New York: Harper & Row, 1951.

Likert, R. A. *New Patterns of Management.* New York: McGraw-Hill, 1961.

Lippitt, G. L. (ed.). *Leadership in Action.* Fairfax, Va.: National Training Laboratories, 1961.

Lippitt, G. L., Langseth, P., and Mossop, J. *Implementing Organizational Change.* San Francisco: Jossey-Bass, 1985.

MacGregor, D. *The Human Side of Enterprise.* New York: McGraw-Hill, 1960.

McLeroy, K. R., Bibeau, D., Steckler, A., and Glanz, K. "An Ecological Perspective on Health Promotion Programs." *Health Education Quarterly,* 1988, *15,* 351–378.

Margulis, N., and Adams, J. "Introduction to Organizational Development." In N. Margulis and J. Adams (eds.), *Organizational Development in Health Care Organizations.* Reading, Mass.: Addison-Wesley, 1982.

Mohr, L. B. *Explaining Organizational Behavior: The Limits and Possibilities of Theory and Research.* San Francisco: Jossey-Bass, 1982.

Orlandi, M. A. "Promoting Health and Preventing Disease in Health Care Settings: An Analysis of Barriers." *Preventive Medicine,* 1987, *16,* 119–130.

Passwater, D., Trisch, L., and Slater S. "Seaside Health Education Conference: Effects of Three 5-Day Teacher Inservice Conferences." *Eta Sigma Gamman,* 1981, *13,* 28–30.

Plovnick, M. S. "Structural Interventions for Health Care Systems Organizational Development." In N. Margulis and J. Adams (eds.), *Organizational Development in Health Care Organizations.* Reading, Mass.: Addison-Wesley, 1982.

Porras, J., and Hoffer, S. "Common Behavior Changes in Successful Organization Development Efforts." *Journal of Applied Behavioral Science*, 1986, *22*, 477–494.

Porras, J. I., and Robertson, P. J. "Organization Development Theory: A Typology and Evaluation." In R. W. Woodman and W. A. Pasmore (eds.), *Research in Organization Change and Development*. Vol. 1. Greenwich, Conn.: JAI Press, 1987.

Randolph, A. "Planned Organizational Change and Its Measurement." *Personnel Psychology*, 1982, *35*, 117–139.

Roethlisberger, F. J., and Dickson, W. J. *Management and the Worker*. Cambridge, Mass.: Harvard University Press, 1939.

Rogers, E. M. *Diffusion of Innovations*. (3rd ed.) New York: Free Press, 1983.

Sashkin, M., and Burke, W. W. "Organization Development in the 1980's." *Journal of Management*, 1987, *13*, 393–417.

Schaller, W. *The School Health Program*. Philadelphia: Saunders, 1981.

Schein, E. H. *Process Consultation: Its Role in Organization Development*. Reading, Mass.: Addison-Wesley, 1969.

Scheirer, M. A. *Program Implementation*. Newbury Park, Calif.: Sage, 1981.

Scheirer, M. A. "Approaches to the Study of Implementation." *IEEE Transactions on Engineering Management*, 1983, *30*, 76–82.

Schiller, P., Steckler, A., Dawson, L., and Patton, F. *Participatory Planning in Community Health Education: A Guide Based on the McDowell County, West Virginia, Experience*. Oakland, Calif.: Third Party Associates, 1987.

Simons-Morton, B. G., Parcel, G. S., and O'Hara, N. M. "Implementing Organizational Changes to Promote Healthful Diet and Physical Activity at School." *Health Education Quarterly*, 1988, *15*, 115–130.

Sommer, R. "An Experimental Investigation of the Action Research Approach." *Journal of Applied Behavioral Science*, 1987, *23*, 185–199.

Tichy, N. M., and Beckhard, R. "Organizational Development for Health Care Organizations." In N. Margulis and J. D. Adams (eds.), *Organizational Development in Health Care Organizations*. Reading, Mass.: Addison-Wesley, 1982.

U.S. Department of Health and Human Services. *Smoking and Health: A National Status Report.* Rockville, Md.: Public Health Service, 1986.

Weber, M. *The Theory of Social and Economic Organization.* New York: Free Press, 1964.

Weisbord, M. R. "Towards a New Practice Theory of OD: Notes on Snapshooting and Moviemaking." In R. W. Woodman and W. A. Pasmore (eds.), *Research in Organizational Change and Development.* Vol. 2. Greenwich, Conn.: JAI Press, 1988.

Yin, R. K. *Changing Urban Bureaucracies: How New Practices Become Routinized.* Lexington, Mass.: Lexington Books, 1979.

Zaltman, G., Duncan, R., and Holbek, J. *Innovations and Organizations.* New York: Wiley, 1973.

Chapter 15

William D. Novelli

Applying Social Marketing to Health Promotion and Disease Prevention

The Allure of Marketing

Marketing in the business world is a powerful, persuasive means of moving goods off the shelf and out of the showroom and selling financial, professional, and personal services. The public sees the facade of this discipline, such as advertising, new product introductions, and sweepstakes and other contests. Behind the facade is careful attention to research, product development, pricing and distribution strategies, and financial analysis.

For a long time, nonbusiness managers have looked at marketing and speculated about its application to social change. As was asked nearly forty years ago, "Why can't you sell brotherhood like soap?" (Rothschild, 1979, p. 11). In more recent times, health professionals have been wont to say, "If they can sell cigarettes, why can't we use the same techniques to *unsell* them?"

Increasingly, the answer is that the principles and practices of marketing *are* being successfully applied to social issues, causes, and ideas. In the forefront of this trend are health organizations, including federal agencies, state and local health departments, nonprofit voluntary agencies (such as the American Lung Association), hospitals, and clinics.

It is a mistake, however, to believe that the marketing approaches of laundry detergent and car companies can be easily and completely transferred to health promotion and disease prevention. While marketing can be applied to health, various adjustments and translations are needed. Health behavior products are often intangible. The prices of these products are sometimes measured in dollars and cents (for example, the cost of joining an exercise program), but more often they are nonmonetary. There may be little or no reinforcement for the health behavior being promoted, and involvement may be so low that the target consumer is uninterested (as with teeth flossing) or so high that attitudes are resistant to change (as with vasectomy) (Bloom and Novelli, 1981).

Despite these and other differences, marketing is proving to be a useful process for problem solving in the health field. The same disciplined, step-by-step approach that makes it appealing in moving commercial goods and services gives it strong appeal among health professionals.

Social marketing is defined by Kotler (1982, p. 490) as "the design, implementation, and control of programs seeking to increase the acceptability of a social idea or practice in a target group(s)." Sometimes the social marketing label is applied to programs that have social change as a *secondary* benefit. For example, when the American Dental Association attracts more patients to enhance the revenues of its members, it may improve the dental care of many people who might not otherwise seek dental services. More often, however, the term is applied to programs engendered by government agencies, hospitals, nonprofit voluntaries, and other organizations concentrating on the primary goals of improving the common good. Examples include prevention of adolescent pregnancy, increasing seat-belt usage, cigarette smoking cessation, promotion of reduced dietary fat, and improved physical fitness.

Derivation of Marketing Theory

Marketing is theory based. It is predicated primarily on theories of consumer behavior, which in turn draw upon the social and behavioral sciences. This eclectic borrowing from other disciplines characterizes both the theoretical underpinnings and many of the practices of today's marketing.

The term *consumer* is used to refer to those targeted individuals whom marketers seek to persuade to purchase or adopt goods, services, causes, or practices. As marketing has evolved, the complexities and conflicts inherent in consumer behavior have become more apparent. The study of consumer behavior seeks to understand these complexities, as well as the influences that create consumer needs and how these needs can be met.

For example, choosing a brand of laundry detergent is a consumer decision that may involve a variety of product attributes and influences in the marketplace. Larger, more important consumer decisions (such as whether to vacation in Europe this year or how to choose an affordable new home) are far more complex. Health-related behaviors, such as following a long-term medical regimen, avoiding pregnancy, deciding whether to get a second opinion on major surgery, or changing lifelong dietary habits, are also complex and based on rational and emotional factors.

In examining and interpreting these factors, consumer behavior theory seeks to explain why people make certain decisions, what decisions they make about buying, trying, joining, voting, and other aspects of the decision process. The analysis of consumer behavior has its antecedents in the following disciplines:

- Anthropology, which provides an understanding of cultural influences on decision making
- Sociology and social psychology, which contribute knowledge about how group behavior affects individual decision making
- Psychology, the analysis of individual behavior, which contributes to insights about consumers' personal characteristics
- Economics, whose theories provide a broad social context regarding resource distribution

Three broad areas may be used as a framework for understanding the determinants of consumer behavior. First, there are environmental influences, which include the cultural and societal context in which consumer behavior occurs. To take one example, women of reproductive age in Cairo, Egypt, Cali, Colombia, and

Cleveland, Ohio, may have quite different environmental influences affecting their decisions about contraception. These include static and shifting social values, urban crowding, rural changes that affect the need for children to do agricultural work, the role and status of women, media influences, membership in subcultures, religious beliefs and practices, and class structure.

Individual influences represent another broad area. Each consumer is unique and operates with some degree of independence, even within rigid social structures. Consumer behavior is learned, and habits and patterns are developed through experience. Attitudes are formed and altered and are part of the cyclical consumer decision process.

A third part of the framework for consumer behavior involves information processing and actual decision making. (These issues are also discussed in Chapters Two and Four.) Consumers recognize needs, analyze conditions, search out information, evaluate alternatives, and take action. This may all take place quickly, on the basis of impulse, or be a conscious, studied, and deliberative process. A woman who is counseled to lose weight and is interested in doing so may happen upon a storefront sign announcing weight management classes, walk in, and enroll immediately. Many factors, or only a few, may have entered into her decision-making process. Alternately, she may have spent weeks searching for information among friends and assessing price, location, the reputation of the class instructor and then decided to hold off on the decision (itself a decision) pending further deliberation (Berkman and Gilson, 1981).

Concepts of Marketing

Exchange Model. The essence of marketing is based on the theory of exchange, which posits that individuals, groups, and organizations have resources that they are willing to exchange for perceived benefits. The "buyer" in this exchange therefore pays a price, such as money, effort, time, or other resources. The "seller" provides an offering, such as a tangible good (for example, contraceptives, oral rehydration solution for infant dehydration); a service (such as nutrition counseling or blood cholesterol testing); or an idea (for example, the control of hypertension). The key to eliciting voluntary exchanges with targeted audiences is to offer benefits that are valued (for example, a longer, healthier life; looking better and feeling better; fewer, healthier children) as being worth the cost or effort.

Although the objectives of social organizations differ from those of profit-motivated groups, the principles of marketing are similar. The essential marketing model of creating voluntary exchanges with carefully targeted marketing strategies remains valid.

Consumer Orientation. Along with the concept of exchange, the other fundamental of marketing is a tight, continuous focus on the targeted market, most often the (health) consumer, but also health providers, legislators, corporate decision makers, educators, or other audiences. The health consumer must be at the center of health education programs and efforts. This intense concentration on the consumer is marketing's greatest asset. It is the most significant contribution that the marketing discipline can bring to any social program.

Marketing Tools. Marketing makes use of research as the basis for identifying audience needs, wants, expectations, satisfactions, and dissatisfactions; segmenting the target audience(s) into homogeneous subgroups; and positioning the product or offering. Along with the offering—whether a health practice or behavior, a cause or an idea—other essential elements of social marketing include price strategies, channel strategies, and communication.

The key to effective marketing is to study and understand the target consumer, to respond to that consumer in designing, introducing, reshaping, and when necessary, discontinuing product offerings and to monitor the market to adjust to consumer and competitive reaction and marketplace trends.

Marketing Integration. In marketing texts, the "marketing mix" is often described as being composed of the "4 *P*'s": product, price, place (distribution), and promotion (communication). Since this nomenclature can sometimes cause confusion, the term *communication* is used in this chapter to mean advertising, public relations, and so on, whereas *promotion* is a term confined more narrowly to such marketing devices as coupons, premiums, and cash incentives. *Distribution* here connotes processes of disseminating a product, program, or idea, whereas *place* refers only to physical location.

While communication is an important part of marketing, all elements of the marketing mix—*product* development and differentiation, *distribution* channel strategies, *pricing* strategies, *placement* strategies, and communication—should be included in a full marketing program to have the best chance at success. Communication includes several key strategies that contribute to an overall marketing plan. The components of communication are discussed in the following section.

Communication

Within the overall marketing mix, *communication* is itself divided into a number of areas (Novelli, 1988c). These include advertising, public relations, direct marketing, promotion, and face-to-face communication.

Advertising. In commercial marketing, advertising is nearly always purchased by buying time or space in the media (newspapers, magazines, television, radio, billboards, bus and subway posters, and so forth). In nonprofit endeavors, advertising is usually public service in which the media donate time to organizations with worthy messages in the public interest.

Many nonprofit organizations depend solely on public service advertising. Because it is so limited in availability, it lacks the basic qualities of commercial advertising: broad reach, message frequency, and therefore the potential for impact. Public service advertising should be viewed as just one element in a full communication effort.

Public Relations. Public relations tactics include the placement of stories, articles, columns, op-ed pieces (the page opposite the editorial page in most newspapers), and letters to the editor in newspapers and magazines. Other media tactics in public relations involve the placement of spokespersons on television and radio news and talk shows and video news releases (VNRs). (A video news release is a type of feature that is produced by an organization in two versions, one with and one without a sound track, and is incorporated by television stations into their programming as appropriate.)

Public relations tactics also are developed for nonmedia uses, including videotapes for teaching and training; speechwriting and speaker placement; classroom materials; books, booklets, and pamphlets; programs for organizations; conferences, conventions, trade shows, and symposia; and special events (for example, walkathons, health screenings).

Public relations activities can communicate longer, more indepth messages than can advertising and add message credibility because the information is embedded in media news, programming, and editorial material. Public relations tactics are also useful for reaching specialized audiences (for example, handicapped individuals or oncology nurses), adding reach and frequency to mass media campaigns, generating interest and excitement (for example, a weight loss contest between two local companies), and dealing with crisis situations such as public concern over contaminated blood supplies in community hospitals.

Direct Marketing. Direct marketing activities are beamed to a targeted audience via one or more media for the purpose of generating a response by phone, mail, or personal visit. Techniques include direct mail, mail order, "response" advertising that contains a phone number or address, and telemarketing.

Direct marketing tactics are useful for reaching narrow or "niche" markets; distributing materials, samples, and literature; delivering sensitive information to public or professional audiences that should be downplayed in the media; generating leads (for example, for volunteers, members, or potential employees or for services or goods); and establishing a long-term relationship with a client, customer, or patient.

Promotion. In marketing communication, promotional methods are used to build on the other communication techniques as a means of activating behavior. Examples of promotional activities are providing coupons, premiums (such as a cookbook for those who participate in a cholesterol screening), cash incentives, and bonus packs (purchase two packages of condoms, get one free); conducting sweepstakes and contests; offering free samples of goods; and providing demonstrations and displays.

The purpose of these promotional devices is to induce consumers, professionals, volunteers, and other targeted audiences to buy, switch to, and try various offerings, often at points of decision such as retail stores, clinics, screening locations, restaurants, vending machines, and cafeterias.

Face-to-Face Communication. The final area of marketing communications is interpersonal or face-to-face communication. This, of course, is the most direct and dynamic way to deliver information and to persuade. It also provides opportunities for feedback from the audience and tailored messages and responses to overcome objections and concerns and to correct misunderstandings. An example of face-to-face communication is a test program conducted by the National Cancer Institute in which nurses were trained to teach breast self-examination to women patients.

Just as the total marketing mix must be integrated, so too should the various elements of marketing communications. To be most effective, marketing communications must be integrated on the basis of common objectives and related strategies. This leads to better program quality control, increased message uniformity, and greater energy for the entire effort (Novelli, 1988d).

The Marketing Process

One of the appeals of marketing to the administrators of social programs is that it offers a systematic, research-based process for problem solving. The same disciplined, stepped approach that makes marketing useful in the private sector also makes it attractive among managers who seek to change social attitudes and behaviors.

The marketing process is circular, or iterative, with the last stage feeding back into the first in a continuous cycle of replanning and improvement. A clear, workable marketing process has six stages, which are to be pursued in sequence until the process begins again. These are (1) analysis (including needs assessment); (2) planning; (3) development, testing, and refining of plan elements;

(4) implementation; (5) assessment of in-market effectiveness; and (6) feedback to the first stage. Figure 15.1 shows these stages, which are designed to take into account consumer wants, needs, expectations, and satisfactions or dissatisfactions; formulate program objectives; utilize an integrated marketing approach and marketing mix (product, price, communication, distribution); and continuously track and respond to consumer and competitive actions (Novelli, 1984).

First Stage: Analysis. The first area of analyis is the marketplace itself. Most social organizations cannot simply search for areas of open opportunity but must consider organizational mandates and goals. Within these parameters, markets are defined, estimates are made of their current and projected size and shape, and existing competitors are analyzed. Market analysis is also concerned with

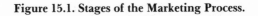

Figure 15.1. Stages of the Marketing Process.

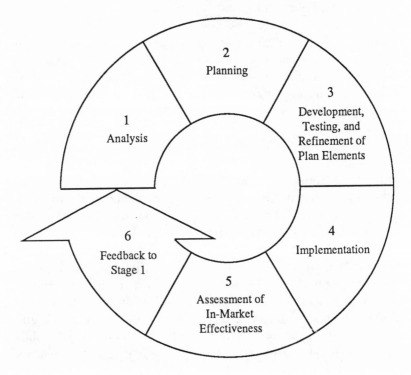

geographical scope, distribution, and outlets. It is important to know how the current market is structured and how current product offerings reach the target consumers. A sense of timing is necessary in market definition. For instance, are uncontrolled hypertensives increasing or decreasing as a percentage of those with high blood pressure? Market trends and growth projections are foundations for budgets, program allocations, and other aspects of a marketing plan. In some instances, as in the rural United States and developing countries, a market analysis should also examine whether such local resources as advertising and public relations agencies, distribution firms, universities (containing faculty with marketing skills), local research suppliers, and printing and packaging firms are available.

The second area of analysis is the consumer who is involved in the marketing exchange. The ultimate target consumer may be an at-risk individual with poor eating habits. But the person who purchases and prepares the food may be as important in the marketing effort as the person who consumes the food. In other instances, the target consumer may be a professional, such as a physician, a corporate executive, or a social worker.

Data on demographic characteristics are usually the easiest to gather. Examples are age, sex, income, education and literacy, social class, family size and life cycle, occupation, religion, race, culture, and ethnicity. Geographic attributes such as region, city size, population density, climate, and mobility may also be significant. A third category of consumer attributes is life-style and behavioral. Consumers may be analyzed according to the benefits they are seeking and their user or behavior status. Finally, media patterns of target audiences are important traits for analysis (Kotler, 1982).

The third area of analysis is the organization itself. Are the necessary financial, management, and staff resources to mount an effective marketing program available? Equally important is whether there is enough commitment by top management to accept a marketing approach and to stick with it long enough for the program to have a chance to succeed. Data collected on these matters, from both secondary and primary research sources, in this first stage of the marketing process serve as the basis for planning.

Second Stage: Planning. The planning phase must result in clear, specific directions for action because virtually all the marketing program's resources will be allocated on the basis of the marketing plan. First, the marketing objectives must be realistic. Most behavior change programs, whether or not good marketing techniques are utilized, realize only small effects, at best. Difficulties often begin with objectives that are too ambitious, too broad, and too hard to translate into action.

Once objectives have been set and audiences identified, strategies can be devised for each element in the marketing mix. The first of these is the product, or offering. One strategy decision is determining product positioning. The idea is to position the offering (for example, an exercise program) at some point on the spectrum of what the target segment wants while avoiding, as much as possible, niches where competitive offerings are located. Other product strategy decisions involve the selection of product characteristics. While it is often difficult to alter the product in social change programs to meet consumer expectations, it may be possible to shape some attributes of the offering that affect consumer perceptions. For instance, the side effects of an oral contraceptive may not be something the social marketer can change, but changing a pill color, package, name, and usage instructions can influence consumer acceptance.

Distribution strategies are also part of the marketing plan. The channels for disseminating the offering to the target market may be direct or may utilize intermediaries such as state agencies, civic or religious organizations, companies, or health providers. Another aspect of developing a distribution strategy is to determine the "outlet" or place at which the offering will be made available to the consumer. In offering smoking prevention programs for children, for example, possible outlets are schools, clubs, and sports facilities.

Price strategies often are the most difficult to set. Consumers' perceptions of monetary, psychic, energy, and time costs must be understood and decisions must be made on how to reduce these costs or otherwise facilitate adoption and maintenance of the behavior being promoted.

The next element in formulating marketing-mix strategies is

communication. A solid communication strategy should contain the primary benefits that the target consumer can expect, supporting points to bolster the promised benefits, the specific action the consumer is encouraged to take, and the tone or image of the communication that is to be conveyed over time. It should also establish the tactics for program advertising, public relations, direct marketing, promotion, and face-to-face communication.

When all the planning is complete, the final step is to incorporate the many components into a single marketing plan, with schedules, milestones for measuring progress, final outcome measures, a total marketing budget, and a budget and schedule for each element in the mix.

Third Stage: Development, Testing, and Refinement of Plan Elements. The initial step in the third stage of the marketing process is product concept development and testing. The concept is the underlying idea for positioning new products or repositioning established ones in relation to the wants, needs, and expectations of the target market. An example of a social marketing product concept might be "A new quit-smoking clinic developed especially for nurses, based on proven methods and offered at convenient hours right here at your hospital."

Pretesting the communication concept(s) provides direction for eliminating weaker approaches and selecting those that appear to have the most appeal. One method for doing this is by means of focus groups (Templeton, 1987). After the selected concepts are transformed into full messages (for example, televison announcements, booklets, posters), they are pretested in nearly final form to assess the target audience's comprehension and reaction. One way to accomplish message testing is through central location (shopping mall) intercepts, a technique in which people typical of the target audience are stopped for short interviews in a highly trafficked location. Unlike focus groups, which yield only qualitative data, a sufficient number of mall intercepts yields more quantitative data that can be used to make generalizations about the target audience. (For a complete discussion of pretesting techniques, see U.S. Department of Health and Human Services, 1989).

Once the communication concepts and messages have been

developed and pretested, all the components of the social marketing program can be assembled as closely as possible to the final form. A small, prototype evaluation can be carried out to obtain a realistic assessment of market reaction before more costly steps are undertaken. The program can then be refined and applied to a test market.

Fourth Stage: Implementation. In the implementation stage of the marketing process, the full social marketing program is put into effect in the entire geographical area to be covered. This requires implementing the marketing plan and monitoring marketplace performance. Distribution channels must be checked to determine whether the offering is reaching the market smoothly. "Retail" monitoring may be necessary to check prices, point-of-purchase (or point-of-decision) displays such as shelf space and inventory, and competitive reaction.

Monitoring "sales" (for example, the number of school districts that accept an American Lung Association curriculum program) may be another part of the implementation phase. Communication must also be monitored. This may involve verifying the placement of paid and/or public service advertising, quantifying the amount of publicity generated, and tracking interpersonal communication. The social marketing organization itself should be monitored, including staff and management performance, funding, communication flow, and decision making.

Fifth Stage: Assessing In-Market Effectiveness. As implementation proceeds, a systematic assessment determines the degree to which the marketing program is meeting its objectives, what midcourse corrections are needed to address deficiencies or capitalize on new opportunities, and how to replan the next cycle of the marketing process. The continuous monitoring of the implementation process and the ongoing assessments in the fifth stage of the market process should fit together into an effective management information system. The purpose of this system is to gather, process, and report timely, adequate, and accurate data for marketing decision making. This should include a comprehensive internal process for storing and retrieving relevant program information and a marketing intelligence network that uses members of the distribution force, intermediaries, field workers, and others to gather and send in useful data.

Program areas requiring assessment usually include the target audience's reaction and response; intermediaries' performance; "retailer" (or other point of exchange) response: communication penetration and impact; and sales, market share, and financial performance.

Sixth Stage: Feedback to Stage 1. There can be no letup in the marketing process. The marketplace changes, programs enter phases of maturity and decline, and the marketing organization may change. The sixth and last stage of the marketing process must therefore feed back into the first. All the information collected should now be carefully reviewed to uncover problems, disclose weaknesses, and identify opportunities. Finally, all of the reviewed and synthesized data should be recycled into the first stage—analysis—to begin anew the continuous and systematic process of refinement and improvement. (For additional reading on market research evaluation, see Andreasen, 1988, and Tull and Hawkins, 1984.)

Challenges to Overcome

A number of general problems confront planners who attempt to transfer the marketing approaches used to sell toothpaste and financial services to promote concepts such as family planning, smoking cessation, and nutrition. An awareness of these problems can help in the formulation of more effective social programs (Bloom and Novelli, 1981).

Market Analysis Problems. Commercial marketers often encounter difficulty in gathering valid, reliable, and relevant data about their consumer targets. But the data-gathering issues facing social marketers tend to be even more difficult. Often, social program planners do not have much secondary data about their consumers. Social marketers also face difficulties in sorting out the relative influence of various determinants of consumer behavior. This is because social behaviors tend to hinge on more than one or two variables and can be difficult for respondents themselves to understand and articulate. Finally, people are more likely to give inaccurate or socially desirable answers on sensitive topics such as sickness, smoking, or contraception than they are on topics such as cake mixes or soft drinks (Colburn, 1988).

Market Segmentation Problems. The process of dividing the market into homogeneous segments and then targeting marketing programs to each key segment is widely practiced by most profit-making and many social marketers. However, social program planners often face pressure not to segment because doing so would mean ignoring certain other segments (Bloom and Novelli, 1981). This often seems discriminatory to social service organizations. To compound the problem, social marketers often lack the behavioral data necessary for identifying key segments. When data exist, social marketers often face the unhappy situation of targeting to those consumers who are the most negative about their offerings—for example, drivers who avoid using seat belts, sexually active teenagers who avoid using contraceptives, or heavy smokers.

Product Strategy Problems. Commercial marketers often have the capacity to shape the products and their characteristics to meet consumer expectations. But marketers of social issues and behaviors have more difficulty in adjusting their offerings, because of legislative, technological, behavioral, or other constraints. Also, social marketers have problems in formulating simple, meaningful product concepts around which a marketing and communications program can be built. Even if a relatively simple product concept can be developed, there remains the problem of selecting a product positioning that will be attractive and acceptable to the many publics of concern.

Pricing Strategy Problems. While commercial marketers usually price their products to maximize financial returns, the complex objectives of social marketers usually compel them to focus on reducing the monetary, psychic, energy, and time costs incurred by consumers engaging in a desired social behavior. This is made difficult by a lack of data to explain consumer perceptions of price and also because little can be done to reduce many of the prices consumers must pay in time, embarrassment, social disapproval, or effort. Much of the time, the social marketer simply tries to convince the target market that the product's benefits outweigh its costs.

Channel Strategy Problems. Developing channel strategies for commercial organizations usually involves the selection of appropriate intermediaries or distributors and designing ways to control and monitor their performance. However, social marketers may have trouble in utilizing and controlling desired intermediaries, such as physicians, the media, community centers, government field offices, or civic organizations. Since they are not likely to have the mandate or the funds to build their own distribution channels or to provide attractive incentives to get cooperation, they must rely primarily on the attractiveness or inventiveness of their appeal, the quality of their training programs, and the goodwill of the intermediary.

Communication Strategy Problems. Social marketers often find that their communications options are somewhat more limited than those of commercial marketers (Bloom and Novelli, 1981). For example, paid advertising may be unavailable because of mandates against government agencies buying media, or the high cost of time and space, or the controversial nature of the message. Many voluntary agencies avoid paid advertising for one program because they fear the media will demand payment for their other programs. This restricts many social marketers to public service announcements, with their inherent limitations in reach and frequency.

Social marketers also face pressures not to use certain types of communication appeals, such as hard sell, fear, or humor, because of the attitudes of their donors, the predisposition of the target audience, and the nature of the subject being promoted. At the same time, social marketers are often dealing with complex behaviors, which require that relatively large amounts of information must be communicated. This makes it imperative to look beyond public service announcements and other broadcast media opportunities toward the use of public relations, direct response, face-to-face strategies, and other types of nonadvertising communication.

Evaluation Problems. Measuring program effectiveness is difficult in any marketing environment but is especially hard for social marketers. In place of immediately quantified measures such as units sold, social agency goals deal with long-term results—for example, reduced morbidity and mortality from breast cancer. Because some goals are distant, they require intermediate measures (awareness, knowledge change, reported behavior) that may not indicate whether long-term objectives are being achieved.

Even when objectives are clear, immediate, and quantifiable, social marketing programs do not typically lend themselves to evaluation that uses common research designs. Randomized experiments or quasi-experiments are difficult to structure because they tend to be costly and because it is often difficult to package social interventions for delivery to some people or regions and not to others. While few social marketing efforts are evaluated with enough rigor for managers to have a clear indication of cause and effect between program and outcome (Bloom, 1980), some public health programs have incorporated significant social marketing efforts and these have been evaluated (for example, Lefebvre and Flora, 1988).

Organizational Problems. Much of the success of a marketing program depends on the nature of the organization in which it operates. Trained marketing managers in key positions, a systematic marketing planning process, and careful monitoring and control are essential ingredients of program success.

Many social organizations have long had communications functions, sometimes called departments of public relations, public information, public affairs, or communications. These departments seem to a social agency the natural place to install and house a new marketing function. Yet such structures may not be conducive to the broader role that marketing must have if any significant impact is to result (Novelli, 1988b).

Perhaps the biggest organizational hurdle of all is the lack of marketing technical assistance. Public health organizations do not yet have the marketing tradition to serve as training grounds. Some organizations, such as the Stanford Five City Program and the Pawtucket Heart Health Program, have successfully incorporated marketing into their models for health promotion and disease prevention (Lefebvre and Flora, 1988). But far more often, outside technical assistance will be needed to incorporate the potent problem-solving techniques of marketing into public health on an effective, broad-scale basis.

These challenges in social marketing are not insurmountable, but they must be recognized and dealt with in sound planning, program implementation and control, and evaluation. Resourcefulness and imagination are needed to strengthen social marketing and continue its acceptance and growth.

Applications

Social Marketing Works. It contributes to successful health and social interventions. Marketing is being applied as part of an overall approach, along with classic health promotion models and other behavioral theory and disciplines. The result is a pragmatic, affordable, systematic blending that yields results. The following two examples illustrate the efficacy of marketing health promotion and disease prevention.

Metro Manila Measles Immunization Campaign. A major objective of the Aquino government in the Philippines is to provide the country's population with access to basic health services. One aspect of this public health initiative is to improve levels of immunization against major childhood diseases, including measles, pertussis, poliomyelitis, diphtheria, and tuberculosis. Only 21 percent of Philippine children under one year of age are fully immunized to prevent these diseases (Abad, 1987).

HEALTHCOM, a marketing-oriented program funded by the U.S. Agency for International Development, works with developing countries in health promotion and disease prevention, with emphasis on child survival. HEALTHCOM professionals viewed the Philippines' need for immunization as an opportunity to provide technical assistance and to help the Philippine Department of Health (DOH) on its long-term efforts to upgrade the marketing and communication skills of its health educators.

The Philippine DOH set a goal for its Expanded Program on

Immunization: to increase complete infant immunization from 21 percent to 50 percent in two years. A pilot campaign was to be implemented in the nation's capital area (Metro Manila) to test-market the campaign approach prior to wider implementation. Measles was selected by the DOH and HEALTHCOM as the program's emphasis because measles vaccination is the last in the immunization series and it was believed that boosting vaccination rates for measles would increase completion of the series. Also, measles had the lowest vaccination rate of the childhood diseases, even though it is widely recognized by most Filipinos. It was reasoned that measles could be used as a "hook" to attract mothers and their children into health centers, where they could be informed about the value of full immunization.

The DOH health educators thought that the primary reason underlying resistance to measles immunization was a widespread belief that the disease is a natural, relatively harmless childhood disease. It seemed clear that there was little understanding by Filipino mothers of the dangers of the disease, including the possibility of infant mortality from measles-related complications.

The targeted behavior set by the HEALTHCOM and DOH planners was to get mothers to have their children immunized against measles when the children were nine and twelve months of age. The primary target audience was identified as women with children under one year old, living in Metro Manila, of lower socioeconomic status. A secondary target audience was family and peers (husbands, parents, friends), who might influence mothers' decisions regarding immunization.

An important part of the campaign was to communicate that measles immunizations were offered every Friday at government health clinics and at three government hospitals in the area. Other information in campaign messages concerned the potential seriousness of the disease and why immunization was so important.

The research elements of the pilot campaign included the following:

• An initial review of past research undertaken on the Expanded Program on Immunization

- Three survey waves of target mothers: a baseline prior to the campaign's start, a midpoint wave, and a postcampaign wave
- Interviews with mothers and staff members in eight health centers
- A day-after recall test among target mothers to assess comprehension, recall, and various diagnostic elements (for example, believability, importance, likes/dislikes) of television commercials twenty-four hours after exposure
- Print and radio messages, which were tested qualitatively, and television and radio advertising that was purchased for the campaign

Publicity was generated as part of the communications effort. Attention was given to face-to-face communication with mothers once they were drawn to the clinics and hospitals. The logistical requirements for proper immunization delivery were reviewed with the DOH/National Capital Region staff, and training and orientation were provided for the staff members of the 331 health centers involved. To track and respond to events and conditions in the health centers during the campaign, a communications monitoring plan was devised and implemented.

The media campaign was launched with the objective of reaching 75 percent of the total target audience twice a week for a three-month period. Three television commercials, three radio promotions ("plugs"), and daily newspaper advertising were used. Other materials included two versions of posters for health centers, T-shirts for health center staff (*Ligtas Ako Sa Tigdas*, or "I am protected from measles"), auto bumper stickers, bunting and streamers for health centers, and a comic book and baby book for each mother. The materials and messages were developed by a Filipino advertising agency working with HEALTHCOM and the DOH.

Results of the pilot program indicated that it was successful in increasing the rate of all vaccinations in the target area, not only measles (Abad, 1988). The tracking studies (surveys) showed improvements in the understanding of the seriousness of measles; awareness of immunization as a protection against measles also increased significantly. Media channels were cited as a primary source of this information. Other changes among target mothers included greater knowledge of the correct age for measles vaccinations and increased understanding of specifics (number and form of doses) about immunization.

In addition, a diffusion effect was observed as an outcome of the emphasis on measles. Vaccination for all infant diseases increased, and general attendance at the health centers rose. This suggested a more active involvement with child health among women of lower socioeconomic strata.

Findings suggest that knowledge and behavior change objectives among target women were met, the DOH staff enhanced communication planning and implementation skills (including working with advertising agency professionals), and health center and hospital counseling and treatment practices improved (Debus, 1988).

National High Blood Pressure Education Program. In the United States each year, hypertension (high blood pressure) contributes to an estimated 250,000 deaths from stroke, coronary heart disease, congestive heart failure, and kidney disease. Approximately one-half of those who suffer a heart attack and about two-thirds of those who suffer a stroke have hypertension. The disease limits the activities of an estimated three million people in the United States. The prevalence of hypertension among blacks is one-third higher than among whites, and the stroke mortality rate among blacks is nearly double that for whites. The stroke mortality among blacks under sixty-five years of age is nearly three times that for whites of the same age (National Heart, Lung, and Blood Institute, 1984).

To address this major health problem, the National High Blood Pressure Education Program (NHBPEP) was established in 1972 by the National Heart, Lung, and Blood Institute (NHLBI). The program is a cooperative effort involving numerous organizations, including federal agencies, state health departments, and private- and public-sector health care organizations.

The goal of the NHBPEP is to reduce death and disability related to high blood pressure through professional, patient, and public education (National Heart, Lung, and Blood Institute, 1982). Strategies include development and stimulation of widespread health promotion and disease prevention activities, the creation and distribution of educational materials and technical assistance, and support to community health programs. The NHBPEP has led the way in examining a wide range of important issues and establishing policies, guidelines, and recommendations. These include appropriate roles of health care professionals in hypertension control, the most effective treatment practices in medical management, high blood pressure control at the work site and in rural communities, high blood pressure in the elderly, the relationship between diet and high blood pressure, controlling the disease in minority populations, and educational strategies for professional and lay audiences (Ward, 1984; Bellicha, 1988).

Since the beginning, the program has applied marketing principles in the use of consumer research, audience segmentation, and the strategic development, pretesting, production, and assessment of public messages. The initial challenge of the program's public education effort was to mount a campaign that would build awareness of the "silent killer" and the dangers of leaving hypertension undetected and untreated. Messages at this early stage encouraged the general public to "know your high blood pressure number as readily as you know your age and your social security number."

Slowly, as public awareness and knowledge increased and screening and detection became more widespread, communication strategies shifted to focus on the need to begin and maintain treatment. The theme for these compliance-with-treatment campaigns first stressed the concept of controlling the disease not only for the hypertensive person but also for those who need and depend on him or her ("Do It for Yourself and All the Loved Ones in Your Life"). Then they evolved into "High Blood Pressure—Treat It and Live" and finally to "High Blood Pressure—Treat It for Life."

Program planners at the NHLBI initiated parallel public, patient, and professional education programs. As the NHBPEP took hold, it seemed clear that the concurrent audience approach was a wise course of action. Not only did it shorten the time needed to effect results, but a certain synergy seemed evident, a synergy in which patients' questions about hypertension increased physicians' (and nurses') response, and health professionals' understanding led to more aggressive counseling and treatment. In marketing terms, health professionanls were "pushing" high blood pressure control through the health care system, while patients were "pulling" the concepts and practices through the same system.

Subsequent public education initiatives addressed the misconceptions of controlling hypertension (for example, that it has symptoms that signal when something should be done). These initiatives should include patient compliance with treatments and support for treatment by family and friends. Educational initiatives also should include skill-building; for example, increasing patients' skills in asking physicians about medications.

Over time, as progress was made, therapy maintenance was demonstrated in a broad variety of social settings. The action steps remained constant: "Take your pills, cut down on salt, exercise, and control your weight."

The National High Blood Pressure Education Program has made substantial progress in educating professional, patient, and public audiences and in controlling hypertension. Data from the *Health Promotion/Disease Prevention Supplement to the National Health Interview Survey* (National Center for Health Statistics, 1985) indicate very high levels of public knowledge about the relationship between high blood pressure and heart disease or stroke. The survey found that 92 percent of the U.S. adult population were aware that hypertension is a cause of heart disease (up from 24 percent in 1973), and 77 percent were aware that high blood pressure increases one's risk of suffering a stroke (up from 29 percent in 1973). A Department of Health and Human Services report states that "Success . . . is attributable in large part to the effectiveness of the National High Blood Pressure Education Program and the many cooperative, complementary efforts of public and private organizations at national, state, and local levels" (Office of Disease Prevention and Health Promotion, 1986, p. 20).

In addition to these changes in awareness and knowledge, behavior change has also occurred. From 1972 to 1986, physician visits for hypertension increased almost 74 percent in comparison to physician visits for all causes, which increased only 9 percent (*National Disease and Therapeutic Index,* 1986). The number of those on medication for hypertension increased from 36 percent in 1973 to 56 percent in 1980, and the number of those in control (less than 160/95 mm Hg) and on medication rose from 16 percent to 34 percent. (The 1973 data are from the 1971–1974 National Health and Nutrition Examination Survey of people twenty-five to seventy-four years of age. The 1980 data are from the 1976–1980 National Health and Nutrition Examination Survey of people eighteen to seventy-four years of age.)

It is clear that progress is being made in the control of coronary heart disease in the United States. The NHBPEP is only one contributor to this progress, although certainly a major one. Within the program, the application of marketing principles and the public education component have been paralleled by other effective approaches.

Conclusion

Evidence based on numerous programs in various settings indicates that the systematic application of marketing principles and practices to social and health issues can contribute to measurable behavior change (Flay and Burton, 1988). Unfortunately, this is as far as one can go in making a claim for social marketing's efficacy. No studies have been conducted across an array of programs to answer such key questions as when does social marketing work best, what elements or conditions contribute to or inhibit its application and success, and which components of the marketing model appear to be most important to success in social and health programs.

While we can say that the marketing of health promotion and disease prevention brings results, marketing is nearly always applied as part of an overall or larger approach in an interdisciplinary combination along with health promotion models based on behavioral theory and disciplines. Thus, social marketing is often part of a hybrid behavior change model.

This hybrid approach most likely occurs because marketing is being learned and applied by planners trained in other disciplines, such as health education and health communication. Where marketing professionals assume planning responsibilities for social and health programs (for instance, hospital marketing directors often come from commercial marketing backgrounds), they also seem to borrow from other planners and models as they learn about health.

Thus, marketing is being embraced not as a stand-alone technology but as part of an interdisciplinary approach to health promotion and disease prevention. This is illustrated in a report issued by the Academy for Educational Development (Rasmuson, Seidel, Smith, and Booth, 1988) on effective health communication initiatives in developing countries: "Public health communication incorporates the theories and methods of several disciplines. Social marketing provides a framework for selecting and segmenting audiences and for promoting products and services. Behavior analysis supplies tools for investigating current practices, defining and teaching new practices, and motivating change. Anthropology reveals perceptions and values which underlie existing practices and which can help sanction new ones" (p. 9).

What steps can health planners take to incorporate social marketing into their operations? Obviously, technical assistance from marketing practitioners can help. But before marketing can take root in a social service organization, it is wise to examine the organization itself, to determine whether conditions that will be hospitable to marketing strategies exist. Here are six questions (Novelli, 1988a) to assist in this organizational analysis:

1. Is research being conducted to understand target markets and make real program decisions?
2. Are there measurement systems that regularly provide data on "customer" (that is, public, patient, and/or professional segments) satisfaction? On emerging consumer needs?
3. Do program managers, at all levels, have regular, in-the-flesh contact with target audiences? (Many corporate marketing divisions require that managers frequently visit the marketplace where consumer decisions are made.)
4. Does every program manager, no matter how high the rank, have a view of the marketplace subject to challenge and input from others?
5. Does the organization have a true and constant focus on the health consumer, or does it tend to look mostly inward, giving

primary attention to operating efficiencies, revenue generation, and other operational issues?

6. Does the organization have the resources (primarily staff and budget) and the management support to take a systematic marketing approach?

If the answer to many of these questions is yes, chances are good that planners and managers can learn and incorporate marketing concepts into program analysis, planning, implementation, and control.

Social marketing has much to offer. The evidence is there; the potential is clear. It is not easy to apply marketing techniques creatively to change health behavior. But it can be done, and the rewards in improved public health can be considerable.

References

Abad, M. *EPI Measles Campaign: Survey.* Manila: Trends, Inc., Oct. 1987.

Abad, M. *EPI Measles Campaign; Metro Pre- and Post-survey Report.* Manila: Trends, Inc., Oct. 1988.

Andreasen, A. R. *Cheap But Good Marketing Research.* Homewood, Ill.: Dow Jones-Irwin, 1988.

Bellicha, T. "The Mass Media Campaign: This Year's Look." Paper presented at National Heart, Lung, and Blood Institute state workshops, Bethesda, Md., and Denver, Colo., Sept. 1988.

Berkman, H., and Gilson, C. *Consumer Behavior: Concepts and Strategies.* Boston: Kent, 1981.

Bloom, P. N. "Evaluating Social Marketing Programs: Problems and Prospects." In R. Bagozzi and others (eds.), *Marketing in the 1980s: Changes and Challenges.* Chicago: American Marketing Association, 1980.

Bloom, P. N., and Novelli, W. D. "Problems and Challenges in Social Marketing." *Journal of Marketing,* 1981, *45,* 79–88.

Colburn, D. "Selling Health—How Do You Warn a Drug Addict About AIDS? When All Else Fails, There's Bleachman." *Washington Post,* September 20, 1988, p. Z8.

Debus, M. *Memorandum on Manila Program Drawn from Unpub-*

lished Trip Reports, Research Findings, and Other Program Data. Washington, D.C.: Porter/Novelli, Oct. 1988.

Flay, B. R., and Burton, D. "Effective Mass Communication Campaigns for Public Health." Paper presented at Conference on Mass Communications and Public Health: Complexities and Conflict, the Annenberg Center, Rancho Mirage, Calif., Sept. 1988.

Kotler, P. *Marketing for Nonprofit Organizations.* Englewood Cliffs, N. J.: Prentice-Hall, 1982.

Lefebvre, R. C., and Flora, J. A. "Social Marketing and Public Health Intervention." *Health Education Quarterly,* 1988, *15,* 299-315.

National Center for Health Statistics. *Health Promotion/Disease Prevention Supplement to the National Health Interview Survey.* AdvanceData no. 113, 1985.

National Disease and Therapeutic Index. Ambler, Pa.: IMS America, 1986.

National Heart, Lung, and Blood Institute. *High Blood Pressure Control: Information and Education Strategies for Messages to Public and Patient Audiences.* Bethesda, Md.: National Heart, Lung, and Blood, Institute, 1982.

National Heart, Lung, and Blood Institute. *Tenth Report of the Director.* Vol. 1: *Progress and Promise.* National Institutes of Health Publication no. 84-2356, 1984.

Novelli, W. D. "Developing Marketing Programs." In L. Frederiksen, L. Solomon, and K. Brehony (eds.), *Marketing Health Behavior.* New York: Plenum, 1984.

Novelli, W. D. "Non-Business/Social Marketing." In V. P. Buell (ed.), *Handbook of Modern Marketing.* (2nd ed.). New York: McGraw-Hill, 1986.

Novelli, W. D. "Marketing Focus: Understanding Consumers, Understanding Ourselves." Paper presented at the SOMARC Asia/ Near East Contraceptive Social Marketing Conference, Pattaya, Thailand, Feb. 1988a.

Novelli, W. D. "Marketing vs. PR: Who's Taking the Prisoners." *Medical Marketing and Media,* 1988b, *23,* 38-48.

Novelli, W. D. "Public Relations." In W. Wells, J. Burnett, and S.

Moriarty (eds.), *Advertising Principles and Practices*. Englewood Cliffs, N.J.: Prentice-Hall, 1988c.

Novelli, W. D. "Stir Some PR into Your Communications Mix." *Marketing News*, December 5, 1988d, p. 19.

Novelli, W. D. " 'Selling' Public Health Programs: How Marketing Applies." *Medical Marketing and Media*, 1989, *24*, 36-44.

Office of Disease Prevention and Health Promotion. *The 1990 Health Objectives for the Nation: A Midcourse Review*. Washington, D.C.: Office of Disease Prevention and Health Promotion, Public Health Service, U.S. Department of Health and Human Services, 1986.

Rasmuson, M. R., Seidel, R. E., Smith, W. A., and Booth, E. M. *Communication for Child Survival*. Washington, D.C.: Academy for Educational Development, June 1988.

Rothschild, M. L. "Marketing Communications in Nonbusiness Situations or Why It's So Hard to Sell Brotherhood Like Soap." *Journal of Marketing*, 1979, *43*, 11-20.

Templeton, J. *Focus Groups*. Chicago: Probus, 1987.

Tull, D. S., and Hawkins, D. I. *Marketing Research: Measurement and Method*. New York: Macmillan, 1984.

U.S. Department of Health and Human Services. *Making Health Communications Programs Work: A Planner's Guide*. National Institutes of Health Publication no. 89-1493, April 1989.

Ward, G. W. "The National High Blood Pressure Education Program: An Example of Social Marketing in Action." In L. Frederiksen, L. Solomon, and K. Brehony (eds.), *Marketing Health Behavior*. New York: Plenum, 1984.

Chapter 16

Lawrence Wallack

Media Advocacy: Promoting Health Through Mass Communication

Mass communication in the United States pervades daily life. The mass media structure the way we think about, discuss, and respond to public health issues on a social as well as an individual level. The mass media, it is often said, may not tell people what to think, but they certainly tell people what to think about. Finding the key to using the mass media to promote health is the health education equivalent of splitting the atom. One common view that is implicit in much health education reasoning is that if we can only get the right message to the right person in the right way at the right time, then the frequency of risky behaviors will surely diminish. This atom, however, cannot be split. The mass media are not the magic bullet of health promotion and disease prevention. The mass media play an important role as part of a comprehensive approach to improving health, but the nature of that role is poorly understood. The purpose of this chapter is to put the use of mass media in perspective and suggest possible roles that might be appropriate.*

*The description of the application of media advocacy was written by Philip Wilbur, Director, Health Advocacy Resource Center, Advocacy Institute, Washington, D.C. The contributions of Russell Sciandra, Janine Sadlik, and Alan Blum, M.D., are also gratefully acknowledged.

The mass media work, but it is unclear how. We are all deeply affected by what we read, watch, and listen to, but the effects are hard to assess and difficult to interpret. It is common to assert that television, our most constant companion, affects children's classroom performance and shortens attention spans but research does not support this assertion. It is common to assert the effectiveness of advertising in promoting alcoholic beverages, high-fat foods, or tobacco products, but the research in these areas is controversial. It is common to assert the effectiveness of public education campaigns on "life-style" issues such as drugs, alcohol, tobacco, and diet, but the evidence is far from compelling. It is almost as if the research would lead us to the conclusion that the mass media have no effect. This, however, would not be accurate either. The mass media are central to our society and have profound effects on health and well-being.

It is best to start with what we do know about the functions of the mass media. The mass media are effective in setting the public agenda and stimulating public discussion. The mass media confer status and legitimacy on issues and thereby make it acceptable and easier to discuss issues. This can be seen in a specific case such as a made-for-television movie on the topic of incest that almost overnight made it acceptable to discuss this issue. It can also be seen in the general case of AIDS, where the word *condom* had never appeared on television and virtually overnight was not only on television but common currency in open discussions. This power to stimulate and frame discussion is a power worth working for.

One of the mistakes commonly made in considering media is an underestimation of the importance of structuring public discussion around an issue. The way a society thinks about cigarette smoking, in the long run, is certainly as important as, and may be even more important than, getting small numbers of people to quit smoking. For the most part, however, we look to the media as a way of directly changing behavior. The underlying assumption is that people adopt risky behaviors because they do not fully understand the consequences of such acts; they just don't know any better. If people really knew the effects of a poor diet or of not using safety belts, then they would not behave in such irresponsible ways. Ignorance is the problem, and the solution is information packaged in the right way. Once the right information and right message are agreed on, then the mass media, particularly television, which is turned on for over 600 million hours every day in 98 percent of U.S. households, are the perfect delivery mechanism. Unfortunately, this approach simply does not work. Even sophisticated variations that incorporate mass communication theory and social marketing concepts, though useful, are limited in effectiveness.

The health educator of the 1990s will need to have expertise in two fundamental approaches to using the mass communication system to promote health. The first approach is an "enhanced" public communication model that uses social marketing concepts as a framework in which to integrate marketing principles and social-psychological theories to better accomplish behavior change goals (Flora, Maibach, and Maccoby, 1989). The second approach uses media access and issue-framing strategies that are more closely associated with political campaigns than traditional public education efforts. The goal of this second approach is not to change individual risk behaviors but to redefine what are typically seen as individual problems into public health or social issues. This leads to increased prospects for the development of supportive or "healthy" public policies and social-environmental change.

Although these two approaches share certain common principles, each evolves from a fundamentally different set of assumptions about the nature of health problems. Public communication campaigns are based on an individual-centered understanding of health as an absence of disease. Media advocacy is linked more to an environmental understanding of health as primarily determined by factors external to the individual. These different assumptions result in divergent strategies for using mass media. Both approaches have strengths vital to the mission of health education and should be combined in a comprehensive approach.

Public Communication Campaigns

Public communication campaigns are a frequent response to health and social problems. Such campaigns come in all levels of sophistication and funding and generally seek to educate large populations about issues thought to be important to individual and community well-being. For the most part, however, these efforts appear to have little demonstrable lasting effect on personal behavior or population disease rates: "The literature of campaign research is filled with failures, along with some qualified successes" (Rogers and Storey, 1988, p. 817).

Public communication campaigns have been shown to stimulate the use of a cancer hot line number, increase the purchase of high-fiber cereals (Levy and Stokes, 1987; Freimuth, Hammond, and Stein, 1988), and in some cases stimulate attempts to quit smoking (Cummings, Sciandra, and Markello, 1987) or reduce smoking (Flay, 1987). In addition, the carefully planned use of mass media has been shown to influence life-style behaviors in a national Finnish study (Puska and others, 1985) and reduce the risk of heart disease in an American study (Farquhar, Maccoby, and Wood, 1985). There is, in fact, substantial optimism among mass communication and health promotion scholars regarding the promise of mass media–based campaigns as a vehicle for health promotion (for example, Flay, 1981; Atkin, 1983; Farquhar, Maccoby, and Wood, 1985).

Social Marketing as a Source of Optimism

Much of the optimism about the use of mass media as a vehicle for changing health behavior results from recent applications of social-psychological theories and social marketing concepts (see Chapter Fifteen). The intervention is developed from a solid base of communication and social-psychological theories, and marketing techniques are used to supplement message development and program implementation (Farquhar, Maccoby, and Solomon, 1984; Lefebvre and Flora, 1988; Flora, Maibach, and Maccoby, 1989). Ideally, social marketing also involves mobilization of local organizations and interpersonal networks.

Social marketing has been suggested as a useful approach to planned social change (See Chapter 15). Careful definition of the problem and clear setting of objectives are important aspects of social marketing approaches. However, the most significant contribution of social marketing has been the strong focus on consumer orientation, the use of formative research, and attention to exchange theory as a way of getting the consumer to comply with the message. None of this should be news to the health educator, but the pressing needs of the practice environment make the application of key principles a luxury.

Consumer orientation means identifying and responding to the needs of the target audience. This is a departure from many past campaigns (and some current ones) in which message and strategy development were centralized with little input from those whom the message was designed to reach. The primary tool to tailor public communication efforts to specific audiences is formative research. Formative research can be applied at all stages of intervention design and implementation. It basically involves the collection of various levels of data to enhance the overall quality and appropriateness of the intervention. For example, small groups representing a potential target audience might be convened to get their ideas about program strategy or to test their reaction to specific messages. Modifications to strategy and content would then be made on the basis of the results from these "focus groups." Other kinds of formative research might include audience segmentation, analysis of the most appropriate channels of communication, or the assessment of preexisting knowledge and attitude levels in target groups.

Exchange theory is critical to the efficacy of social marketing approaches. The basis of exchange theory is that people are willing to exchange some resource (such as money or time) for a benefit (such as a product or product attribute). As Lefebvre and Flora (1988) note, the marketing process attempts to facilitate a voluntary exchange that provides the consumer with tangible benefits at a minimal cost of money, physical or emotional effort, or group support. If in the end the campaign is not able to facilitate this voluntary exchange successfully, the likelihood of effectiveness will be slight.

Social marketing has limitations that affect its usefulness. First, exchange theory has not been very successful in social marketing applications. The limited success of typical health promotion programs that seek to exchange increased health status, positive image, or presumed peer approval for delayed gratification (diet, smoking cessation), increased physical effort (exercise), risk of social rejection (abstinence from drugs), or physical discomfort (withdrawal from cigarettes) raises significant questions regarding the applicability of exchange theory to this area.

Second, the developmental research that is the hallmark of social marketing requires time, money, and skill. Oftentimes at least one of these key factors is missing, and the result can be limited effectiveness. Health agencies can seldom support extensive research or provide adequate time for optimal campaign planning and may see no need for it anyway.

Third, the apparent successful examples of the social marketing approach often reflect the "Mercedes Benz" model conducted in university or well-funded demonstration settings. The generalizability to more usual settings is debatable. More common is the use of the media on a shoestring budget, use not made by media specialists but by those with limited training. While social marketing applications will undoubtedly contribute to better campaigns, it is not clear that this necessarily means better health outcomes.

Fourth, social marketing largely assumes the negative aspects of the media environment to be a given and does not attempt to alter the pervasive antihealth education messages implicit in advertising and television programming. In a way, social marketing violates one of the basic principles of the advertising that it seeks to emulate: placing one's message in a fertile and supportive environment.

Fifth, some people view social marketing as basically a reductionist approach to understanding health, which tends to reduce serious health problems to individual risk factors. This approach may contribute little to reducing the incidence of disease (Syme, 1986; Winkelstein and Marmot, 1981; Slater and Carleton, 1985). In addition, the strong focus of public communication campaigns on individual risk factors may serve to deflect attention away from environmental factors beyond the control of the individual (such as social class) that have been shown to be a major determinant of health.

Social marketing involves acquiring better knowledge of the audience, better message strategies, improved message placement and media mix, and better ways of monitoring audience response to the campaign. These are all positives and will enhance the use of mass media to alter key behaviors. Yet, while it makes for a better application, the effectiveness of social marketing remains limited.

Media Advocacy

Media advocacy is a relatively new concept that has been most closely associated with the smoking control movement. In addition, consumer groups concerned with alcohol, nutrition, and AIDS issues have contributed to the growing number of cases from which the principles of media advocacy are beginning to emerge. "Media advocacy," according to Michael Pertschuk, one of the architects of this approach, "is the strategic use of mass media for advancing a social or public policy initiative" (Advocacy Institute, 1989, p. 8). Media advocacy utilizes several important community organization concepts, including empowerment, citizen participation, and involvement in issue selection. (See Chapter Twelve).

Media advocacy promotes a range of strategies to stimulate broad-based media coverage in order to reframe public debate to increase public support for more effective policy-level approaches to public health problems. It does not attempt to change individual risk behavior directly but focuses attention on changing the way the problem is understood as a public health issue. For example, a media advocacy approach might develop a strategy to stimulate media coverage regarding the ethical and legal culpability of alcohol companies that promote deadly products to teenagers. The purpose is to shift attention from defining alcohol problems as solely the property of individuals and highlight the role of those who shape the environment in which individual decisions about health-related behavior are made.

All media coverage of health, whether news, entertainment, or public service, will tend to increase awareness and knowledge regarding health issues. Social marketing, social advertising (such as Partnership for a Drug Free America), and public communication campaigns in general serve this purpose. The essence of media advocacy, however, is to move beyond this function and stimulate public participation in the policy-generating process (American Cancer Society, 1987). For example, media advocacy in the area of nutrition would carefully use media to reframe the problem of diet from one of poor individual eating habits (an awareness and knowledge problem) to one of public policy (regulation of saturated fat in food, promotion of clear nutrition labeling). The goal is to empower the public to participate more fully in defining the social and political environment in which decisions affecting health are made.

Media advocacy is issue oriented. It recognizes that the mass media are often the forum for contesting major policies that affect health. Unfortunately, the public debate tends to be narrowly defined by ideological (individual-focused explanations) and practical (limited time to present complex issues) considerations of media coverage and the concerns of vested interest groups. Overcoming these barriers represents a major challenge for media advocacy. It attempts to move from the individual-simple to the social/political-complex part of the problem definition continuum.

A number of skills are essential for the media advocate. These include research, "creative epidemiology," issue framing, and gaining access to media outlets. Research is important in becoming a reliable and credible media advocate. The advocate must not only know the key studies, significant data, and contested issues regarding the particular topic but must also know the characteristics of the various media outlets. For example, the nutrition activist might regularly screen the local newspaper to identify which reporters cover relevant issues or whether the paper has taken editorial positions on food and health.

Creative epidemiology is the use of research and existing data to gain media attention and clearly convey the public health importance of an issue. It does not imply a loose use of data or misleading presentation of the facts. On the contrary, because creative epidemiology will stimulate media coverage and, perhaps, generate controversy, it must be scientifically sound. For example, an American Cancer Society videotape explains that "1000 people quit smoking every day—by dying. That is equivalent to two fully loaded jumbo jets crashing every day, with no survivors." Creative epidemiology frames data to be interesting for the media and more understandable and meaningful to the general public.

Framing the issue to be consistent with policy goals is a complex and sophisticated endeavor. The corporate world is very skilled at using valued symbols to their advantage. For example, legitimate criticism of the marketing practices of tobacco and alcohol producers becomes an "attempt at censorship" or an "assault on the First Amendment." The corporate world provides funds for local community groups, thus buying friends and goodwill. In addition, substantial support is provided to art and cultural events in order to purchase "innocence by association" (Advocacy Institute, 1989). The tobacco industry uses a range of strategies to capture symbols such as freedom of choice, freedom of speech, patron of the arts, and many others to stake out the high moral ground and gain widespread support.

Successful framing of an issue puts the framer in a more advantageous position. The framer can determine, to a great extent, the terms of discussion. The tobacco industry has carefully crafted an image of itself as an advocate of civil rights, protector of free speech, and good community citizen. Antismoking groups have been successfully characterized as zealots, health nuts, and health fascists. The industry was very successful at this until recently when antismoking activists reframed the issues by stripping the industry of its positive symbols. Tobacco producers became "merchants of death," "hitmen in three-piece suits," and exploiters of youth, women, and minority groups. A number of strategies were developed to expose and publicize tobacco industry ties to cultural events, shaming through public exposure those who accept industry money, and continually making explicit the link between death and tobacco. These strategies are described in greater detail later in this chapter.

Successful reframing uses two primary strategies. First, it often focuses attention on industry practices, not the behavior of the individual, as the problem. This results in increased support for regulatory measures that can have a substantial public health impact. Second, it seeks to delegitimize the industry by exposing industry practices that are exploitive and unethical. Advertising and marketing practices that exploit children and place profits before health and safety provide raw material for the media advocate.

Increasing access to the mass media is fundamental to media advocacy. Historically, health educators have been heavily dependent on the willingness of the media to provide time or space. In a sense, the media were allowed to define which issues would be aired and how the discussion would be structured. The availability of public service time is declining as media outlets increase efforts to sell all available time. Even public service time now figures into bottom-line calculations (Brown, 1987). By using creative epidemiology and framing strategies, it is possible to have greater control over how the media cover an issue. To be effective, it is necessary to take advantage of free and paid media.

It is useful to rethink the concepts of free and paid media. This usually is interpreted to mean the difference between a public service announcement, which may air at any time of the day or night, and a purchased spot where one can assure desired audience exposure to that spot. In reality there is a wide assortment of good free time for the media advocate to use. For example, the media advocate can create news in a number of ways. It is possible to build on breaking news stories. For example, by creating "local reaction" many communities mobilized media coverage around the release of the surgeon general's twenty-fifth anniversary report on smoking and health. The media advocate can also create news by presenting small research studies of local or national interest. For example, the Center for Science in the Public Interest drew attention to the issue of alcohol advertising and children by conducting a small study that showed that children could name more brands of beer than presidents of the United States. This received national attention. The media advocate can build on related news opportunities. For example, when tons of Chilean fruit were banned because they contained a small amount of cyanide, local antismoking activists used this to point out to the media that it would take bushels of tainted grapes to equal the cyanide in the sidestream smoke of just one cigarette.

There are numerous ways that the media advocate can increase media coverage of an issue. For example, news coverage can be extended by providing op-ed pieces to newspapers and stimulating letters to the editor. In addition, print and electronic journalists can be cultivated to gain access for follow-up stories with local perspectives. Cultivating access should be viewed as a long-term, cumulative strategy that will improve with every successful effort.

Media advocacy has several limitations. First, this approach has not been adequately defined, and no set of principles has been developed. It is an evolving approach that has emerged from grass roots and public interest groups. Second, the skills involved in media advocacy are probably more varied than those of the social marketer. The media advocate needs to understand the media culture, including what is news and how it can be framed to gain media interest and citizen support. Third, the necessary time for research and cultivating media gatekeepers may be beyond the bounds of those working in public agencies. Fourth, media advocacy is linked to an environmental approach that focuses primarily on the social and political aspects of health and is less concerned with direct behavior change. This focus makes it difficult to get and hold media attention, which tends to highlight the personal and individual aspects of health problems.

Media advocacy is an aggressive approach to using mass media to promote health. It involves sophisticated use of valued symbols and arguments in order to refocus attention on the social-structural aspects of public health problems. The effectiveness of media advocacy has not been established, and researchers are just beginning to outline basic principles. There are, however, impressive case studies from the smoking, nutrition, AIDS, and alcohol fields that indicate this to be a promising approach.

The application presented next is an example of how media advocacy can be used to heighten community awareness and encourage public participation.

Utica Alvin Ailey Protest

An example of media advocacy is provided by activities conducted in Utica, New York, to protest cigarette company support for the arts. A National Cancer Institute project, COMMIT (*COMM*unity *I*ntervention *T*rial), was designed to test ways to reduce the number of heavy smokers through community-level approaches. One of the key objectives is to increase community awareness about smoking so that people understand it as a public health issue and not just an individual issue. One of the eleven test communities in the COMMIT program is Utica, New York.

One of the ongoing goals of the Utica COMMIT project is to reframe their community's perception of cigarette companies as upstanding corporate citizens and community leaders to enemies of society and "merchants of death." As a means of accomplishing that goal, the project devised a media advocacy initiative centering around a protest of a Philip Morris–sponsored local performance of the Alvin Ailey American Dance Theater.

The protest was a response to Philip Morris's ongoing strategy of "buying" social legitimacy through its sponsorship of various cultural events. The COMMIT project consisted of efforts to attain as much publicity as possible around a fairly simple "media event."

The media event itself was nothing more than the distribution of a pamphlet to theater patrons as they entered the Stanley Theater the night of the performance. The pamphlet was a simple yet carefully researched example of creative epidemiology. To reframe Philip Morris's public role from patron of the arts to merchant of death and disease, the front page of the pamphlet contained the following bold message: "Philip Morris brings you more than art . . . they also bring you cancer, heart disease, emphysema, stroke, bronchitis, 135,729 deaths every year." This message also reframed the slogan that appears on all advertisting that accompanies Philip Morris–sponsored cultural events, "Philip Morris brings you the arts."

The death toll cited on the front of the pamphlet was significant in that it was not the more frequently cited number of 390,000 cigarette-caused deaths in the United States each year. Instead, the cited figure represents the deaths caused specifically by Philip Morris products (total number of deaths divided by Philip Morris's market share). The resulting figure was more compelling in that it directly linked Philip Morris itself with an estimated number of deaths.

On the inside of the pamphlet, this connection was made even clearer by a chart labeled "Annual Deaths in U.S. Caused by Philip Morris, Inc.," which listed the number of Philip Morris-caused deaths by disease (for example, lung cancer = 43,185, heart disease = 45,230).

Most of the pamphlet was used to explain the social consequences of cigarette company sponsorship of public events: "When cigarette companies sponsor sports teams or racing cars, they are buying exposure on television and other media to which they otherwise would not have access. . . . When they sponsor the arts, such as tonight's presentation by the Alvin Ailey Dance Company, they buy prestige and respectability. What they spend on the arts is only a fraction of the three billion dollars they spend every year on cigarette advertising and promotion, but it is enough to enhance their image as public benefactors. They hope you will forget where the money came from."

To emphasize the ability of Philip Morris to "buy respectability," the concept of creative epidemiology was applied to the corporation's finances: "In 1988, its profits amounted to *$190,000 per hour.*"

The pamphlet was also used to ask patrons to talk to their children about the hazards of smoking and to "let them know that throwing a few dollars to the artists and dancers doesn't make Philip Morris a socially responsible company."

The pamphlet concluded with a request to patrons to "Help Alvin Ailey Dance Company break its dependence on the cigarette industry: Make a contribution to support the company, but make it contingent on not accepting tobacco money in the future." This request again involved the patrons in the reframing process. The focus of the request was also important since any perceived attack on the Ailey company would likely have backfired on the sponsors of the protest. By focusing on the dance company's "dependence" on the industry, the protest framed the company as a victim of Philip Morris's exploitation and kept the focus of the protest on the enemy—the cigarette industry.

Because of a rainstorm the night of the performance, only one doctor, a local surgeon, showed up to distribute pamphlets and talk to the media. One other person was recruited to help distribute the pamphlets, and the manager of the theater offered to set up a table in the lobby for the pamphlets. Because the Stanley Theater only has one entrance and because the surgeon was well known in the community, the effort was sufficient to make the message of the protest clear to both dance patrons and the media.

A press release summarizing the protest and the pamphlet were distributed to the local newspaper and radio and television stations two days before the performance with an embargo that was lifted the night of the performance. In addition, personal contact was made with people representing the area's one newspaper, two television stations, and approximately ten radio stations. Utica COMMIT had learned that this personal contact was a crucial part of any successful media initiative.

Soon after Utica COMMIT was established, it began notifying relevant media contacts whenever there was a local tobacco-related event or story or when it could offer a local spin on a national or statewide story. By the time of the Ailey protest, Utica COMMIT had established relationships with contacts at each of the area's radio and television stations and with several writers and editors at the local newpaper. These relationships had developed to the point where, shortly after the Ailey protest, several media contacts were calling on a regular basis asking for news leads.

These relationships paid off when the protest received coverage on both of Utica's television stations, each of which interviewed the surgeon, and in the local newspaper, where it received coverage in the review of the performance itself. The final two paragraphs of Jonas Kover's review in the *Utica Observer Dispatch* (May 11, 1989) summarized the protest and quoted the local surgeon on his motivation for participating ("because cigarettes are helping to kill people").

The review was important not only because it represented access to a media channel not normally utilized by health advocates but also because it articulated the theme of Utica COMMIT's ongoing goal of identifying cigarette companies as enemies of the public's health.

This media advocacy initiative was a success in gaining access to the media, including media channels that do not normally cover public health issues, and in using that coverage to frame a community event in a way that focused on the practices of the cigarette industry rather than on the behavior of individual smokers. In addition, and significantly, the protest was crafted in a way to directly involve the public in the reframing process.

The coverage was achieved because Utica COMMIT had creatively provided the media with a story to cover. As one leader noted, "To gain the media's attention, you can't just say something, you have to *do* something. The protest gave the media something to cover and gave us a chance to have our message heard."

By accomplishing the goals of this single event, Utica COM-

MIT helped make the local environment more receptive to pro-health messages and initiatives while making it harder for cigarette companies to sustain an environment in which their advertising and promotion practices are seen as acceptable or even beneficial.

Conclusion

A recent major study on the future of public health defines the mission of public health as, "fulfilling society's interest in assuring conditions in which people can be healthy" (Institute of Medicine, 1988, p. 7). Too often, we use the mass media to focus on disease conditions and not the conditions of disease. Social marketing is important in providing information and skills regarding the need to alter life-style behaviors to change disease conditions. However, unless public health focuses on eliminating the conditions of disease and promoting conditions of health, our efforts to improve health will have limited effect. The use of mass media in a structured, thoughtful way to change health behavior is useful but in no way sufficient to have a meaningful effect on aggregate health status.

Media advocacy can be used to shift the focus from disease conditions to conditions of disease. Public health problems are conceived as socially, not individually, produced. It is important to deal with this concept of social production. The decisions society makes "upstream" will go a long way toward determining the "downstream" body counts. Media advocacy can illuminate the upstream activities of governments and commercial interests and help restructure public debate.

Media advocacy provides an exciting new approach. At the least, it suggests that power over health status will come from gaining greater control over the social and political environment in which decisions that affect health are made. It invites citizens to participate more fully in this arena. Participation, after all, is key to health education practice.

In the long run, social marketing and media advocacy must be more balanced. Many health education efforts seek to give people better information so that they can beat the odds and have a healthy and successful life. Real change will come with programs that change the odds to make it more likely that people have sufficient opportunity to be healthy and succeed (Schorr, 1988). Health educators should continue to use social marketing in the most creative way to get people the right information to help them beat the odds. In addition, health educators must commit to media advocacy to emphasize the importance of working to change the odds.

References

Advocacy Institute. *Smoking Control Media Advocacy Guidelines.* Bethesda, Md.: National Cancer Institute, National Institutes of Health, 1989.

American Cancer Society. *Smoke Signals: The Smoking Control Media Handbook.* New York: American Cancer Society, 1987.

Atkin, C. "Mass Media Information Campaign Effectiveness." In R. Rice and W. Paisley (eds.), *Public Communications Campaigns.* Newbury Park, Calif.: Sage, 1983.

Brown, L. "Hype in a Good Cause." *Channels,* 1987, 7, 26.

Cummings, M., Sciandra, R., and Markello, S. "Impact of a Newspaper Mediated Quit Smoking Program." *American Journal of Public Health,* 1987, 77,1452–1453.

Farquhar, J., Maccoby, N., and Solomon, D. "Community Applications of Behavioral Medicine." In W. Gentry (ed.), *Handbook of Behavioral Medicine.* New York: Guilford Press, 1984.

Farquhar, J., Maccoby, N., and Wood, P. "Education and Communication Studies." In W. Holland, R. Detels, and G. Knox (eds.), *Oxford Textbook of Public Health.* New York: Oxford University Press, 1985.

Flay, B. "On Improving the Chances of Mass Media Health Promotion Programs Causing Meaningful Changes in Behavior." In M. Meyer (ed.), *Health Education by Television and Radio.* Munich, Germany: Saur, 1981.

Flay, B. "Mass Media and Smoking Cessation: A Critical Review." *American Journal of Public Health,* 1987, 77, 153–160.

Flora, J., Maibach, E., and Maccoby, N. "The Role of Mass Media Across Four Levels of Health Promotion Interventions." In L. Breslow, J. Fielding, and L. Lave (eds.), *Annual Review of Public Health.* Palo Alto, Calif.: Annual Reviews, 1989.

Fox, K., and Kotler, P. "The Marketing of Social Causes: The First 10 Years." *Journal of Marketing*, 1980, *44*, 24-33.

Freimuth, V., Hammond, S., and Stein, J. "Health Advertising: Prevention for Profit." *American Journal of Public Health*, 1988, *78*, 557-561.

Institute of Medicine. *The Future of Public Health*. Washington, D.C.: National Academy Press, 1988.

Kotler, P., and Zaltman, G. "Social Marketing: An Approach to Planned Social Change." *Journal of Marketing*, 1971, *35*, 3-12.

Lefebvre, C., and Flora, J. "Social Marketing and Public Health Intervention." *Health Education Quarterly*, 1988, *15*, 229-315.

Levy, A., and Stokes, R. "Effects of a Health Promotion Advertising Campaign on Sales of Ready to Eat Cereals." *Public Health Reports*, 1987, *102*, 398-403.

Maccoby, N., Farquhar, J., Wood, P., and Alexander, J. "Reducing the Risk of Cardiovascular Disease: Effects of a Community-Based Campaign on Knowledge and Behavior." *Journal of Community Health*, 1977, *3*, 100-114.

Puska, P., and others. "Planned Use of Mass Media in National Health Promotion: The 'Keys to Health' TV Program in 1982 in Finland." *Canadian Journal of Public Health*, 1985, *76*, 336-342.

Rogers, E., and Storey, J. "Communication Campaigns." In S. Chaffee and C. Berger (eds.), *Handbook of Communication Science*. Newbury Park, Calif.: Sage, 1987.

Schorr, L. *Within Our Reach*. New York: Doubleday, 1988.

Slater, C., and Carleton, B. "Behavior, Lifestyle, and Socioeconomic Variables as Determinants of Health Status: Implications for Health Policy Development." *American Journal of Preventive Medicine*, 1985, *1*, 25-33.

Syme, L. "Social Determinants of Health and Disease." In J. Last (ed.), *Public Health and Preventive Medicine*. East Norwalk, Conn.: Appleton & Lange, 1986.

Winkelstein, W., and Marmot, M. "Primary Prevention of Ischemic Heart Disease: Evaluation of Community Interventions." In *Annual Review of Public Health*. Palo Alto, Calif.: Annual Reviews, 1981.

Chapter 17

Karen Glanz

▲ ▲ ▲

Perspectives on Group, Organization, and Community Interventions

The chapters in Part Four have presented five models of health behavior intervention at the group, organization, and community levels. The aim of these chapters is to demonstrate the utility and promise of each theory or framework in health education and health promotion. This chapter discusses the similarities among the theories, draws common themes, and critiques their usefulness for research and practice in health promotion.

The central theme of Part Four is that we need to understand, predict, and know how to work with people through the social structures that are the context for their health behavior. The concepts of social networks, role relationships, change within and among systems, and communication channels are apparent across each of the chapters.

Two general domains help define the scope of the models that are included in this section: social action or activation and processes for changing attitudes and behaviors. The former is usually characterized by "internal" or *intra*group stimuli for change, whereas the latter are more likely to inform external change agents about how to facilitate changes that they deem desirable. None of the models is "pure" in this sense, but all roughly break down into these categories.

387

Social action or *activation* is central to community organization, organizational development, and media advocacy, though the emphasis differs in each of these models. As Minkler notes in Chapter Twelve, several of the key concepts in community organization practice relate directly to the notion of a community creating the conditions for change: empowerment, community competence, and the principles of participation and "starting where the people are." Two of the three models of community organization proposed by Rothman—locality development and social action—stress consensus, cooperation, group identity, and mutual problem solving.

Organizational Development (OD) Theory aims to improve organizational performance and the quality of work life. Its roots are in the human relations or humanistic psychology perspective. It is concerned with members of organizations and involves problem diagnosis by gathering information directly from the members or workers, through formal surveys, interviews, and other methods. OD interventions include strategies such as team building, group development, and T-groups to promote interpersonal exchanges. As Goodman and Steckler point out in Chapter Fourteen, face-to-face contact and group interaction are integral to this approach.

Media advocacy uses the mass media strategically to advance a social or public policy initiative (Advocacy Institute, 1989). It focuses attention on changing the way a problem is understood as a public health issue. It focuses heavily on activation of forces in a social system (that is, media coverage) that can help to stimulate public concern and action.

Processes for facilitating large-scale *changes in attitudes and behaviors* are the province of Diffusion of Innovation Theory, social marketing, and Stage Theory of organizational change. Each of these frameworks offers guideposts for professionals wishing to promote specific changes in individuals within a larger society and in organizations. A key concept in diffusion of innovations is the spread of ideas, products, and behaviors within a society or from one society or social system to another. Social marketing adopts techniques from the commercial marketing arena to promote ideas and practices for socially worthy causes such as improved health practices. Stage Theory is closely allied to diffusion of innovations because it focuses on understanding and matching the organizational stages of change with efforts to introduce or encourage organizational change.

Cyclical Nature of the Change Process

In some theories and theory-based models for organizational and social change, the overall change process is conceptualized as a cycle of defining needs or problems, developing and implementing intervention strategies, and assessing the impact of these efforts. This cyclical model mirrors the same process that is proposed for individual models of change and more generally for program development and evaluation in health education. Both the decision-making frameworks of Janis and Mann (1977) and others, and the consumer information processing framework set forth by Bettman (1979) conceptualize individual learning, decisions, and action in a parallel manner. General models for health education program planning and development advocate the use of planning, implementation, and evaluation phases with feedback for future planning as likely to enhance the success of practice (see, for example, Dignan and Carr, 1987; Green and others, 1980; Green and Lewis, 1986).

The cyclical change process is depicted in the two chapters in this section that address organizational change theories and social marketing. In Chapter Fifteen, Novelli describes social marketing as including five stages: analysis; planning; development, testing, and refining of plan elements; assessing in-market effectiveness, and feedback to the first stage. He notes that a central challenge in successful social marketing is effective management of this change process.

In their chapter (Fourteen) on organizational change theories, Goodman and Steckler analyze both Stage Theory and OD Theory in terms of the cycle of change. They describe seven steps in Beyer and Trice's (1978) Stage Theory: sensing of unsatisfied demands, search for possible responses, evaluation of alternatives, decision to adopt a course of action, initiation of action within the system, implementation of the change, and institutionalization of the change. Their stages appear to conclude with institutionalization, or long-term maintenance/adoption of change, rather than with evaluation and feedback. However, Everett Rogers's (1983) description of stages of the innovation process in organizations indicates that implementation of change *involves evaluation that often results in redefining or restructuring* the innovation and its fit for the organization and clarifying the innovation before it becomes routinized, or institutionalized. Thus, while the "end point" of the change process in Stage Theory is ideally that of change becoming institutionalized, evaluation occurs during the early stage of implementation. If an innovation is evaluated unfavorably and cannot be adapted to suit the organization's needs, it will not survive to be routinized. If the problem that stimulated the innovation persists, this evaluative information will feed back to an earlier stage and be used in the consideration of new alternatives.

Within OD Theory, Goodman and Steckler describe the four steps of Implementation-Procedure Theory as diagnosis, action planning, intervention, and evaluation. These steps are equivalent to the stages of the marketing process and closely related to those of Stage Theory. Stage Theory becomes a useful complement to OD Theory because well-timed "matching" of OD interventions to the evolving stages of organizational change can improve the likelihood of successful adoption and institutionalization.

The change cycles and processes that are well accepted for individual change models and program development are well suited to large-scale and institutional change efforts. We next examine the approaches to defining needs or problems that emerge from the macro intervention models in this section.

Approaches to Defining Needs and Problems

The roots of change efforts for health enhancement lie in the initial phase of needs assessment or problem definition. Several issues reflect the philosophy and methodology of designing health promotion strategies: *Who* will decide what is a problem? What is the relative importance of professional (outsider/change agent) definition of needs and lay/community (insider/target audience) expression of needs? *What methods* yield accurate and useful information? Will the methods be quantitative, qualitative, or a combination of both? How much time and what resources are available to define needs and problems, and with what level of detail?

Three models described in the preceding chapters in Part Four reflect a continuum of "insider" or target audience definition of needs to an "outsider-initiated" problem diagnosis: community organization, OD Theory, and social marketing. Actually, each of these models reflects the need to be community, consumer, or participant oriented—where the models differ is in their relative emphasis on who should express or gather information for needs assessment.

As Minkler notes, a key principle of community organization is "starting where the people are." In other words, individuals must experience a *felt need* before they will learn or change. In a strict sense, the community must identify needs and issues to be addressed. *Ownership* and *participation* are important to the success of change efforts. However, when professionals are working with communities, the ideal may not match the reality of "setting their own goals." The mission of the practitioner's organization and the availability of earmarked resources or technical data may modify the priorities that are identified by community members when it comes to designing action strategies.

While ownership and participation are also important in OD Theory, identification of problems or gaps in organizational functioning is most often conducted with the help of an outside consultant. The most traditional form of problem diagnosis is accomplished with surveys of the organization's members. The factors assessed are likely to include the organization's mission, goals, policies, procedures, and structures; social and interpersonal factors; desired outcomes; and readiness to take action. Because OD usually is initiated with the assumption that there are problems, or the potential for improvements, in intraorganizational functioning, it is logical to seek the assistance of an outside party. Matters of interpersonal conflict, challenging management authority, and job stability make it unlikely that a valid appraisal of problems will emerge from a self-analysis conducted entirely *within* the organization.

Social marketing emphasizes the consumer orientation to understanding the audience, but at the same time it includes *marketplace analysis* (of market structure and the competition), and *organization analysis* (what the resources and commitment of the sponsoring organization can support). *Audience analysis* and segmentation strategies to assess the characteristics of individuals and groups who are the targets for change include analysis of demographic, geographic, life-style and behavior, and media-use patterns. Multiple methods are often used, including quantitative market surveys, central location intercept interviews, and focus groups. The aim of such needs assessment in social marketing is to provide the practitioner (that is, the sponsoring organization or its marketing/communications specialist) with sufficient information to design and deliver appropriate programs to promote its cause, product, or practice. With its roots in commercial marketing, social marketing tends to sound far less "client centered" or "community oriented" than community organization. However, the concept of *social* marketing implies that socially beneficial aims are the focal product. (But not everyone will agree that they are beneficial; causes such as family planning and fluoridation are not universally agreed to be desirable!)

In addition to the continuum from "inside" to "outside" problem assessment in these three models, there is a continuum of data-gathering methods from qualitative to quantitative. Although community organization, OD, and social marketing may each use a combination of "soft" and "hard" data, the relative emphasis on qualitative information and quantitative data usually varies across the models.

Different approaches to needs assessment are suited to different models of health behavior and to diverse approaches to stimulating change. Most important, researchers and practitioners whose work is informed by one or more models should bear in mind the source of data and data-gathering methods when interpreting such information for intervention design.

Dynamic Models of Change

One of the most important crosscutting themes of the change models in Part Four is that models for understanding and influencing organizational, community, and social change are dynamic rather than static. It has often been said that the only thing that is constant is that there will always be change. The change processes that include feedback loops and ongoing evaluation imply that future interventions should be based on reactions to previous programs and to new social situations as well.

Changes in organizational structures and institutional policies that are *not* the results of planned change can powerfully affect the context of health promotion. For example, changes in the delivery and financing of health services can profoundly affect patient health behaviors, such as the decision to seek professional care, choice of a particular provider, and the volume of use of services. The effects of increasing bureaucratization and corporatization of medicine can influence the behaviors of professionals, support staff, and patient-provider relations (Greenley and Davidson, 1988). The case example that Goodman and Steckler present in Chapter Fourteen about changes in delivery of health services underscores these issues.

Relatively little is known about the area of secular health promotion, that is, various behavior change and political and social action efforts to promote health and prevent disease *outside* of those activities associated with professional health education and health promotion (Elder and Sallis, 1988). Also, environmental changes such as shifts in the food supply can radically alter the barriers and opportunities for promoting healthy behaviors (Glanz and Mullis, 1988). Such naturally occurring change processes must be incorporated into researchers' and practitioners' adaptations of macro change models.

Legislation, community organization, and social norms may converge to support important health promotion causes, and these dynamics provide leverage points for practitioners and natural laboratories for researchers. Hingson, Howland, and Levenson (1988) reviewed the recent progress in reducing drunken driving and alcohol-related traffic fatalities. They note that more than 500 legislative reforms were passed from 1980 to 1985 and more than 400 local chapters of citizen groups such as Mothers Against Drunk Driving (MADD) were founded during that time. Concurrently, published news stories about the problem of drunk driving increased fiftyfold during this period. The opportunities for media advocacy were thus increased by legislation and community organizing activities. As Hingson and others (1988, p. 665) point out, laws "function to disseminate and reinforce social norms about drunk driving" and outcome measures should also "examine attitudes about the laws and their reinforcement, perceived dangers of drunken driving, and social pressure not to drink." Advocacy both during the development of legislation and following its implementation can help accelerate social change for health improvement.

The principles of media advocacy are useful for illustrating the dynamic nature of macro models of change for health behavior, for they are based on seizing critical opportunities to advance social or public health policy initiatives. Among the principles of media advocacy are the admonitions to be flexible and opportunistic, to take the initiative, and to keep it local and relevant. Strategies for gaining access to the mass media include timely reaction to the general news environment, identifying policy initiatives that are newsworthy, and creating news with created events (Advocacy Institute, 1989).

Professionals working in health promotion and education must be constantly vigilant, must stay current with what has been tried, and must understand what forces in the social environment bear attention when planning and evaluating intervention strategies. The evaluation of "side effects" or unintended/unanticipated results of our efforts should be framed within the context of emerging salient social and health issues.

Similarities Between Models

Each theory and model in Part Four of *Health Behavior and Health Education* is distinctive in its perspective, emphasis, and research base. At the same time, there are many similarities between the models, as well as similarities to the intrapersonal and interpersonal models of health behavior presented earlier in this book. This section highlights some of those similarities and the related differences in the models: (a) social marketing and diffusion of innovations, (b) organizational change theories and diffusion of innovations, (c) community organization and organizational change, (d) diffusion of innovations and social learning theory, and (e) diffusion of innovations and communication-persuasion models of attitude change. This chapter does not offer in-depth analyses of these related models because each comparison would require a chapter in itself (and this has been done in other books).

Social Marketing and Diffusion of Innovations. Social marketing is defined as "the design, implementation, and control of programs seeking to increase the acceptability of a social idea or practice in a target group(s)" (Kotler, 1982, p. 490). Diffusion of innovations is concerned with understanding how new ideas, products, and social practices spread within a society or from one society to another (Rogers, 1983). An initial perusal of these definitions suggests that social marketing and diffusion of innovations have the same goals, with social marketing having a more proactive, intervention stance and diffusion frameworks being primarily interested in description and explanation. Both frameworks and areas of study are concerned with the dissemination and utilization of innovations. Rothman, Teresa, Kay, and Morningstar (1983, p. 10) note that "social marketing and diffusion research are virtually one and the same, yet perceived value differences have kept these fields quite separate. . . . [T]he difference is that the diffusion people approach their subject from a humanistic or nonprofit point of view, while the social marketing writers draw upon a body of literature that originally had overriding profit-making motivation. . . . [This] has made them seem incompatible." The label *social marketing* may be incompatible with the values of some nonprofit organizations and human services workers, but when the resultant strategies are applied to social causes, the methods used are likely to be no different from those that could be drawn from diffusion frameworks. Social marketing springs from a free market approach, which recognizes that resources and exchanges are essential to the survival of organizations (Winett, 1986). Similarly, innovations must compete in society (or the marketplace) for survival, and those that are not widely adopted become extinct. In sum, while the origins of social marketing and diffusion, the relative emphasis on *understanding* and *changing,* and much of the terminology employed distinguish these two areas from each other, in many ways "diffusion and social marketing as areas of study meld" (Rothman, Teresa, Kay, and Morningstar, 1983, p. 10). Their broad aims are similar, and their key concepts are compatible and often parallel.

Organizational Change Theories and Diffusion of Innovations. In his 1983 book, Rogers notes the need for diffusion of innovation frameworks to focus on innovations in organizations. He argues that a better understanding of collective and authority innovation decisions is an important base of understanding for those wanting or needing to aim at groups to achieve changes in ideas and practices. He spells out the stages of the innovation process in organizations and indicates the importance of attention to those stages for successful adoption of innovations. The two overarching stages which he proposes, initiation and implementation, are the same as those described by Zaltman, Duncan, and Holbek (1973) and other theorists of organizational change. Stage Theory is one of the two central frameworks that Goodman and Steckler have set forth in this book as important conceptual bases for organizational change. Their preferred articulation of the model is that of Beyer and Trice (1978). However, this model and the organizational-level diffusion approach spring from the same tradition in the organizational behavior literature. They vary mainly in the level of specificity in defining stages and in the selected terminology for describing key stages in the innovation process.

Both diffusion and organizational change research have fallen short on studies of *processes* of change, and various writers have acknowledged the need to examine systems from within as they consider and adopt new ideas and practices. One recent study of medical innovations examined organizational innovation from *both* an intraorganizational and an interorganizational perspective. Fennell and Warnecke (1988) chronicle the development of cancer treatment networks in an effort to link organizational theory with the more long-standing "person-centered" model that has dominated diffusion theory. In doing so, they combine contingency theory with a resource dependency perspective to explain why some organizations might initially consider an innovation, refine it to fit their own context, and then implement it.

Community Organization and Organizational Change. Chapter Twelve on community organization presents key principles and models of community organization, along with the theoretical foundations that form its base. There is no single theory of community organization that applies adequately to health promotion work (Solomon and Maccoby, 1984). Rather, one must borrow from other theories; some of these theories are integral to the organizational change frameworks articulated in Chapter Fourteen. They include Social Support Theory, community development, and network analysis, which are most pertinent to OD Theory as a component of organizational change. Another important consideration relates to the final phase of Stage Theory that Goodman and Steckler present. That phase, institutionalization, involves an organization's adopting an innovation, a new idea or practice, as an ongoing part of its structure and activities. The relationship to community organization lies in the virtual necessity of considering community organization principles (and, very likely, OD methods) in order for institutionalization to be possible.

Diffusion of Innovations and Social Learning Theory. Albert Bandura's 1986 volume on Social Learning Theory (which he renamed Social Cognitive Theory) includes a chapter on social diffusion and innovation. In it, Bandura notes that "understanding how new ideas and social practices spread . . . has important bearing on personal and social change" (1986, p. 142). Even before this relatively recent attention to diffusion, the linkages between social learning and diffusion were set in place. The most apparent difference, which is reflected in the structure of this book, is that diffusion concepts and research emphasize the macro nature of social change, whereas social learning emphasizes intrapersonal and interpersonal factors, that is, the micro level.

Winett (1986) has succinctly outlined some of the similarities and differences between social learning and diffusion. Similarities include the focus on behavior change, the importance of interpersonal networks for behavior change, the essential role of information exchange, and movement toward two-way influence processes (a recent emphasis in diffusion theory). Social learning and diffusion differ in their research traditions, as reflected in the dominant measurement methods and research designs. Diffusion measurement is usually aggregate, whereas social learning emphasizes individual- or interpersonal-level variables. Moreover, diffusion research primarily involves naturalistic field surveys, whereas social

learning research designs are primarily experimental and often conducted in the laboratory. It is the differences in research methods
and design that mirror the distinct conceptual perspectives of these
two paradigms and exemplify the way in which macro models of
behavior change depart from intrapersonal and interpersonal
approaches.

Diffusion of Innovations and Communication-Persuasion. Diffusion frameworks are useful in understanding how the mass media
contribute to the spread of innovations in populations. The phases
of diffusion can also be examined as phases of psychological change
in individuals. These parallels are described in Green and McAlister's (1984) discussion of how macro-interventions are distinct from
micro-interventions to support health behavior. The correspondence draws parallels between models of communication and persuasion and information processing at the individual level, and the
corresponding organization or community frameworks of adoption.
Individual-level phases of exposure and attention correspond to the
diffusion concept of *awareness*. Comprehension for individuals relates to *interest* in a macro model. And belief, decision, learning,
and action roughly parallel the *trial* and *adoption* phases in a population. Communications can be designed to promote effects on individuals at each stage of the individual models and disseminated to
promote optimal diffusion in a social system.

Research Issues

Each of the theories and action models presented in Part Four of
Health Behavior and Health Education is complex and multimodal
and aims to influence not only large groups of individuals but
organizational structures as well. An assessment of the impact of
interventions based on these frameworks requires more complex
and less controlled designs than those at the intrapersonal or interpersonal level. Such evaluations may also require unusually large
numbers of people in order to allow detection of statistically significant differences if organizations are used as the unit of randomization
and analysis. Further, access to information at the organizational
level may be difficult to obtain and even harder to validate given the

divergent perspectives of managers and workers or members and constituents/clients of an organization.

Additional research challenges involve the study of community change and societal change as two-way processes, the need to attend to personal influence as well as the content of interventions, and the need to plan for and integrate both qualitative and quantitative data sources. Because the magnitude of comprehensive evaluations of these interventions is beyond the funding and skills of many health education providers, the adequate documentation of *processes* will take on increasing importance.

Conclusion: Macro Level Frameworks in Context

Societal, community, and institutional factors are critical to promoting health because they can provide a fertile environment for health enhancement as well as directly shape individuals' health behavior. The power of policy is evident in health education settings such as workplaces and schools. For example, a recent study found that school smoking policies in two California counties were associated with decreased amounts of smoking in adolescents (Pentz and others, 1989). Broad social changes have also been linked to individual behavior and perceptions. The impact of these social historical events on individuals is complex: It appears to interact with individual receptivity to change as reflected in life stages and other key developmental markers. The impacts can be seen, for example, in changes in women's work, family roles, and health-related behaviors as they differentially impact each generation of women (Stewart and Healy, 1989).

Macro-level approaches can complement intrapersonal and interpersonal theoretically derived methods of health education and health promotion. Blended models suggest integrated strategies for reaching various units of practice in community-wide programs (Solomon and Maccoby, 1984). Some health issues, for example, environmental protection through control of air pollution, hazardous waste, and water contamination, cannot be influenced through individual-level efforts alone. However, they may be affected positively through methods based on individual behavior analysis frameworks *combined with* social marketing to promote wide dissemination (Geller, 1989).

The integration of group, organization, and community intervention frameworks with individual and interpersonal models of health behavior has potential for real-world impact that exceeds the use of any one approach. Our most challenging public health problems require increased attention to organizational and environmental factors. Because behavior is highly influenced by settings, rules, organizational policy, community norms, and opportunities for action, changes in these factors are promising targets for change. Individual change will follow successful organizational and environmental changes (Winett, King, and Altman, 1989).

The theories and methods of community organization, stage theory, organizational development, diffusion of innovations, social marketing, and media advocacy provide a strong foundation for understanding and positively influencing health behavior. Advances in research will clarify the mechanisms of these theories' operation and refine our understanding of how best to use them. Health education and health promotion strategies will achieve greater success through informed application of these frameworks for social action and activation and community attitude and behavior change.

References

Advocacy Institute. *Smoking Control Media Advocacy Guidelines.* Bethesda, Md.: National Cancer Institute, National Institutes of Health, 1989.

Bandura, A. *Social Foundations of Thought and Action: A Social Cognitive Theory.* Englewood Cliffs, N.J.: Prentice-Hall, 1986.

Bettman, J. R. *An Information Processing Theory of Consumer Choice.* Reading, Mass.: Addison-Wesley, 1979.

Beyer, J. M., and Trice, H. M. *Implementing Change: Alcoholism Policies in Work Organizations.* New York: Free Press, 1978.

Dignan, M. B., and Carr, P. A. *Program Planning for Health Education and Health Promotion.* Philadelphia: Lea & Febiger, 1987.

Elder, J. P., and Sallis, J. F. "Secular Health Promotion." In *Health*

Promotion in California: A Compendium of Papers from Cali-
fornia Health Promotion Consensus Project. Berkeley, Calif.:
Western Consortium for Public Health, 1988.

Fennell, M. L., and Warnecke, R. B. *The Diffusion of Medical*
Innovations: An Applied Network Analysis. New York: Plenum,
1988.

Geller, E. S. "Applied Behavior Analysis and Social Marketing: An
Integration for Environmental Protection." *Journal of Social*
Issues, 1989, *45,* 17-36.

Glanz, K., and Mullis, R. M. "Environmental Interventions to Promote Healthy Eating: A Review of Models, Programs, and Evidence." *Health Education Quarterly,* 1988, *15,* 395-415.

Green, L. W., and Lewis, F. M. *Evaluation and Measurement in*
Health Education and Health Promotion. Mountain View,
Calif.: Mayfield, 1986.

Green, L. W., and McAlister, A. L. "Macro-Intervention to Support
Health Behavior: Some Theoretical Perspectives and Practical
Reflections." *Health Education Quarterly,* 1984, *11,* 322-339.

Green, L. W., and others. *Health Education Planning: A Diagnostic*
Approach. Mountain View, Calif.: Mayfield, 1980.

Greenley, J. R., and Davidson, R. E. "Organizational Influences on
Patient Health Behaviors." In D. S. Gochman, (ed.), *Health Be-*
havior: Emerging Research Perspectives. New York: Plenum,
1988.

Hingson, R. W., Howland, J., and Levenson, S. "Effects of Legislative Reform to Reduce Drunk Driving and Alcohol-Related Traffic Fatalities." *Public Health Reports,* 1988, *103,* 659-667.

Janis, I. L., and Mann, L. *Decision Making.* New York: Free Press,
1977.

Kotler, P. *Marketing for Nonprofit Organizations.* Englewood
Cliffs, N.J.: Prentice-Hall, 1982.

Pentz, M. A., and others. "The Power of Policy: The Relationship
of Smoking Policy to Adolescent Smoking." *American Journal*
of Public Health, 1989, *79,* 857-862.

Rogers, E. M. *Diffusion of Innovations.* (3rd ed.). New York: Free
Press, 1983.

Rothman, J., Teresa, J. G., Kay, T. L., and Morningstar, G. C.

Marketing Human Service Innovations. Newbury Park, Calif.: Sage, 1983.

Solomon, D. S., and Maccoby, N. "Communication as a Model for Health Enhancement." In J. D. Matarazzo and others (eds.), *Behavioral Health: A Handbook of Health Enhancement and Disease Prevention.* New York: Wiley, 1984.

Stewart, A. J., and Healy, J. M. "Linking Individual Development and Social Changes." *American Psychologist,* 1989, *44,* 30–42.

Winett, R. A. *Information and Behavior: Systems of Influence.* Hillsdale, N.J.: Erlbaum, 1986.

Winett, R. A., King, A. C., and Altman, D. *Health Psychology and Public Health.* New York: Pergamon Press, 1989.

Zaltman, G., Duncan, R., and Holbek, J. *Innovations and Organizations.* New York: Wiley, 1973.

PART FIVE

▲▲▲

NEXT STEPS AND BEYOND

Chapter 18

Irwin M. Rosenstock

The Past, Present, and Future of Health Education

It would be the height of folly to predict the future needs of health education research and practice, at least without the assistance of an outstanding California astrologer or the Great Kreskin. Yet some clear trends have emerged over recent decades, trends that are well worth remembering if we hope to make progress. George Santayana put it well in his (frequently mangled) quotation: "Those who cannot remember the past are condemned to repeat it." Let us then remember some of the past.

It was not much longer ago than the years preceding World War II when our approach to health education could be summarized in a single statement: Give the people the facts, and the people will act. Act they may have but not necessarily because of the facts we gave them. We were naive enough then to believe that we all had a common understanding of the meaning of the word *fact*. In those days, we did not even appreciate the complex processes involved in giving people facts. We were not concerned with influence processes that might make facts more or less acceptable; we did not consider alternative ways of providing facts; we did not distinguish facts from attitudes or opinions. We did not worry about how causal attribution of facts might influence their believability; we did not consider that people might vary in their acceptance of the threat of disease except as a consequence of their sheer ignorance of the truth. We did not believe that there was a compliance problem. We did not fully appreciate the need for skill training in education. We did not appreciate that innovations often, and often fortunately, diffuse slowly. While these points of view reflected an innocence about influence processes, they had in common a reliance on cognitive processes. The mind (however simplistically it was regarded) was regnant.

As indicated earlier, behaviorism began its ascendancy at the turn of the century; however, although still tenacious in many halls of academia, strict behaviorism has been rejected by social psychologists and health educators, influenced by the work of people such as Wolfgang Kohler (1925); Edward Tolman (1932); Kurt Lewin (1936); Lewin, Dembo, Festinger, and Sears (1944); and their students. These scientists forged the rudiments of a modern cognitive psychology. While Lewin owed much to Tolman, it is Lewin who is best remembered by behavioral scientists, including health educators, for his landmark studies on the dynamics of decision making, which were initiated before and during World War II and continued by his many followers thereafter.

Most behavioral science researchers and practitioners owe a debt of gratitude, often unacknowledged, to Tolman and Lewin. While there are many other potential heroes, this is my chapter and these are my heroes. Another hero should be added to this list, Mayhew Derryberry, who introduced behavioral science theory and method to the activities in health education of the U.S. Public Health Service. Not only did he provide proof of the tenet that health education practice draws from behavioral science theory and that behavioral science theory must be tested in health education practice, but in so doing, he employed, trained, and influenced a large number of health educators and behavioral scientists, some of whom are still active in the field and many of whom transmitted his wisdom and philosophy to succeeding generations.

In considering future trends in health education research and practice, some themes seem most worthy of continued effort.

The World of the Perceiver

The cognitive focus is here to stay, at least for the foreseeable future. Nearly every chapter in this book emphasizes the important role of knowledge, beliefs, and attitudes in influencing behavior, and I believe we must continue to delve ever deeper into the phenomenological world of the actor or actors whose behavior we are trying to understand and influence.

We have learned that knowledge of certain kinds is often important, sometimes essential, to behavior change but that it is rarely if ever sufficient. Giving people the "facts" may be required before they will act, but facts alone will rarely stimulate action in most people. But what kinds of knowledge and beliefs are required for action? Proponents of the Health Belief Model will emphasize the need for knowledge of the likelihood of contracting a disease and the severity of the failure to act as well as knowledge of the means available to avert or minimize the threat at acceptable cost. Intention to act, according to the Theory of Reasoned Action, is based on appreciation of the subjective norms surrounding the recommended behavior as well as attitude toward the behavior. Multi-attribute Utility Theory relies on "grounding" explanatory efforts to the concerns of target populations. I will later return to the emphasis on grounding.

We will properly continue to devote effort to explaining how people make choices that may affect their health. In this regard, one hopes that we will focus on prospective research, eliminating or reducing to a minimum retrospective studies that link current or past behavior with even more remote determinants. Controlled intervention studies are preferred to explanatory studies. While health education theory has not achieved a satisfactory level of validation, we have progressed far enough to test our theories iteratively in the real world. To be sure, if our interventions fail, we have to entertain three not so entertaining hypotheses: first, that our measures or our designs were flawed—always a distinct possibility; second, that our interventions were not implemented correctly; or third, that our interventions were ineffective, the least-appealing alternative. Yet that, of course, is the way of science—we observe, we hypothesize, we experiment, and on rare occasions, we uncover data in support of our hypotheses, which then become knowledge. If, as occurs more frequently, our hypotheses are disconfirmed, the process begins again.

Integration of Risk-Factor Interventions

It is increasingly clear that maximum effectiveness in behavior and life-style modification probably occurs through a combination of educational and environmental interventions, and research of the future should identify the ideal combination of those interventions under different conditions (U.S. Department of Health and Human Services, 1986). As an example, public education to use seat belts has produced disappointing results at best. Similarly, laws mandating the use of seat belts have also demonstrated limited success. We have seen educators on the one hand and environmentalists on the other each profess the importance of their specialized interventions. It should be clear, however, that the proper combination of the two approaches is likely to be more successful than either one alone. No matter how serious the penalty for failing to obey the law, it will be disobeyed by some of those unfavorable to the proposition. Similarly, those favorable to the proposition may need legal or social support to strengthen their resolve to act.

If one reviews the history of the disappearance of the spittoon, it is clear that the virtual elimination of spitting in public required both the legal sanctions to prohibit public expectoration and the modification of social values, which changed spitting from an acceptable activity to a socially reprehensible one. A similar process occurs in the case of smoking. The importance of the view expressed here is accented in the ecological perspective on health promotion proposed by McLeroy, Bibeau, Steckler, and Glanz (1988). In their model it is argued compellingly that "appropriate changes in the social environment will produce changes in individuals, and that support of individuals in the population is essential for implementing environmental changes" (p. 351). But much more work is needed to develop the proper combinations of educational and environmental interventions necessary to assist society both in modifying the environment and in modifying health beliefs and behaviors in desired directions.

One might argue (as some have) that direct educational intervention with target groups should be foresworn altogether in favor of an exclusive emphasis on the social and physical environment. There is, however, a reason for emphasizing education in behavior change strategies that is at least of equal importance to its expected effectiveness. In the long run, we want people to behave in what they regard as their own self-interest. We want them to exercise a substantial degree of voluntarism in their behavior. We want people to use seat belts because they see potential benefits in doing so, not merely to avoid receiving a traffic citation. We want people to abstain from smoking not only because continuation is expensive and in some areas prohibited but also because they see smoking abstinence as having personal health or aesthetic benefits. In short, most of us want an informed public behaving voluntarily in its own self-interest, where behavior is made more likely by the enactment of supporting law and by the evolution of supporting social standards.

Personal Responsibility for Health

Among those who emphasize a reliance on environmental interventions to promote healthful changes are some whose approach is influenced by a desire to avoid blaming the victims for problems presumably not under their personal control. According to this view, those who are sedentary, who smoke, who abuse alcohol, who have poor dietary practices should not be blamed for having their problems. At the same time we are constantly bombarded by messages directing us to take responsibility for our own health.

There is no necessary inconsistency between avoiding victim blaming and taking responsibility for one's own life (Rosenstock, 1988). This view grows out of work on models of helping and coping with problems, developed by Brickman and others (1982). In these models two critical questions are asked about responsibility for a problem, whether it be a health problem, an educational problem, or any other problem of social welfare. The questions are (1) who is to blame for causing the problem and (2) who is responsible for solving it. By posing these two questions, it is possible to derive four models in which responsibility for having caused the problem and responsibility for solving the problem may each be attributed either to the victim or to a source outside the victim.

In the *moral* model, people are held responsible for both problems and solutions. The prototypic view is "You got yourself into this—now get yourself out." Others are not obligated to help because problems are of one's own making. It is this orientation that leads people to blame the victim.

In the *enlightenment* model, people are "enlightened" about the cause of their problems—they themselves are the cause; improvement is possible, but only if they submit to the discipline of authoritative agents. Enlightened people learn that their impulses to drink, smoke, or overeat are out of control, but unlike in the moral model, they believe that help can come only by submitting to the discipline of authority. Alcoholics Anonymous is one of the most successful examples of an enlightenment model.

In the *medical* model, people are not blamed for the origin of their problems, nor are they held responsible for solutions to their problems. A typical example would be a bacterial infection. The cause is not attributed to affected patients, nor do we ordinarily expect them to recover by acts of will, as in the moral model, or by putting their faith in a higher power or in others with similar conditions, as in the enlightenment model. Rather, we prescribe a course of antibiotics. The individual is not blamed for having the condition but is expected to recover promptly if the condition is diagnosed and treated by an expert. The only responsibility of the victim or the victim's guardian is to follow the provider's advice.

Finally, in the *compensatory* model, people are not blamed for causing their problems, but they are held responsible for compensating for their handicaps by acquiring the power or skills to overcome the problems. Alcoholics, smokers, and obese people are not blamed for their problems, but they are held responsible for acquiring the skills necessary to control their urges. In acquiring the skills, the victims may enlist the aid of experts, but the experts are not responsible for the solution; the people with the problems are responsible.

The compensatory model is illustrated in the often-quoted statement of Jesse Jackson, "You are not responsible for being down, but you are responsible for getting up." Individuals may, of course, need help in getting up, but it is their responsibility to do so.

By using a compensatory model, it is therefore possible to avoid blaming victims for having a problem while seeing to it that they assume responsibility for seeking a solution to the problem. Research is needed, however, to ascertain which problems are amenable to a compensatory approach, which clients and providers can adopt that approach, and whether clients and providers can be taught to adopt a compensatory approach.

In another context Marlatt and Gordon (1985) are engaging in exciting work on the prevention of relapse to undesirable, addictive life-styles, using a compensatory model as a framework. Such work is of great importance and should be encouraged.

Induction and Deduction

Most modern scientists believe that a combination of inductive and deductive approaches affords the most proficient route to progress. We make observations, we develop inductive (grounded) hypotheses as a product of those observations, we generate hypotheses in the form of deductions from those induced hypotheses, and finally, we test the deductions. Where the tests disconfirm the deduced hypotheses, we regroup, reformulate, recalibrate, retest, and so on. Where tests do not disconfirm the deduced hypotheses, we regard the findings as knowledge and we move on to new intellectual pursuits. (Where our hypotheses are consistently disconfirmed we may be encouraged to move on to new employment.)

It is widely regarded as efficient to generate testable hypotheses from actual observations, and I heartily concur in this view. Problems arise, however, when investigators adopt a know-nothing attitude that rejects prior knowledge and requires new basic exploratory research before any subsequent hypothesis-testing investigation is allowed to begin. Such an approach may be appropriate for the American-trained investigator who wishes to test explanatory hypotheses about health behavior of members of a little known culture, but the strict grounding requirement seems unnecessary and even wasteful when studying subgroups of frequently investigated populations. Moreover, grounded theory is often less grounded than it seems. The questions asked, even the topics covered, reflect hypotheses held by the investigator on what is important and what is not.

I would be among the last to argue that any behavioral science findings relevant to health have been so perfectly validated as not to merit further critical study. But I would be among the first to argue that where substantial evidence in favor of a hypothesis has been accumulated, it would be more efficient to move on to experimental interventions derived from that hypothesis than to start from scratch with still another explanatory study that cannot be initiated until grounded hypotheses are generated out of still more exploratory, relatively unstructured research.

There may be a more subtle difference than is at first evident between those who lean toward a reliance on induction and those who prefer deduction. I suggest that grounded theory is preferred by scientists seeking to identify differences among people, whereas testing of deductions is preferred by those seeking to identify similarities among people. The former may be likened to clinicians seeking to make a differential diagnosis, whereas the latter are seeking the common elements in a process. Advocates of grounded theory in this view want to know why two people who are similar in many respects behave in different ways; deductive scientists want to know why people who are different in many respects behave in the same way. The grounded theory approach seems to represent a clinical point of view, whereas the deductive approach represents a public health point of view. The public health educator who can demonstrate an impact on a substantial though minority proportion of the public may feel and may be regarded as very successful. In baseball, a batter can fail 70 percent of the time and still be a hero and a millionaire. In public health, if we can show a 30 percent improvement in some educational effort, we too may be regarded as highly successful (though our financial reward may not reflect that success). The approach I am caricaturing comes close to reflecting an infinite regress in which the more we learn, the less we know until, ultimately, we know nothing at all. At that point, we really need a grounded theory approach.

It is interesting that many of the adherents of grounded theory are becoming converted to meta-analysis, an expensive and time-consuming form of literature review. Certainly, the strengths and weaknesses of this approach are worthy of discussion and further investigation. With the exponential rise in published materials, it is worthwhile to explore all techniques that hold hope of lightening the load of the scholar who seeks truth while swimming awash in seas of scientific Siwash and high-dudgeonedly drowning in data. It has yet to be demonstrated, however, that meta-analysis is advancing our knowledge in proportion to its costs.

Providers and Patients

The importance of the provider-client relationship for compliance is well established. What is not yet known convincingly is how to "activate" patients and how to help providers develop a role of mutual participation or to adopt a compensatory model of helping. Such new roles for both the laity and professionals may develop slowly without outside intervention as a function of increasing levels of education in the public and as a function of the introduction of greater behavioral science sophistication into the training of health professionals. Research on ways of expediting the process are to be encouraged.

Evaluation of Health Promotion

Evaluation is necessary for planned change to strengthen our programs. But what should be evaluated? Using the familiar distinctions described by Windsor, Baranowski, Clark, and Cutter (1984) and by Green and Lewis (1986), one could focus on formative or summative evaluation and within those categories, process evaluation, impact evaluation, and health outcome evaluation.

As a matter of good administrative practice, some process data should be gathered to assure that needed resources are available and that program activities are carried out in the amount and manner that was planned. When it is also possible to conduct pilot studies during the formative stage, data may suggest ways of strengthening the program at little or no extra cost. It is, however, the topic of summative evaluation that I wish to address, with a note on the analysis of cost-effectiveness.

Consider first the distinction between program impact evaluation and health outcome evaluation. Impact evaluation assesses a program's effectiveness in achieving desired cognitive and behavioral effects in a target group. How much smoking did we prevent in a school-aged population over a specified period of time? In what proportion of cases did we prevent relapse to obesity for a year?

During our program, how many members of our target group learned how to practice safe sex and how to minimize transmission of AIDS in intravenous drug use? The answers to such questions reflect impact evaluations.

We may, on the other hand, ask questions about health outcomes. Have our efforts resulted in improved morbidity and mortality outcomes? Have we reduced cardiovascular death rates? Have we succeeded in reducing the extent of disability in a target group? Some would argue, as Kaplan (1985, p. 577) does, that "Health status is the only reasonable focal point for clinical health promotion activities" and that "Variables often studied by health educators are important only in relation to health status. . . . [R]isk factors should not be confused with the outcomes."

In an ultimate sense, Kaplan's argument is, of course, correct. There would be little point in preventing smoking if it could not be shown that smoking prevention has beneficial individual and social effects. Yet arguments such as Kaplan's are too simple. Of course, Kaplan has in mind a broader definition of health than the prevention of specific diagnoses; he certainly includes functional ability, even happiness, as part of his conception. Nevertheless, we need to acknowledge differences in the time spans required to demonstrate effects, and we must therefore recognize the legitimacy of health promotion goals that are not intended to have even a short-run effect on behavior let alone an effect on health status.

Because one cannot expect behavioral changes to affect health outcomes in the short run, it seems reasonable to focus short-term evaluations of health promotion on impact evaluation, including attitude and behavior change. Thus, the Stanford three-community study (Farquhar and others, 1977) demonstrated reduction in community risk factors through behavior change before it was possible to report changes in mortality rates. The short-term focus is also endorsed by Green, Wilson, and Lovato (1986). To take another example, it is naive to believe that increasing the minimum legal drinking age from eighteen to twenty-one has an immediate or even short-run substantial effect on the amount of alcohol consumed by eighteen- and nineteen-year-olds. It is even more naive to expect a short-run effect on alcohol-involved automobile fatalities. We would, however, expect a gradual change in social norms to set a standard of behavior resulting in a long-term reduction in drinking rates among younger people, with health benefits accruing further in the future.

In other cases, a health promotion intervention may not even have behavioral change as an immediate objective but rather may be directed toward increasing readiness to accept subsequent health recommendations. Roberts (1975, p. 53) observes that "While [mass] media may not tell us what to think, they have a significant effect on telling us what to think about." Thus, while members of the public may hold various opinions about whether smoking should be prohibited in all public places and whether drunk drivers should be jailed, nearly all are thinking about those issues. The media and other interventions may therefore have more of an agenda-setting role than a persuasive role, and setting the agenda may well contribute to the ultimate persuasion process. Accordingly, while one should properly decry the paucity of well-controlled evaluations of health promotion activities, it is equally problematic to evaluate a program before its time. The ultimate goal of all health programs is to maintain or improve health status, but not all health programs can be properly evaluated against that criterion at any given point in time.

Cost-Effectiveness: Is Prevention Better than Cure?

For years, health educators were challenged to prove that health promotion is cost-effective or, more specifically, that prevention is cheaper than cure. I would urge educators not to accept that seductive challenge. Russell (1986) addresses costs, benefits, and effects of preventive and curative medical interventions, though not of environmental interventions, in a provocative book. She argues that prevention is not always less expensive than providing medical care and may at times be more expensive. Preventive measures are usually directed toward large numbers of people, only some of whom would become ill in the absence of such interventions. As a result, it may cost less to treat the few who become ill than to provide even a low-cost preventive measure to large population groups. As Russell (1986, p. 112) says, "Choosing investments in prevention is thus an economic choice like any other. Prevention offers good things at some additional cost." Thus, while cost-effectiveness analysis can provide useful information for program planning, it is restricted primarily by its value-free approach.

A few years ago, the University of Michigan completed its replacement hospital project, including equipment, road construction and landscaping, and related items at a cost of $285 million, a sum that seemed shockingly high to me—high, that is, until I learned that the cost of a single B1 bomber is $285 million, and each additional B1 bomber costs the same amount. Of course, it may be argued that the university hospital cannot fly, but then again neither can the B1 bomber fly reliably, according to many news reports. The B2 (Stealth) bomber, at about twice the cost of the B1 bomber, is now said to be capable of flying for two hours, though its invisibility makes us wonder how we can know for sure. Moreover, and more seriously, military experts usually expect three experimental planes to crash; one hopes that the B2 bombers will beat those odds.

The point of this irony is to illustrate that whether an item is regarded as expensive depends on one's values. It seems likely that the health establishment and the military establishment would hold quite different views about the relative cost-effectiveness or cost-benefit ratios of a university hospital and a B1 bomber, or half a B2 bomber.

Most people will argue that good health does have intrinsic value and is worth paying for, but we are reminded of the need to analyze what its actual costs are and to think about how much we are willing to pay for it. However, "even when prevention does not save money, it can be a worthwhile investment in better health, and this—not cost saving—is the criterion on which it should be judged" (Russell, 1986, p. 5). Warner (1987) also distinguishes cost-effective programs from cost-saving programs. Screening for and treating hypertension over a lifetime to prevent heart disease may well cost as much as bypass surgery; indeed, it may cost even more to produce the same level of quality-adjusted years of life. But when proper weight is given to the suffering of the victim of heart disease and to problems of postsurgical rehabilitation, prevention may seem preferable.

While cost-effectiveness analysis provides a tool and method for systematic thinking about resource allocation, we may not yet have sufficient data or analytic techniques to permit valid conclusions. Requirement for proper application of this approach may include selecting proper discount rates, allocating valid costs to such items as "time" required to engage in an activity and the "side effects" of an activity. Health educators are urged to assess the costs of their accomplishments but to avoid the trap of arguing for the dollar benefits of health promotion. Rather, demonstrating the benefits in terms of quality of life and prevention of suffering seems more appropriate.

Role of Government in the Support of Research

Science evolves slowly and progressively. The parallel with evolution is apt because natural selection may favor the fittest of the theories and principles in health education and health behavior. But natural selection cannot be improved upon by the meddling of men or by the willfulness of women. Just as no group of biologists could have planned the development of the human being as it exists today, so it is that no funding agency can create the solutions to important social problems, though it can certainly provide the resources necessary to find solutions. The trend over the past three decades toward support of directed research rather than investigator-initiated research may in the long run be self-defeating. Traditionally, we have relied on the ingenuity and creativity of individual scholars and small groups of scholars to illuminate the dimensions and causes of social problems and to provide the keys to dealing with those problems. To be sure, many of the efforts of such scholars require financial and social support, but it should be support of the investigator's ideas, not the ideas of the funding agencies.

There do come times in the course of human history, however, when it is appropriate to launch an all-out attack on a social problem of vast importance by using the combined resources of many disciplines and financial resources that can only be provided by government or by consortia of major philanthropic agencies. The issue that needs careful thought and resolution is how to determine the optimal allocation of resources to investigator-initiated research and to agency-initiated research.

One must consider not only the costs of supporting one approach or another but also the opportunity costs associated with any endeavor. The best recommendation is that funding agencies ought to reserve a fixed, substantial percentage of their grant funds to investigator-initiated research, particularly in topical areas where technology is still primitive enough to require considerable additional study before it can be reasonably expected to have a substantial impact in the field.

The field of public health attracts many activists—activists who are impatient—who want solutions to major problems now. Their zeal is laudable and should be encouraged. But where the needed technology lags far behind understanding the problem, we should devote major resources to strengthening the technology before we test it in long-term community studies.

Training of Health Educators

When I entered the field of public health in 1951, few people with training and interest in the behavioral sciences had actual experience in community health work. Nor could many people be identified with equal interest in research and practice. Over the following twenty-five years, less than an eye blink in historical time, the situation changed radically. Most of the authors of the chapters in this book are qualified to design, conduct, and evaluate intervention programs to create social change and are interested in implementing those strategies in the field. I am gratified to note that the pattern of producing health educators qualified to do research is increasing and is becoming the standard for the field, at least for doctoral- and master's-degree graduates. I am proud to have been part of the movement in this direction. And I encourage its continued development.

References

Brickman, P., and others. "Models of Helping and Coping." *American Psychologist,* 1982, *37* (4), 368–384.

Farquhar, J. W., and others. "Community Education for Cardiovascular Health." *Lancet*, 1977, *1*, 1191–1195.

Green, L. W., and Lewis, F. M. *Measurement and Evaluation in Health Education and Health Promotion.* Mountain View, Calif.: Mayfield, 1986.

Green, L. W., Wilson, A., and Lovato, C. Y. "What Changes Can Health Promotion Achieve and How Long Do These Changes Last? The Trade-Offs Between Expediency and Durability." *Preventive Medicine*, 1986, *15*, 508–521.

Kaplan, R. "Behavioral Epidemiology, Health Promotion, and Health Services." *Medical Care*, 1985, *23*, 564–583.

Kohler, W. *The Mentality of Apes.* San Diego, Calif.: Harcourt Brace Jovanovich, 1925.

Lewin, K. *Principles of Topological Psychology.* New York: McGraw-Hill, 1936.

Lewin, K., Dembo, T., Festinger, L., and Sears, P. S. "Level of Aspiration." In J. Hunt (ed.), *Personality and the Behavior Disorders.* New York: Ronald Press, 1944.

McLeroy, K. R., Bibeau, D., Steckler, A., and Glanz, K. "An Ecological Perspective on Health Promotion Programs." *Health Education Quarterly*, 1988, *15*, 351–377.

Marlatt, G. A., and Gordon, J. R. (eds.). *Relapse Prevention.* New York: Guilford, 1985.

Roberts, D. F. "Attitude Change, Research and the Motivation of Health Practices." In A. J. Enelow and J. B. Henderson (eds.), *Applying Behavioral Science to Cardiovascular Risk.* Dallas, Tex.: American Heart Association, 1975.

Rosenstock, I. M. "Adoption and Maintenance of Lifestyle Modifications." *American Journal of Preventive Medicine*, 1988, *4*, 349–352.

Russell, L. B. *Is Prevention Better Than Cure?* Washington, D.C.: Brookings Institution, 1986.

Tolman, E. C. *Purposive Behavior in Animals and Men.* East Norwalk, Conn.: Appleton & Lange, 1932.

U.S. Department of Health and Human Services. *Integration of Risk Factor Interventions.* Washington, D.C.: Office of Disease Prevention and Health Promotion, Public Health Service, 1986.

Warner, K. E. "Selling Health Promotion to Corporate America:

Uses and Abuses of the Economic Argument." *Health Education Quarterly*, 1987, *14*, 39–55.

Windsor, R., Baranowski, T., Clark, N., and Cutter, G. *Evaluation of Health Promotion and Education Programs*. Mountain View, Calif.: Mayfield, 1984.

Chapter 19

John P. Kirscht

▲ ▲ ▲

Some Issues for
Health Behavior
and Health Education

The preceding chapters in general and Professor Rosenstock's commentary (Chapter Eighteen) on health education in particular are broad and inclusive. They contain a great variety of themes and thought-provoking observations. Without doubt, it is not possible to discuss this work in any detail, and I must opt for noting a few themes, hoping that my remarks do not appear too superficial or random.

What is your choice of theory? This is not simply a matter of preference or an expression of a personality disposition toward representations of the world. Rather, theoretical predilections represent the way in which applied problems are conceived and addressed, the importance given to different sorts of interventions, views regarding what health education is and should be, and even the proper process for conducting research and evaluation. Surely, it is correct to say that a cognitive focus will be with us in the foreseeable future. This delicate reference to (say) health beliefs indicates the continuing application of expectancy value constructs, the marked interest in social learning theory in cognitive appraisal, and the continuing viability of information-processing paradigms. We should not, however, fall victim to blaming the psychologists for the attention given to cognitive dispositions. There is a real place for emphasis

421

on cognitive factors and cognitive change in health education research and practice.

Nonetheless, many writers note that psychological framing of issues may preclude or diminish more comprehensive views of the system within which health and health behavior are operating. Sociological and organizational theories are just as vital to our understanding of events; they also suggest different modes of intervention (although a favorite cliché of mine is that the Health Belief Model doesn't prescribe how to change anything). I think it is healthy to see the development of broad frameworks that include several levels of reality (see Gochman, 1988). Cigarette smoking, for example, can be viewed in individual, social group, cultural, institutional, political, or economic terms.

What may not appear as a related issue is the stance one takes on the proper roots for health education practice. Yet it is associated with "What's your theory?" An emphasis on the social and cultural connectedness of those to whom programs are offered appears to contrast with a more individualistic perspective. Focus on the environment in which health activities take place may be set over against conceptualizing around cognitive dispositions. Yes, of course, the physical and social environments are important, but researchers and practitioners choose up sides, depending on the presumed centrality of different factors. A notable exception is the eclecticism of Green (1984).

Allusion to grounded theory is also symptomatic of some divisions in our ranks. The dispute may well be groundless. On one hand, data do not speak for themselves, and on the other, it is often easy to assume that we know how people think or how social groups function. As Rosenstock notes, data do not transcend the process through which they were collected. Yet it seems to me that the real issue is the utility of conceptualizations. Grounded or not, the question is still "Will it fly?"

Discussion of attributions concerning responsibility for the occurrence of health problems or for their solution (see Brickman and others, 1982) brings back thoughts that crept out after my reading some of Baric's writings (1975). It was a novel idea to me that health education is (can be seen as), among other things, a normative enterprise. Because sickness and health have social consequences and definitions, it does follow that the work of conscious intervention is a norm-creating or norm-sustaining process. When the underlying judgments are taken on the high ground, health education can be regarded as a moral enterprise. By high ground, I mean with worthy aims and sufficient reason. Thus, dietary prudence is recommended to promote a better long run and to serve what we think are the best interests of the society rather than to sell oat bran or to register our disapproval of those who indulge in gastronomic excess. While it is true that there is no health education version of the curia or the office of propaganda, moral ventures run the risk of judging the members of the congregation. So there is tension between the knowledge that behaviors, situations, and policies are likely to affect health in negative ways and the proscription on blaming or the prescription for leaving as much freedom as possible.

As a concept that calls attention to forces that the individual cannot control, victim blaming is useful; it has been overworked, however, and applied to situations in which attributions of personal responsibility are even implied (Green, 1987). Brickman and others (1982) and Rosenstock (in this book) call attention to a helpful distinction between attributions concerning causes and those concerning solutions. A critical analysis of the assumptions, choices, and unintended effects of health education programs is necessary and desirable. But the use of the victim-blaming idea as an epithet that closes down dialogue is counterproductive.

Chapter Eighteen contains several references to health promotion, in the contexts of combined intervention strategies, evaluation, and cost-effectiveness. Interest in health promotion has provided a rallying point for a diverse set of professionals who can relate to a more positive emphasis that is not per se the turf of physicians. There is even a national mandate. Explosive growth in programs illustrates the extent to which the time has come. Health promotion is the crusade of the 1990s, and health educators are in the vanguard. In this heady set of events, all the issues that have marked the history of health education are present and lively. Theoretical and attributional disputes abound.

By now, there are critical and thoughtful commentaries on the health promotion juggernaut, and some sense of unease has developed (Gottlieb, Burdine, and McLeroy, 1987). First, there is uncertainty regarding what can be promoted with good faith. In large part, this is a function of the nature of information about the relationship of behaviors to outcomes. In turn, this uncertainty brings out the analytic difficulties concerning how (and when) to frame questions about effects and the arbitrariness of assigning values to states of people and states of the world. In addition, the evidence for the value of recommendations is quite uneven, depending on the behavior. Few would hesitate to say "don't smoke" to one and all. More hesitancy occurs when the issue is weight reduction for those who are moderately overweight. In many health-risk appraisal instruments, there are very "soft" items that may suggest values for change far beyond any data (for example, getting into arguments or satisfaction with one's life). Second, commercial interests and promoters have seized territory in the health promotion arena. Some are circumspect in marketing and claims; others are not. At the least, conflicting claims and borderline practices make problems for those who are trying to act in the public interest. Popularity is a two-edged sword. It is wonderful to be wanted (a state not always experienced by those in public health) but not so wonderful to counsel caution and the need for more evidence. Third, and related, evaluations of health promotion programs to this point leave results that in the aggregate are shaky. Many health educators do not want to hear this academic-sounding jeremiad. To be sure, prevention as a concept is a cornerstone of public health and of health education. It is an article of faith that I share. In Dr. Rosenstock's long history of activity in public health, there is a consistent advocacy of prevention and of research to understand preventive orientations. With the complexity of linkages among practices and outcomes, however, can we tolerate the tensions created by withholding judgment, acting on the basis of the best information available, calling for stronger evidence? One must steer a course between the true believers and the bottom-liners.

In several of the preceding chapters, the terms *health education theory* and *health education practice* are both used. Over the years, I've noticed that the phrase "theory and practice" rolls off the tongue of my colleagues very easily. What is the relationship between the two? It has been my assumption that theory in health education is used to generate workable models that serve as templates for programs. That is not to say that the program is a strict translation of the model; nor is it to say that the models are necessarily highly coherent. Yet at some level, the enactment of health education is guided by a more-or-less explicit plan.

It has also been my assumption that health education theory is largely derived from the social and behavioral sciences (Wallston and Wallston, 1984). How does that process work? Is there anything systematic about it? We have a situation in which the social science disciplines pursue their own academic agenda. Some of the people trained in those disciplines develop interests, however fleeting, in health-related subject matter and try to operationalize concepts and relationships in the context of the subject matter. Others move more directly into careers that are focused on problems of health education. In the latter situation, evolution occurs, among other ways, when the applied but originally certified social scientist trains health education researchers or derived social scientists who are then in an interdisciplinary mode. Clearly, some social science specialties have evolved as much more applied. For example, both medical sociology and health psychology are major areas of specialization, with many connections to health education.

To make a bad analogy, this system was not set up to produce the health education equivalent of polio vaccine by a certain time. As in many other areas, the arrangement just happened, and there is no "they." Social scientists who work on health issues have some responsibilities to their colleagues in the health fields. First, the social scientist must keep up with the relevant theory in the basic discipline so as to present it accurately. Of necessity, this requires continuing mastery of appropriate literature, including findings from research. Second, the applied social scientist needs to translate the concepts accurately in making applications. It is in making appropriate concepts operational that we face a major challenge. On one hand, there are always many ways in which the measurement of a given concept can be accomplished (and, in fact, there may well be disagreements about the proper dimensions to represent, as in the literature on social support); on the other hand, it behooves us to know enough about the health issues to be plausible. There is some real potential for tension between the health professional's view of a problem and the social scientist's desire for a context in which models can be studied. Even more, when the development and evaluation of interventions are involved, a number of discontinuities between the goals of the different actors can occur. Testing a theory-driven intervention in the context of adding to knowledge may not be very high on the priority list of a health professional with a pressing problem to solve. Even academic health educators may not appreciate the sometimes passionate and irrational involvement of, for instance, psychologists with their theories.

Even now, the future of health education theory and practice is being formed in the health crisis of our time: the AIDS epidemic. Seldom do such dramatic and demanding challenges come along. In this situation, there seems to be virtual unanimity concerning the need for education. Moreover, the requirements for educational and persuasive efforts are complex. There are groups, not always well identified, at considerably higher risk than others. Among these are people who are stigmatized already; a substantial pool is infected. In the case of AIDS, we cannot even compare prevention with cure. In spite of what some wish to believe, there is, of course, social connectedness among wide segments of society, creating the need to deal with virtually the entire social fabric. From the point of view of health education, the central areas of concern are behaviors and beliefs related to infection. Preventing the transmission of the virus is a major concern. Other concerns include dealing with the social and psychological consequences of risk and infection, both on those who face the threat directly and on others. How useful are models from the social sciences in terms of responding to the issues posed to health education by AIDS?

Profound changes have already occurred if one looks at what is happening in gay communities or even the rapid diffusion of information in the larger population (Becker and Joseph, 1988). Nevertheless, very difficult tasks remain. A key question is the degree to which changes that occur are due to planned efforts derived from theoretical considerations. It may be a bit surprising that "behavior change" as a category of knowledge really does not exist. Behavior modification deals with specific and rather narrow aspects of changing behavior. Our theories tend to focus on the independent, or causal, factors. Thus, what can readily be said about principles of changing behavior is fairly simple-minded or of limited practical value (as in the theoretical solution to the submarine menace in World War II: "Boil the seas"). I do think that there is an extraordinary effort going on to develop and apply useful educational interventions involving a broad array of health professionals and social scientists. It is to be hoped that the opportunities present now will initiate another era that is as fruitful as the one that began with pioneering work in the 1950s.

References

Baric, L. "Conformity and Deviance in Health and Illness." *International Journal of Health Education*, 1975, *18* (suppl.), 1–12.

Becker, M., and Joseph, J. "AIDS and Behavioral Change to Reduce Risk: A Review." *American Journal of Public Health*, 1988, *78*, 394–410.

Brickman, P., and others. "Models of Helping and Coping." *American Psychologist*, 1982, *37*, 368–384.

Gochman, D. (ed.) *Health Behavior: Emerging Research Perspectives.* New York: Plenum, 1988.

Gottlieb, N., Burdine, J., and McLeroy, K. (eds.). "Ethical Dilemmas in Health Promotion." *Health Education Quarterly*, 1987, *14* (entire issue 1).

Green, L. "Modifying and Developing Health Behavior." In L. Breslow, J. Fielding, and L. Lave (eds.), *Annual Review of Public Health, No. 5.* Palo Alto, Calif.: Annual Reviews, 1984.

Green, L. Letter to the Editor. *Health Education Quarterly*, 1987, *14*, 3–5.

Wallston, B., and Wallston, K. "Social Psychological Models of Health Behavior: An Examination and Integration." In A. Baum, S. Taylor, and J. Singer (eds.), *Handbook of Psychology and Health, Vol. 4.* Hillsdale, N.J.: Erlbaum, 1984.

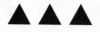

Chapter 20

The Editors

▲ ▲ ▲

Moving Forward:
Research and Evaluation Methods
for Health Behavior
and Health Education

Here, we will discuss a number of methodological issues that emerge from Rosenstock's chapter (Chapter Eighteen) and from points raised by other contributors. These include the need for real-world testing of theories, the importance of multilevel evaluation, the role of cost-effectiveness studies, the importance of multivariate analyses, and the accessibility of research to practitioners. Our goal is not to provide definitive answers but to address matters that belong on the health education research agenda as the year 2000 approaches.

Testing Theory in the Real World

Theories should be tested iteratively in the real world, as Rosenstock notes. First, health education professionals can use promising theories to craft interventions that can be applied and tested in clinical and public health settings. Evaluations should include both the appropriate data to assess the impact of interventions of interest and measures that permit an assessment of theories. This will contribute to both theory development and action for improved public health. By testing theory through evaluating interventions, investigators

428

can identify new variables that may enhance the predictive value of theories. For example, Rosenstock emphasizes the importance of adding the concept of self-efficacy to the Health Belief Model. Future studies will do well to include this concept and examine the extent to which it improves the overall predictiveness of the model. The laboratory of health education is the real world, and that is where theory needs to be tested and refined.

Importance of Multilevel Evaluation

Rosenstock urges the collection of process, impact, and outcome indicators, building upon the early work of Donabedian (1968) and health education researchers as well (Green and Lewis, 1986; Windsor, Baranowski, Clark, and Cutter, 1984). Much is to be learned about whether and why programs are successful (or not successful) when data are collected systematically at all three levels. It still is rare to find research reports in the published literature that have collected and presented data at each of the three levels.

Impact data, of course, can provide information about whether a program has changed health behavior. But process data can help to answer the question"why?" or "why not?" Process data are particularly important because seldom do evaluation studies, even large-scale ones, provide unequivocal evidence of major effects (Green and Lewis, 1981).

Outcome data provide answers to bottom-line questions about changes in morbidity, mortality, and quality of life. Most health education programs are outside the context of large, costly epidemiological studies and do not collect outcome data systematically. In the future, research could be strengthened by increased use of health data registries, such as cancer and stroke registries, to track the incidence of disease in defined populations. Death registries can also provide useful data.

Triangulation Between Qualitative and Quantitative Methods

Rosenstock discusses the induction-deduction dichotomy and urges researchers not to ignore what is known in favor of unstructured research. The best posture may be to encourage researchers and practitioners alike to pursue the middle ground, using both inductive and deductive techniques as appropriate. For example, in the preliminary stages of some research or intervention development efforts, nothing could be worse than assuming one knows the target audience. The use of focus groups and open-ended exploratory interviews can give the health educator a window to the world of the target audience. But that is not sufficient. Deductive methods help assure that conclusions are based on a larger context and are therefore generalizable to some known group. The most meaningful data are often those that emerge from a combination of quantitative and qualitative methods.

There are several ways in which quantitative and qualitative methods can be combined. As in the above example, qualitative methods can be used to help develop quantitative measures and instruments. Also, qualitative methods might help to explain quantitative findings. Third, quantitative methods can be used to embellish a primarily qualitative assessment, as when an anthropologist conducting an in-depth ethnography complements his findings by using survey results (Steckler, McLeroy, and Goodman, 1989).

Increasingly, formal methods will be developed to triangulate information obtained from quantitative and qualitative studies. These methods will go far beyond the simplistic notion that qualitative data merely add texture or substance to the quantitative data. Rather, methods increasingly will specify precisely how and when the two sets of data can be combined and compared. The increased systematic integration of these two types of data will result in more formal methods for refining the theoretical frameworks. These processes have already been advanced greatly by the recent development of text-editing programs for qualitative data that allow on-line coding and the calculation of measures of central tendency for different levels of coding.

Multivariate Analyses

Increasingly, sophisticated analytical methods are needed to test the explanatory power of health behavior and health education theories. These methods are accessible and knowable to both investigators and practitioners. The importance of their ongoing dissemination underscores the need for graduate, postgraduate, and continuing education offerings, as well as establishment of collaborative relationships with knowledgeable statistical experts.

Multivariate analyses are useful for testing the theoretical frameworks presented in this book. Such analyses allow health professionals to estimate more precisely a theory's ability to predict and explain the processes, impacts, and outcomes of theory-driven interventions. At one of the most sophisticated levels of multivariate analyses, analysts use structural equations in which both theoretical and measurement models are tested (Blalock, 1982). LISREL is one statistical program available for doing this (Joreskog and Sorbom, 1979).

Although causal modeling is particularly relevant to testing the types of theoretical frameworks proposed in this book, it is done infrequently in health education research. The goal of causal modeling is to specify, test, and fit the data that represent the underlying theory driving the program. It forces the investigator to translate carefully the assumptions and relationships between the variables in the model. Loose ideas are thus translated into tight connections that link the world of conceptual thought to empirical reality (Blalock, 1969).

Future developments in multivariate methods will include increased refinements in the existing methods for testing both the measurement and theoretical models as well as combinations of data analytic strategies. Increasingly, investigators will turn to these methods in continuing development of their theoretical frameworks.

Submodel Analyses

Although the complex theories in this book require multivariate analyses to cast maximum insight on the study findings, not all answers will come from such sophisticated methods. There will be substantial continuing need for testing subcomponents and microelements in these theories as well. For example, methods of operationalizing and mobilizing social support at the work site may be best examined close up and not merely as part of the larger theoretical framework in which they are cast in Chapter Nine by Israel and

Schurman. When Consumer Information Processing (CIP) theory is tested in research, empirical tests usually examine processes within a given element and/or relationships between a subset of selected variables rather than the CIP model as a whole (Glanz and Rudd, 1987, p. 4). And as Rosenstock points out in Chapter Three, many studies testing the predictive value of the Health Belief Model (HBM) rely primarily on series of univariate analyses testing each major HBM component.

The use of multivariate analytical methods and submodel analyses complement each other to allow multiple perspectives on theories, both in their entirety and as frameworks composed of distinct elements. Optimal theory development and practical use of findings will emerge when both types of analyses are conducted.

Importance of a Multitheory Approach

One of the recurrent themes of this book is that theories seldom should stand alone. Intrapersonal, interpersonal, and organizational or community theories often must be combined for optimal health behavior change. One of the true methodological challenges before us is to create multitheoretical public health programs and to evaluate carefully their effects from multiple perspectives. When woven together, theories may have an even greater predictive ability than when used alone, and they may lead to programs with greater practical power to stimulate change.

We should create study designs and measures carefully so that we gain a much clearer understanding of what combinations of theories are most powerful for addressing what problems and reaching which populations. The contextualist perspective described in Chapter Two (McGuire, 1983) suggests that scientists represent the meaning of theories by making explicit their limiting assumptions or conditions under which the predicted results will occur. This fosters development of a solid foundation for integrating theories and is preferable to a state in which theory melding is performed intuitively. We need to create the hybrids carefully and then evaluate their viability.

Role of Multisite Clinical Trials

As we move increasingly to a multitheory, multilevel understanding of behavior change, we must move likewise to greater use of multi-institutional studies, akin to the clinical trials that form the basis of much modern medical research. To achieve adequate power to detect behavior changes at different levels of intervention may require the participation of several institutions, organizations, or communities. In this and other contexts, sharing of data collection instruments and data sets will improve our knowledge about the success of interventions and the power of theory that guides them.

Research and Evaluation in the Practitioner's World

The preceding discussion addresses matters of importance for an evolving health education research agenda. It focuses primarily on technical issues of research design, measurement, and data analysis. However, for practitioners whose skills and responsibilities are primarily in the realm of program development and administration, research and evaluation are important because they help create improved programs and *not* as scientific endeavors per se. These practitioners are key *consumers* of research and often are "evaluating practitioners" (Green and Lewis, 1986). Three issues are of primary importance in bringing meaningful research and evaluation into these practitioners' worlds: using mixed findings, coping with resource constraints, and collaborating with scientific experts.

Using Mixed Findings. Research reports that present their findings mainly as "number crunching" are difficult for practitioners to use. Practitioners' efforts to interpret research results can be blocked by relying too heavily on statistical inference and quantitative techniques as decision criteria. It is incumbent on practitioners to interpret the *practical* or *clinical* significance of health education and health behavior research in light of the logic of theory and the potential success of attempting to apply the ideas and strategies represented in the research. This must often be done by the practitioner as informed consumer of research. The informed consumer's challenges may include pursuing supplementary information about the content and methods of intervention programs reported in published articles.

Coping with Resource Constraints. Rarely, if ever, is health education conducted with unlimited resources. This limitation affects research as well as practice and is critical to the practitioner's understanding of research findings. Health education intervention studies often have large budgets for both their intervention *and* research components. The practitioner working with a modest budget should realize that it may be impossible to duplicate the programs studied in large formal evaluations. He or she must often adapt elaborate programs to the limits of his or her practice environment and rely on creative fund-raising, voluntary effort, and scaled-down, realistic program goals.

Collaborating with Scientific Experts. Often researchers create intervention programs with the express aim of testing intervention strategies. Many practitioners routinely engage in program evaluation mainly for the purposes of program refinement and organizational decision making. When practitioners and scientists work together, there are opportunities to advance science and practice at once, with synergistic effects.

Such collaborations require sensitivity on both sides: Researchers must learn to appreciate the political and administrative realities of program operations, and practitioners need an open mind to innovative approaches to program implementation and data collection. The balance between science and practice demands compromise, creativity, appreciation of others' skills, and a willingness to cooperate and to learn. The precision of research and the unpredictability of health education practice can coexist when scientists and program staff respect one another's goals and views.

When research and practice in health education and health promotion can be linked in collaborative projects, professionals and the field are equal beneficiaries.

References

Blalock, H. M., Jr. *Theory Construction.* Englewood Cliffs, N.J.: Prentice-Hall, 1969.

Blalock, H. M., Jr. *Conceptualization and Measurement in the Social Sciences.* Newbury Park, Calif.: Sage, 1982.

Donabedian, A. "Promoting Quality Through Evaluating the Process of Patient Care." *Medical Care,* 1968, *6,* 181–202.

Glanz, K., and Rudd, J. *Effects of Quality of Care Information on Consumer Choice of Physicians and Hospitals.* Washington, D.C.: Office of Technology Assessment, U.S. Congress, 1987.

Green, L. W., and Lewis, F. M. "Issues in Relating Evaluation to Theory, Policy, and Practice in Continuing Education and Health Education." *Mobius,* 1981, *1,* 46–58.

Green, L. W., and Lewis, F. M. *Measurement and Evaluation in Health Education and Health Promotion.* Mountain View, Calif.: Mayfield, 1986.

Joreskog, K. G., and Sorbom, D. *Advances in Factor Analysis and Structural Equation Models.* Cambridge, Mass.: ABT Books, 1979.

McGuire, W. J. "A Contextualist Theory of Knowledge: Its Implications for Innovation and Reform in Psychological Research." *Advances in Experimental Social Psychology,* 1983, *16,* 1–47.

Steckler, A., McLeroy, K., and Goodman, R. M. Personal communication, July 1989.

Windsor, R. A., Baranowski, T., Clark, N., and Cutter, G. *Evaluation of Health Promotion and Education Programs.* Mountain View, Calif.: Mayfield, 1984.

Name Index

Subject Index

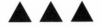

A

A Su Salud Project, 175-178, 243, 247-248

Academy for Educational Development, 366

Action planning, in implementation, 323-324, 331

Adoption stage, in organizational change, 327, 329-330, 331, 334

Adult education, and participation and relevance, 271-272

Advertising, in social marketing, 347

Advocacy. *See* Media Advocacy

Advocacy Institute, 370*n*, 376, 378, 385, 388, 394, 400

AIDS epidemic: and community organization, 253, 257, 266; and health education, 3, 80, 141, 426; and media advocacy, 371, 376

Albuquerque, substance abuse program in, 273-274

Alcohol and Substance Abuse Prevention Program (ASAP), 274

Alcoholics Anonymous, 410

Alma Ata Declaration, 261

Alvin Ailey American Dance Theater, and anti-smoking protest, 380-384

Ambient stressors, concept of, 197

American Cancer Society, 376, 377, 385

American Dental Association, 343

American Health Foundation (AHF), 297, 298, 301, 304, 308, 310

American Lung Association, 342, 354

Analysis stage, in social marketing, 350-351, 355-356

Antecedents, in Attribution Theory, 93-95

Attention and perception, for information processing, 122

Attitudes: defined, 65; group models for changing, 388-389; in Theory of Reasoned Action, 68, 70

Attributions: alteration of focus of, 101; alteration of incorrect, 100-101; of characteristics of individual, 101-102; creation of correct, 99-100

Attribution Theory: analysis of, 92-114; antecedents, processes, and consequents in, 93-95; applications of, 102-108; assessment of, 145-148; background on, 92-93; constructs in, 93-98; development of, 93; and informational power, 225; and interventions, 98-102; and medication compliance, 105-108; and optimum explanatory style, 98; overview of, 34, 35-36; research directions for, 108-109

Awareness stage, in organizational change, 326-327, 330, 334